37.95

# DECISION MAKING IN SPEECH-LANGUAGE PATHOLOGY

# Decision Making in Speech-Language Pathology

David E. Yoder, Ph.D.

Professor
Department of Medical Allied Health Professions
University of North Carolina School of Medicine
Chapel Hill, North Carolina

Raymond D. Kent, Ph.D.

Professor
Department of Communicative Disorders
University of Wisconsin
Madison, Wisconsin

1988

B.C. Decker Inc • Toronto • Philadelphia

Publisher

**B.C. Decker Inc**
3228 South Service Road
Burlington, Ontario   L7N 3H8

**B.C. Decker Inc**
320 Walnut Street
Suite 400
Philadelphia, Pennsylvania   19106

Sales and Distribution

United States
and Possessions

**The C.V. Mosby Company**
11830 Westline Industrial Drive
Saint Louis, Missouri   63146

Canada

**The C.V. Mosby Company, Ltd.**
5240 Finch Avenue East, Unit No. 1
Scarborough, Ontario   M1S 5P2

United Kingdom, Europe
and the Middle East

**Blackwell Scientific Publications, Ltd.**
Osney Mead, Oxford OX2 OEL, England

Australia

**Harcourt Brace Jovanovich**
30–52 Smidmore Street
Marrickville, N.S.W. 2204
Australia

Japan

**Igaku-Shoin Ltd.**
Tokyo International P.O. Box 5063
1–28–36 Hongo, Bunkyo-ku, Tokyo 113, Japan

Asia

**Info-Med Ltd.**
802–3 Ruttonjee House
11 Duddell Street
Central Hong Kong

South Africa

**Libriger Book Distributors**
Warehouse Number 8
''Die Ou Looiery''
Tannery Road
Hamilton, Bloemfontein 9300

South America
(non-stock list
representative only)

**Inter-Book Marketing Services**
Rua das Palmeiras, 32
Apto. 701
222–70 Rio de Janeiro
RJ, Brazil

Printed and bound in Canada

Decision Making in Speech–Language Pathology                    ISBN 0-941158-91-8

Library of Congress catalog card number:     87-50974

10  9  8  7  6  5  4  3  2  1

**MARY RUTH ALTHEIDE, B.S., O.T.R.-L.**

Private Practice, Chapel Hill, North Carolina

**NOMA B. ANDERSON, Ph.D.**

Assistant Professor, Department of Communication Arts and Sciences, Howard University, School of Communications, Washington, D.C.

**JAMES R. ANDREWS, Ph.D.**

Professor and Chair, Department of Communicative Disorders, Northern Illinois Univeristy, De Kalb; Teaching Associate in Surgery, University of Illinois, College of Medicine, Rockford, Illinois

**MARY A. ANDREWS, M.S.**

Instructor, Department of Communicative Disorders and Human and Family Resources, Northern Illinois University; Clinical Member and Approved Supervisor, American Association for Marriage and Family Therapy, De Kalb, Illinois

**KATHRYN A. BAYLES, B.S., M.S., Ph.D.**

Associate Professor, Department of Speech and Hearing Sciences, University of Arizona College of Medicine, Tucson, Arizona

**DANIEL S. BEASLEY, Ph.D.**

Professor and Associate Dean of the Graduate School, Memphis State University, Memphis, Tennessee

**MARY R. BECKER, M.A.**

Supervisor, Communication Disorders Department, Rancho Los Amigos Medical Center, Downey, California

**DAVID R. BEUKELMAN, Ph.D.**

Professor, Department of Special Education and Communication Disorders, University of Nebraska, Barkley Memorial Center, Lincoln, Nebraska

**DIANE M. BLESS, Ph.D.**

Professor of Communicative Disorders, University of Wisconsin, Madison, Wisconsin

**JUNE HAERLE CAMPBELL, M.A.**

Lecturer and Supervisor of Stuttering Therapy, Speech and Language Pathology Program, Northwestern University, Evanston, Illinois

**KAREN A. CARLSON, M.A.**

Department of Communicative Disorders, University of Wisconsin, Madison, Wisconsin

**STEPHEN A. CAVALLO, M.S., B.S., Ph.D.**

Assistant Professor, Department of Speech Arts and Communicative Disorders, Adelphi University, Garden City, New York

**ROBIN S. CHAPMAN, Ph.D.**

Professor of Communicative Disorders, University of Wisconsin, Madison, Wisconsin

**LI-RONG LILLY CHENG, Ph.D.**

Coordinator of Bilingual/Multicultural Program, Department of Communicative Disorders, San Diego State University, San Diego, California

**MICHAEL R. CHIAL, Ph.D.**

Professor, Department of Audiology and Speech Sciences, Michigan State University College of Human Medicine, East Lansing, Michigan

**MICHAEL J. CLARK, Ph.D.**

Associate Professor, Department of Speech Pathology and Audiology, Western Michigan University, Kalamazoo, Michigan

**RODGER M. DALSTON, Ph.D.**

Associate Professor of Surgery and Dental Ecology and Director, Speech and Language Pathology, Oral-Facial and Communicative Disorders Program, University of North Carolina School of Medicine, Chapel Hill, North Carolina

**DONNA J. DePAPE, M.S.**

Head, Communication Aids and Systems Clinic, University of Wisconsin, Waisman Center, Madison, Wisconsin

**FRANK DeRUYTER, Ph.D.**

Director, Communication Disorders Department,
Rancho Los Amigos Medical Center,
Downey, California

**STAN DUBLINSKE, Ed.D.**

Director, State and Regulatory Policy Division,
American Speech-Language-Hearing Association,
Rockville, Maryland

**MARC E. FEY, Ph.D.**

Associate Professor, Department of Communicative
Disorders, The University of Western Ontario Faculty
of Medicine, London, Ontario, Canada

**REBECCA FISCHER, B.A., M.Sc.**

Coordinator, Mama Lere Parent-Infant Center,
Bill Wilkerson Hearing and Speech Center,
Nashville, Tennessee

**DEAN C. GARSTECKI, Ph.D.**

Professor and Head, Audiology and Hearing
Impairment Program, Northwestern University,
Evanston, Illinois

**GARY D. GILL, Ph.D.**

Faculty Associate and Director of Clinics,
Department of Communicative Disorders, University
of Wisconsin, Madison, Wisconsin

**RICHARD M. GOLDSTEIN, M.S.**

Teaching Assistant, Department of Rehabilitation,
Psychology, and Special Education, University of
Wisconsin, Madison, Wisconsin

**HUGO H. GREGORY, Ph.D.**

Professor and Head, Speech and Language
Pathology; Director of Stuttering Programs,
Northwestern University, Evanston, Illinois

**LEE J. GRUENEWALD, Ph.D.**

Director, Integrated Student Services, Madison Metro
School District, Madison, Wisconsin

**VERA GUTIERREZ-CLELLEN, M.A.**

Research Fellow, Temple University School of
Medicine, Philadelphia, Pennsylvania

**W. MICHAEL HAIRFIELD, D.D.S., M.S.**

Assistant Professor of Dental Ecology and Attending,
Oral-Facial and Communicative Disorders Program,
University of North Carolina School of Medicine,
Chapel Hill, North Carolina

**SUSAN S. HARRINGTON, M.S.**

Teaching Assistant, Department of Counseling
Psychology, University of Wisconsin,
Madison, Wisconsin

**GAIL A. HARRIS, M.S.**

Doctoral Candidate, University of Arizona College of
Medicine; President, Harris-Robinson & Associates,
Tucson, Arizona

**DAVID E. HARTMAN, Ph.D.**

Head, Speech Pathology and Clinical Assistant
Professor, Department of Neurology, University of
Wisconsin, Madison; Attending Staff, Gundersen
Clinic–Lutheran Hospital, La Crosse, Wisconsin

**MEGAN M. HODGE, M.S.**

Active Staff, Department of Communication
Disorders, Glenrose Rehabilitation Hospital,
Edmonton, Alberta, Canada

**CELIA R. HOOPER, Ph.D.**

Clinical Assistant Professor and Clinic Director,
Division of Speech and Hearing Sciences,
University of North Carolina School of Medicine,
Chapel Hill, North Carolina

**AQUILES IGLESIAS, Ph.D.**

Associate Professor, Temple University School of
Medicine, Philadelphia, Pennsylvania

**THOMAS S. JOHNSON, Ph.D.**

Professor and Head, Department of Communicative
Disorders, Utah State University, Logan, Utah

**KATHLEEN A. KANGAS, M.S.P.A.**

Clinical Supervisor, Department of Audiology and
Speech Sciences, Purdue University,
West Lafayette, Indiana

**ORV C. KARAN, Ph.D.**

Senior Scientist and Psychologist, Waisman Center
on Mental Retardation and Human Development,
Madison, Wisconsin

**JANE F. KENT, M.S.**

Assistant Researcher, University of Wisconsin,
Madison, Wisconsin

**RAYMOND D. KENT, Ph.D.**

Professor, Department of Communicative Disorders,
University of Wisconsin,
Madison, Wisconsin

**O.T. KENWORTHY, B.A., M.A., Ph.D.**

Former Assistant Professor, Division of
Hearing and Speech Sciences, Vanderbilt University
School of Medicine, Nashville, Tennessee;
Director of Audiology, Providence Speech and
Hearing Center, Orange, California

**LINDA M. LAFONTAINE, M.A.**

Supervisor, Communication Disorders Department,
Rancho Los Amigos Medical Center,
Downey, California

**VICKI LORD LARSON, Ph.D.**

Professor and Assistant Dean of Graduate Studies
and University Research, University of Wisconsin,
Eau Claire, Wisconsin

**LYLE L. LLOYD, Ph.D.**

Professor of Special Education and Audiology and
Speech Sciences, Purdue University,
West Lafayette, Indiana

**JERI A. LOGEMANN, Ph.D.**

Professor, Department of Communicative Sciences
and Disorders, Northwestern University,
Evanston, Illinois

**BARBARA MAJOR, M.S.**

Research Specialist and Ph.D. Student, University of
Arizona College of Medicine, Tucson, Arizona

**RUTH E. MARTIN, M.H.Sc.**

Ph.D. Student, Department of Communicative
Disorders, University of Wisconsin,
Madison, Wisconsin

**NANCY L. McKINLEY, M.S.**

Adjunct Instructor, Department of Communication
Disorders, University of Wisconsin,
Eau Claire, Wisconsin

**JAMES E. McLEAN, Ph.D.**

Senior Scientist, Bureau of Child Research, Parsons
Research Center, University of Kansas,
Parsons, Kansas

**MALCOLM R. McNEIL, Ph.D.**

Professor, Department of Communicative Disorders,
University of Wisconsin; Attending Staff,
Waisman Center on Mental Retardation and Human
Development, Madison, Wisconsin

**JON F. MILLER, Ph.D.**

Professor, Department of Communicative Disorders
and Coordinator, Behavioral Research Unit,
Waisman Center on Mental Retardation and Human
Development, University of Wisconsin,
Madison, Wisconsin

**MARY PAT MOELLER, M.S.**

Coordinator of Aural Rehabilitation, Boys Town
National Institute, Omaha, Nebraska

**FRANK E. MUSIEK, Ph.D.**

Professor, Dartmouth Medical School; Director of
Audiology, Dartmouth-Hitchcock Medical Center,
Hanover, New Hampshire

**RONALD NETSELL, Ph.D.**

Professor, Department of Otolaryngology and Human
Communication, Creighton University School of
Medicine; Director, Center for Speech and Language
Disorders, Boys Town National Institute for
Communication Disorders in Children,
Omaha, Nebraska

**MARIANA NEWTON, Ph.D.**

Associate Professor, Department of Communication
and Theatre, Division of Communication Disorders,
University of North Carolina; Former Director,
University of North Carolina Speech and Hearing
Center, Greensboro, North Carolina

**DANIEL J. ORCHIK, Ph.D.**

Chief of Audiology, Shea Clinic and Deafness
Foundation, Memphis, Tennessee

**MARY JOE OSBERGER, Ph.D.**

Assistant Professor, Department of Communicative
Disorders, University of Wisconsin,
Madison, Wisconsin

**DAVID E. PALM, Ph.D.**

Attending Staff, Department of Audiology, Gundersen
Clinic, La Crosse, Wisconsin

**SALLY J. PETERSON-FALZONE, Ph.D.**

Clinical Professor, Center for Craniofacial Anomalies,
University of California School of Medicine,
San Francisco, California

**PATRICIA B. PORTER, Ph.D.**

Associate Professor, Department of Medical Allied
Health Professions, University of North Carolina
School of Medicine; Director, Clinical Programs,
University of North Carolina Clinical Center
for the Study of Development and Learning,
Chapel Hill, North Carolina

**BARRY M. PRIZANT, Ph.D.**

Assistant Professor, Department of Psychiatry and
Human Behavior, Division of Child and Adolescent
Psychiatry, Brown University Program in Medicine;
Director, Department of Communication Disorders,
Emma Pendleton Bradley Hospital and Allied Health
Associate, Department of Psychiatry, Women and
Infants Hospital, Providence, Rhode Island

**ANNE H. B. PUTNAM, Ph.D.**

Associate Professor, Department of Rehabilitation Medicine, University of Alberta Faculty of Medicine; Consultant in Speech Physiology, Department of Communication Disorders, Glenrose Rehabilitation Hospital, Edmonton, Alberta, Canada

**MARGARET M. ROSIN, M.S.**

Clinical Instructor, University of Wisconsin; Supervisor, Speech/Language Services, Waisman Center Clinical Service Unit, Madison, Wisconsin

**ROBERTA SCHWARTZ-COWLEY, M.Ed.**

Adjunct Faculty, Department of Emergency Health Services, University of Maryland School of Medicine and Adjunct Faculty, Department of Speech-Language Pathology and Audiology, Loyola College; Director, Speech-Communication Disorders Program of the Shock Trauma Center, Maryland Institute for Emergency Medical Services Systems and Montebello Rehabilitation Hospital, Baltimore, Maryland

**LAWRENCE D. SHRIBERG, Ph.D.**

Professor, Department of Communicative Disorders, University of Wisconsin, Madison, Wisconsin

**CHRISTINE SLOAN, Ph.D.**

Associate Professor, Dalhousie University School of Human Communication Disorders, Halifax, Nova Scotia, Canada

**LEE SNYDER-McLEAN, Ph.D.**

Associate Scientist, Bureau of Child Research, Parsons Research Center, University of Kansas, Parsons, Kansas

**SHIRLEY N. SPARKS, M.S.**

Associate Professor, Speech Pathology and Audiology, Western Michigan University, Kalamazoo, Michigan

**RACHEL E. STARK, Ph.D.**

Professor, Audiology and Speech Sciences, Purdue University, West Lafayette, Indiana

**MARK J. STEPANIK, M.S.**

Adjunct Faculty, Department of Speech Pathology and Audiology, Loyola College; Assistant to the Director, Speech-Communication Disorders Program, Maryland Institute for Emergency Medical Services, University of Maryland Medical Systems, Baltimore, Maryland

**SHELLEY STOWERS, M.S.P.H., O.T.R.**

Portland Oregon School System, Portland, Oregon

**EDYTHE STRAND, M.A., Ph.D.**

Lecturer, Department of Communicative Disorders, California State University, Stanislaus, Turlock, California; Owner-Director, Strand-Kelley Speech Pathologists Inc., Modesto, California

**ORLANDO L. TAYLOR, Ph.D.**

Dean and Graduate Professor, Howard University, School of Communications, Washington, D.C.

**DOLORES KLUPPEL VETTER, Ph.D.**

Professor, Communicative Disorders, University of Wisconsin, Madison, Wisconsin

**MERYL J. WALL, Ph.D.**

Chairperson and Associate Professor, Department of Speech Arts and Communicative Disorders, Adelphi University, Garden City, New York

**DAVID J. WARK, Ph.D.**

Associate Professor, Department of Audiology and Speech Pathology, Memphis State University, Memphis, Tennessee

**DONALD W. WARREN, D.D.S., Ph.D.**

Kenan Professor and Director, Oral-Facial and Communicative Disorders Program, University of North Carolina; Attending, Oral-Facial and Communicative Disorders, The North Carolina Memorial Hospital, Chapel Hill, North Carolina

**BERND WEINBERG, Ph.D.**

Professor, Department of Audiology and Speech Sciences, Purdue University, West Lafayette, Indiana

**GARY WEISMER, Ph.D.**

Associate Professor, Department of Communicative Disorders, University of Wisconsin, Madison, Wisconsin

**SUSAN ELLIS WEISMER, Ph.D.**

Faculty Associate, Department of Communicative Disorders and Department of Curriculum and Instruction, University of Wisconsin, Madison, Wisconsin

**TERRY L. WILEY, Ph.D.**

Professor and Chairman, Department of Communicative Disorders, University of Wisconsin, Madison, Wisconsin

**MARY LOVEY WOOD, Ph.D.**

Owner/Director, Austin Speech, Language, and Learning Clinic, Austin, Texas

MARILYN SEIF WORKINGER, Ph.D.

Staff Speech Pathologist and Section Manager, Marshfield Clinic, Marshfield, Wisconsin

BARBARA WURTH, M.S., L.P.T.

Private Practice, Bethlehem, Pennsylvania

DAVID E. YODER, Ph.D.

Professor, Department of Medical Allied Health Professions, University of North Carolina School of Medicine, Chapel Hill, North Carolina

KATHRYN M. YORKSTON, Ph.D.

Associate Professor, Rehabilitation Medicine, University of Washington School of Medicine, Seattle, Washington

# PREFACE

Above all else, *Decision Making in Speech-Language Pathology* is an attempt to systematize the observations and actions that clinicians take in the assessment and management of speech and language disorders. The focal point of each chapter is a decision tree that depicts graphically the data-gathering and logical steps in the clinical process. Each tree is accompanied by a brief text that explains the decisions embodied in the tree. The 84 chapters are condensations, distillations, and a synthesis of clinical knowledge. Although the chapters do not cover every problem that the speech-language pathologist may encounter in a clinical practice, the coverage is, we hope, sufficiently broad to make this book a generalist's compendium of expert opinions.

*Decision Making in Speech-Language Pathology* is not a cookbook. That is, it is not a set of recipes to be followed invariantly in the hope of conducting the perfect assessment or management of a client. The clinician who uses these decision trees will find them more useful as guidelines and prompts than as definite programs for clinical action. The balance between the systematization of a clinical science and the prescription of inflexible clinical protocol is sometimes delicate. As a clinical field matures, it becomes accountable in large part through the specification of its methods, both for the purpose of consistent application and for the purpose of demonstrated accomplishment. Unless and until a clinical field can specify its methods, the knowledge of that field cannot be validated scientifically. On the other hand, excessive or inflexible specification of clinical procedures can thwart their very purpose. Allowances must be made for individual differences, complicating environmental factors, multiple etiologies, and unknown conditions. Cookbooks cannot deal with the unknown or the uncertain, but clinical decision making frequently encounters them.

It may be asked, and probably should be asked, if expert knowledge can be reduced to an algorithm and a few pages of text. Certainly, much of an expert's knowledge cannot be so reduced. There is no substitute for clinical experience with hundreds or thousands of cases. But the expert's conceptualization of assessment and management can be summarized and systematized. The expert can specify the most critical observations, the major or most frequently occurring alternatives in assessment or management, and the need to consider alternative tests, classifications, and interventions. This core knowledge can be imparted in a decision tree and a few hundred words of text. The exact structure of a decision tree is rarely absolute, and readers should not feel under an obligation to follow the diagram lines like roads marked on a map. The critical information to be taken from the chapters is the clinical logic. The tree diagrams are concise representations of that logic.

David E. Yoder, Ph.D.
Raymond D. Kent, Ph.D.

# CONTENTS

The decision tree is the focus of every chapter. The circled letters on the tree refer the reader to the corresponding part of the text. Several general references are included with each chapter. The sample decision tree on this page outlines in a general way the principles used in the chapters that follow.

As do most of the decision trees in this book, the tree for evaluating behavioral management begins with appropriate consideration of background and referral information. Management must take into account the client's history, information provided by the referral source (if any), and assessment results. Typically, a plan of management will be based on at least these factors. Using these data, the clinician determines the general management goals, limiting and facilitating factors, prognostic indications, and social, psychological, physical, and educational or vocational aspirations that are pertinent to development of a management plan.

A.  Almost every management plan requires that the clinician identify the behavior to be developed, increased, reduced, eliminated, or otherwise modified. Perhaps subgoals will be determined as part of a general goal of management.

B.  Selection of the task or target behavior should be made with due consideration to several factors, including the client's daily activities, achievement goals, related behaviors (which may be facilitative or interfering, adaptive or maladaptive), and pertinent correlates in the physical, psychological, and social domains (e.g., medical treatment, ongoing physical disability, peer or family support, vocational or educational involvement, and self-esteem). These factors are important not only for initial planning but also for later evaluation and planning of the management program, and for generalization and for maintenance of the managed behavior.

C.  The general management goal is then defined in terms of a clearly specified task or target behavior that becomes the focus for a stage of management. Isolation and definition of such a focus can require special thought when the behavior in question is complex or multidimensional. For example, in the case of language impairment, the clinician may need to identify a particular linguistic structure as an early focus for intervention. Or, in the case of a stutterer, the clinician may need to target one particular type of dysfluency.

D.  With many clients and behaviors, the clinician has to identify relevant stimulus and response characteristics. For example, with a language impairment in a child, the clinician may need to compose appropriate linguistic materials for a model and to identify specific language responses from the child to be measured, counted, reinforced, and so on. As another example, the clinician who decides to improve a dysarthric individual's prosody must select speech materials that adequately convey the dimension to be changed (such as rate, stress, or intonation) and must define some feature of the client's response (such as rate in syllables per second, success in signalling an intended stress contrast, or performance in matching a target intonation contour) that can be related to the intended behavioral change. It is also impor-

tant to determine the setting, duration, and frequency of treatment.

E.  Component analysis may be indicated for several reasons, but especially to determine those properties of management that are most significant in its efficacy. Frequently, this aspect of evaluation is carried out after a management procedure has been shown to be successful at least to some degree.

F.  If the result of management is not satisfactory, the clinician can consider several steps for the next action. One is to return to A to reevaluate the management strategy. Perhaps the initial plan was misconceived and the failure of the management plan shows that a new approach is needed. Or it may be that the general approach is valid, but either (1) the task or target behavior needs to be changed, or (2) the stimulus and response characteristics need to be revised. It also is possible that the prognosis for management was unduly optimistic. Obviously, several factors may have to be weighed in determining why a management plan was not successful.

This example shows the principles of clinical decision making as cast into the form of an algorithm or decision tree. The structure of the tree gives structure to the clinical process and the design of the tree is a joint product of clinical experience and logical thinking.

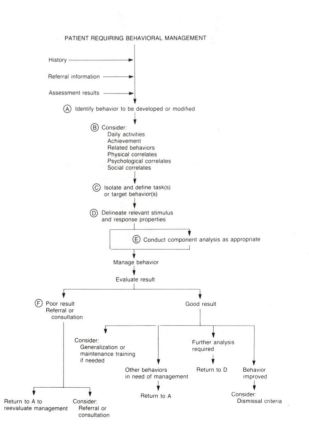

PATIENT REQUIRING BEHAVIORAL MANAGEMENT

History

Referral information

Assessment results

(A) Identify behavior to be developed or modified

(B) Consider:
Daily activities
Achievement
Related behaviors
Physical correlates
Psychological correlates
Social correlates

(C) Isolate and define task(s) or target behavior(s)

(D) Delineate relevant stimulus and response properties

(E) Conduct component analysis as appropriate

Manage behavior

Evaluate result

(F) Poor result
Referral or consultation

Good result

Consider:
Generalization or maintenance training if needed

Further analysis required

Other behaviors in need of management

Return to D

Behavior improved

Return to A

Return to A to reevaluate management

Consider:
Referral or consultation

Consider:
Dismissal criteria

# I: Auditory Function

These chapters discuss basic procedures for the assessment of auditory function and the management of auditory disorders. Although speech-language specialists typically do not conduct audiologic evaluations, they are involved in the management of some auditory disorders, and they need to understand audiologic practice in relation to speech and language functions. This section, then, is not intended to give a complete coverage of audiologic evaluation and management. Rather, it is designed to cover basic issues in clinical decision making relative to auditory function. Some of the chapters overlap somewhat in content, but they differ in overall perspective and in their concentration on a particular age range of clients.

# AUDIOLOGIC EVALUATION

*Terry L. Wiley, Ph.D.*

A. Prior to the administration of formal audiologic tests, a complete case history should be documented. This may be obtained through an interview with the client or parent or may be obtained through prior communication with the client in anticipation of the audiologic evaluation. The case history should include identifying information, behaviors and observations that may suggest hearing impairment, birth history, health status, family history of hearing impairment, social and occupational demands on hearing, and other relevant background. In addition, the results of other evaluations that may be relevant to the audiologic profile should be reviewed. These may include test findings from medical (e.g., neurology, radiology, otolaryngology) and nonmedical (e.g., psychology, speech-language) specialists.

B. If a hearing impairment is suspected or is a primary complaint, the audiologist may elect to administer a hearing-handicap inventory, which is designed to fully document the person's self-assessment of the hearing impairment. Data from the inventory may be useful in selecting subsequent diagnostic tests and in (re)habilitative programming.

C. If a hearing impairment is not suspected, there may still be a reason to suspect the presence of an otologic problem that requires further evaluation. A significant number of young children, for example, may experience otic disease (e.g., middle-ear infections) with little or no hearing loss. The presence of other symptoms such as tinnitus, vertigo or otalgia also require medical consultation.

D. There may be reason to suspect an auditory processing disorder with or without a complaint or history of hearing loss. Persons with pathologies restricted to the central auditory nervous system typically evidence no significant loss in hearing sensitivity. However, they may evidence learning disabilities and other educational problems that require further evaluation (see the relevant chapters in Section II).

E. The test procedures that comprise a basic audiologic evaluation depend on the presenting problem but, in general, consist of otoscopic inspection, tone thresholds for air- and bone-conduction signals, acoustic-immittance measures (tympanometry, ipsilateral and contralateral acoustic-reflex thresholds), and speech audiometry (thresholds and speech-recognition measures) for both ears. Background on these procedures and other topics within this chapter is available in Jerger and Jerger (1981), Katz (1985), Martin (1986), and Wiley (1980). In addition to the need for tailoring the evaluation to significant presenting problems, specific test procedures and materials may be required depending on the age and capabilities of the client. Infants, young children, clients with developmental disabilities and geriatric patients are examples of clients that often require modifications in standard test procedures (p 6, 14, 18).

F. If there is no evident hearing impairment, there may still be reason to suspect an otologic or neurologic problem. Children with middle-ear disease, for example, may evidence no appreciable hearing loss. Such cases may evidence abnormal acoustic-immittance measures, however, and require further diagnostic follow-up. Similarly, a potential otoneurologic abnormality may be suggested from the basic test results in the absence of significant hearing loss. A lesion to the eighth cranial nerve and/or the auditory brainstem, for example, may cause no significant loss in hearing sensitivity.

G. If a hearing impairment is evident or an otoneurologic disorder is suspected, the next step in the diagnostic process is aimed at defining the primary anatomic locus of the disorder. Lesions to specific locations within the auditory system often result in typical test profiles for a battery of audiologic procedures. This process is often termed differential diagnosis because test results are often contrasted with those for normals or for normative results in patients with confirmed lesions to specific auditory structures. In the case of sensorineural hearing loss, for example, the purpose is often one of differentiating results typical of lesions primary to the cochlea from those suggestive of eighth-nerve pathology. Examples of test measures that may be included here are auditory evoked potentials, acoustic-reflex decay and latency, tone decay, electronystagmography, and degraded speech-recognition tasks.

H. If the results are positive for otoneurologic disorder, the client should be referred for appropriate medical follow-up. This may include otologic, neurologic, radiologic, and other relevant evaluations. Such referrals may be warranted even in the absence of significant audiologic findings, particularly if the patient presents significant nonaudiologic symptoms (e.g., tinnitus, vertigo, otalgia) or has not been evaluated medically previous to the audiologic evaluation.

I. With or without otoneurologic referrals, there may be a need for further audiologic testing and follow-up. In the case of significant medical problems, this may take the form of monitoring procedures to evaluate the success or progress of surgery or other medical treatment. In the absence of needed medical treatment there may be a need for additional audiologic management such as evaluation of the patient's candidacy for a hearing aid, selection of a hearing aid or assistive listening device, auditory (re)habilitation programming, educational recommendations, periodic diagnostic monitoring audiometry, and other relevant concerns.

J. In addition to audiologic follow-up for hearing-impaired persons, it may be necessary to refer such individuals for other services such as educational and psychologic evaluation and counseling, social work, speech-language evaluation and therapy, genetic counseling, and vocational guidance. Even in the case of clients who present no history or test results evident of hearing loss or otoneurologic disorder, other referrals may be in order.

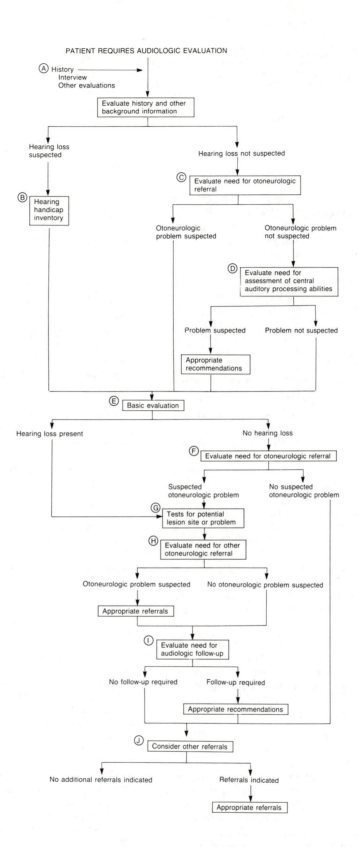

PATIENT REQUIRES AUDIOLOGIC EVALUATION

(A) History
Interview
Other evaluations

Evaluate history and other background information

Hearing loss suspected

Hearing loss not suspected

(C) Evaluate need for otoneurologic referral

(B) Hearing handicap inventory

Otoneurologic problem suspected

Otoneurologic problem not suspected

(D) Evaluate need for assessment of central auditory processing abilities

Problem suspected

Problem not suspected

Appropriate recommendations

(E) Basic evaluation

Hearing loss present

No hearing loss

(F) Evaluate need for otoneurologic referral

Suspected otoneurologic problem

No suspected otoneurologic problem

(G) Tests for potential lesion site or problem

(H) Evaluate need for other otoneurologic referral

Otoneurologic problem suspected

No otoneurologic problem suspected

Appropriate referrals

(I) Evaluate need for audiologic follow-up

No follow-up required

Follow-up required

Appropriate recommendations

(J) Consider other referrals

No additional referrals indicated

Referrals indicated

Appropriate referrals

In the case of a child who presents significant developmental and educational problems, for example, the fact that hearing impairment has been ruled out may signal the need to explore other causes for the presenting problems.

## References

Jerger S, Jerger J. Auditory disorders: a manual for clinical evaluation. Boston: Little, Brown, 1981.

Katz J. Handbook of clinical audiology. 3rd ed. Baltimore: Williams & Wilkins, 1985.

Martin FN. Introduction to audiology. 3rd ed. Englewood Cliffs, NJ: Prentice-Hall, 1986.

Wiley T. Hearing disorders and audiometry. In: Hixon TJ, Shriberg LD, Saxman JS, eds. Introduction to communication disorders. Englewood Cliffs, NJ: Prentice-Hall, 1980:490.

# THE HEARING-IMPAIRED PRESCHOOL CHILD: ASSESSMENT

*O. T. Kenworthy, B.A., M.A., Ph.D.*
*Rebecca Fischer, B.A., M.Sc.*

The hearing-impaired preschool child is identified through a comprehensive program of services including in-service training, public service announcements, case finding (e.g., a high-risk registry), and actual testing, or screening. The intent of such a program is to promote case finding; heighten community awareness; facilitate prevention; aid case selection; provide systematic tracking, referral, and follow-up; and facilitate appropriate intervention. Such a program is also predicated upon a well-developed network of linkages between various professional and community services and resources. By contrast, screening is one subcomponent of identification whereby affected cases are selected from an otherwise asymptomatic population. The outcomes are binomial and can be obtained through history taking, observation, or direct testing, depending upon the age of the child.

A. Communicative assessment establishes the child's degree of functional ability as an interlocutor. Emphasis is placed on establishing the child's capabilities and on facilitating optimal performance. Systematic determination of what the child can do is a more informative report than test failure. Consequently, mitigating factors such as visual impairment, oral-motor control and seating/positioning variables must be ruled out. Preferably, this should be accomplished prior to beginning the screening or assessment cycle. For children 2½ to 7 years of age, Robbins and Klee (1984) offer a protocol for assessing oral-motor function. Prior to 2½ years of age, feeding behaviors may present the most practical index of oral-motor behavior, although in older children the relation of feeding behaviors to speech motor control is unclear.

B. Hearing screening is occasionally conducted during the neonatal period. There is little to contraindicate the practice, providing additional behavioral testing is performed at a later follow-up visit. The question of whether direct testing in the neonatal period is cost efficient or effective remains a matter of controversy.

C. The procedures for auditory assessment are prioritized and listed in a desired order of presentation. The symbol key for the various procedures is as follows: ABR = auditory brainstem response; BOA = behavioral observation audiometry; DISCRIM = auditory discrimination, including difference limen measures (Erber, 1981), as well as speech sound discrimination; SPAR = acoustic reflex testing, including sensitivity prediction protocols; VRA, VRISD, VROCA = visual reinforcement audiometry procedures described by Wilson (1978) Tymp = tympanometry.

D. Traditionally, speech–language screening has not been done prior to 2 years of age. Recent improvements in screening instruments and procedures, such as the Early Language Milestone (ELM) Scale (Modern Education Corporation, Tulsa, Oklahoma, 1983), allow for earlier testing. Given that the primary presenting symptom in most cases of childhood hearing impairment is delayed speech, this is an important advancement in the identification and assessment process.

E. As a complement to the screening process, it becomes necessary to qualify the degree of the child's communicative ability. Miller (1981) has provided a conceptual framework and experimental procedures which accomplish this task for language production. Procedures for language comprehension are forthcoming. (See Hasenstab, 1982, for a review of formal speech and language tests applicable to hearing-impaired children.) The one additional aspect that is not addressed directly by Miller is the question of differences in performance based upon mode of presentation. Moog and Geers (1984) offer some nonstandardized procedures for evaluating mode.

F. Several measures of parent concerns and attitudes are reviewed in Gill and Copeland (1982).

Development of these materials was supported in part by a grant from the Robert Wood Johnson Foundation, but opinions expressed herein are solely those of the authors.

## References

Geers A, Moog J. Predicting spoken language acquisition in deaf children. St. Louis, MO: Central Institute for the Deaf, 1984.

Gill D, Copeland E. Early childhood assessment: recommended practices and selected instruments. Springfield, IL: Illinois State Board of Education, 1982.

Hasenstab MS. Language evaluation. In: Hasenstab MS, Horner J, eds. Comprehensive intervention with hearing-impaired infants and preschool children. Rockville, MD: Aspen Systems Corp, 1982:137.

Miller JF. Assessing language production in children. Baltimore, MD: University Park Press, 1981.

Robbins J, Klee TM. Assessment of oral-motor functioning in children. Unpublished working paper. Nashville, TN: Vanderbilt University, Division of Hearing and Speech Sciences, 1984.

Wilson W. Behavioral assessment of auditory function in infants. In: Mininfie F, Lloyd L, eds. Communicative and cognitive abilities—early behavioral assessment. Baltimore, MD: University Park Press, 1978:37.

HEARING-IMPAIRED PRESCHOOL CHILD IDENTIFIED

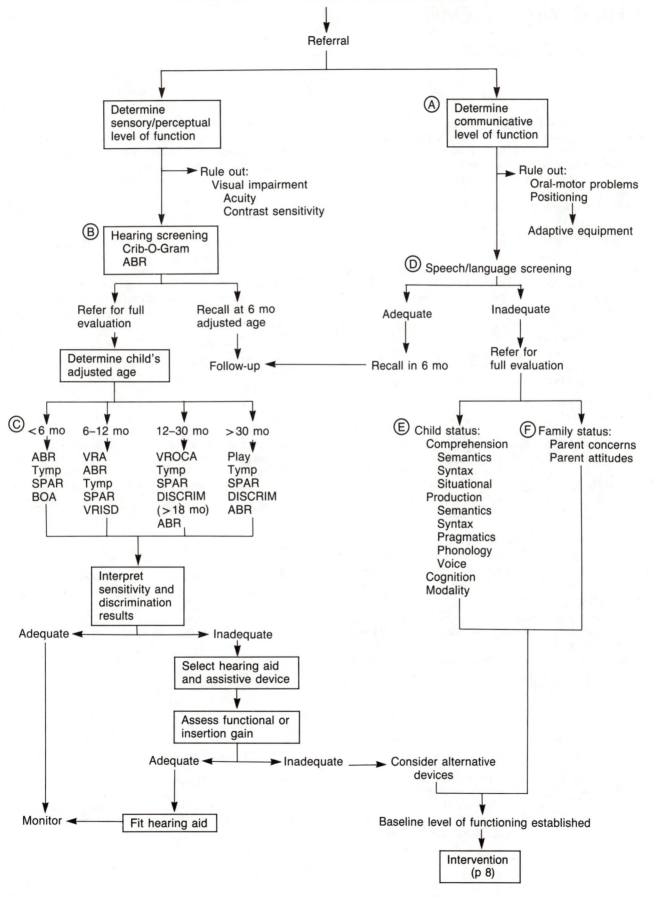

# THE HEARING-IMPAIRED PRESCHOOL CHILD: MANAGEMENT

*Rebecca Fischer, B.A., M.Sc.*
*O. T. Kenworthy, B.A., M.A., Ph.D.*

The establishment and evaluation of an appropriate intervention plan is presumed to be a multidisciplinary team function that incorporates the parents as active team members. Consequently, it is necessary to hold staffings at critical decision-making points throughout the process, particularly when baseline behavior or progress is in question. Refer to page 7 for determination of baseline behavior.

A.  To maximize the child's use of residual hearing, it is desirable for both the parent and child to monitor hearing aid function. The parent is instructed by the clinician, and over a period of time the child learns to perform some of the tasks included in the protocol. The clinician occasionally observes the parent's instruction to the child and models any desired modifications. Periodic electroacoustic evaluation also serves as an important supplement to the daily procedure. For the child who demonstrates minimal gain from amplification systems, employment of other sensory systems or devices, such as signing and/or tactile aids, should be considered.

B.  Establishing communication skills in the hearing-impaired child is viewed here as elaborating upon existing skills, given what is known about normal language acquisition. In addition to developing communication, early intervention programming may include goals in the areas of personal-social behavior, cognition, and gross and fine motor skills. Criteria for program selection include the child's developmental level, the presence of other handicapping conditions, family support, severity of hearing loss, and availability of program options within the community. Following placement in an appropriate educational setting, short-term objectives are selected, subskills are trained, and resulting behaviors generalized to multiple contexts.

C.  Involving parents and siblings in therapy and providing opportunities to share experiences enables the clinician and family to explore the affective impact of the hearing loss. Another important aspect of family dynamics is the interaction pattern between parent and child. Cole and St. Clair-Stokes (1984) offer a protocol for analyzing videotaped samples.

D.  Assessing the rate of progress requires a systematic framework for evaluation, as well as developmental guidelines for determining *change* in the child's performance. Failure to observe closure between the child's chronological age and his or her level of spontaneous language performance should lead to immediate reevaluation of program targets and methods, particularly the mode of presentation. Also, while the use of assessment tools referenced to hearing-impaired children is appropriate for a child placed in a self-contained classroom, instruments normed on the *hearing* population are useful when considering mainstreamed placement for a hearing-impaired child. Criterion-referenced evaluations are valuable for the multi-handicapped child who requires a program designed to meet functional needs.

E.  For hearing-impaired infants and their families, a pragmatically-based program emphasizing the development of interactional skills and utilizing naturally occurring situations seems most appropriate. Occasionally, weaknesses in specific aspects of language and speech development may dictate modifications of the approach or implementation of alternative intervention programs. It is crucial that new procedures are discussed with the family, changes in roles and responsibilities are clearly defined, and progress is carefully monitored.

F.  Most hearing-impaired infants and their families are best served, at least initially, by individual therapy sessions. Placement in child-centered programs such as normal-hearing nurseries, self-contained classes for the hearing-impaired, or other special education programs may be appropriate for older preschoolers. In general, a slow rate of progress indicates the need for placement in a more structured setting. Regardless of placement, it is essential that parental guidance continue and that families are encouraged to remain closely involved with all aspects of the child's educational program.

G.  Traditionally, intervention strategies were driven by philosophical commitment to a modality of choice. More recently, modality choices have been influenced by concerns over communication competence of the child-caregiver dyad (e.g., Greenberg, 1980), as well as natural tendencies and rate of progress evidenced by the child.

## References

Bendet RM. A public school hearing aid maintenance program. Volta Review, 1980; 82:153.

Cole E, St. Clair-Stokes J. Caregiver-child interactive behavior: a videotape analysis procedure. Volta Review, 1984; 86:200.

Davis JM, Hardick EJ. Rehabilitative audiology for children and adults. New York: John Wiley and Sons, 1980:139,245.

Greenberg M. Mode use in deaf children: the effects of communication method and communication competence. Appl Psycholinguistics 1980; 1:65.

Luterman D. Counseling parents of hearing-impaired children. Boston: Little, Brown, 1979.

Weiss A, ed. Language disorders and hearing impairment: implications from normal child language. Topics Lang Disord; 6:3.

HEARING-IMPAIRED PRESCHOOL CHILD

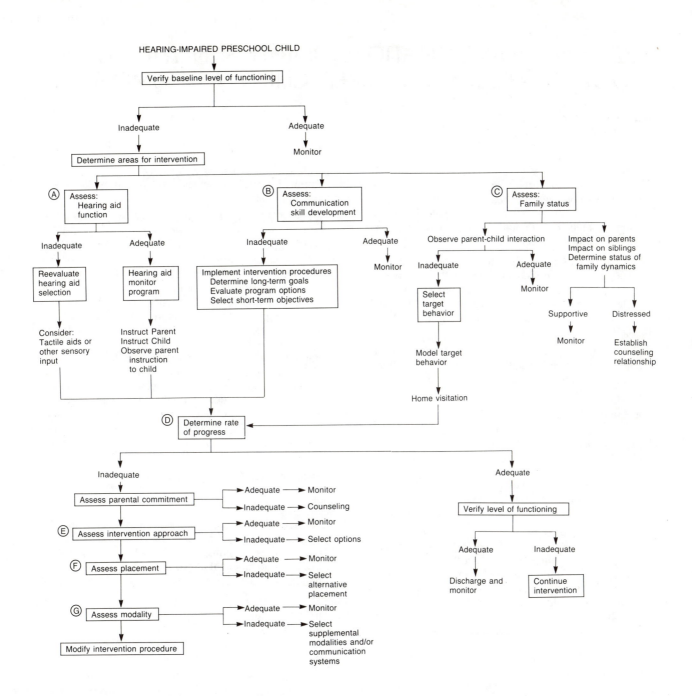

# EXPRESSIVE COMMUNICATION PROBLEMS IN THE SCHOOL-AGE HEARING-IMPAIRED CHILD: ASSESSMENT

*Mary Pat Moeller, M.S.*
*Mary Joe Osberger, Ph.D.*

A. Determine onset of hearing loss, age of identification, initiation and consistency of hearing aid use, educational history (no attempt is made here to evaluate the appropriateness of type of communication methodology), and degree of family involvement.

B. Determine the degree of hearing loss and appropriateness of personal amplification; rule out the presence of middle ear problems. Assess speech perception skills with tests such as Monosyllable-Trochee-Spondee (MTS) test and Test of Auditory Comprehension (Erber, 1982; Ross, 1982).

C. Assess both receptive and expressive language skills using a battery of formal and informal procedures. Measures should be sensitive to a wide range of linguistic and cognitive skills in a heterogeneous population.

D. Vocabulary skills are assessed with standardized picture identification tests (Peabody Picture Vocabulary Test). Informal probes are used to assess the child's conceptual knowledge, classification skills, use of words in context, and ability to discover the meaning of unfamiliar words. Performance on expressive vocabulary measures may suggest word-finding and retrieval problems (Moeller et al, 1983).

E. Syntactic and grammatic skills are assessed with formal measures, such as the Test of Language Development, Child Language Ability Measures, Test of Grammatical Comprehension, and the Test of Syntactic Abilities. The effect of the hearing impairment on the child's perception of morphologic and syntactic elements, which are often obscure in spoken-signed English, should be determined. The length and syntactic complexity of an utterance may affect a child's processing and comprehension of conceptual information. Spontaneous expressive language samples should be analyzed for level of syntactic rule mastery (Osberger, 1986).

F. Academic demands increase in semantic abstraction and requirements for verbal problem solving as children progress through school. Hearing-impaired students often rely on key-word comprehension strategies beyond an age that is appropriate, and thus they fail to attend to structure and content in processing information. It is critical to assess the child's ability to manipulate conceptual and linguistic information to solve problems. Recommended standardized tests are the Inventory of Language Assessment Tasks, Test of Concept Utilization, Test of Problem Solving, and the Word Test or Language Processing Test. Informal procedures are used to assess question comprehension, logical reasoning skills, inferential knowledge, flexibility in problem solving, and influence of abstraction on comprehension.

G. Informal procedures are used to assess discourse skills, such as comprehension of story detail (Ross, 1982), topic identification, maintenance and shifting, use of clarification and repair strategies, level of context sensitivity, and formulation skills.

H. A formal measure, Phonetic Level Evaluation (Ling, 1976), and informal procedures are used to determine if the child can sustain phonation without excessive or inappropriate changes in fundamental frequency (Fo). Informal procedures are used to determine adequacy of word stress, phrase structure (production of phrases with no pauses and appropriate intonation contour), intonation patterns (appropriate variation in Fo as a function of linguistic context). Articulatory skills are assessed with nonsense syllables (Phonetic Level Evaluation) and standardized picture articulation tests, such as the Goldman-Fristoe Test of Articulation, to determine error patterns of consonants and vowels. Informal measures should be used to determine the effect of phonetic and lexical context on phoneme production and the ability to imitate and discriminate speech targets through audition only. Intelligibility is assessed with rating scales or the Speech Intelligibility Evaluation Test.

I. Refer for diagnostic teaching or additional testing to rule out presence of speech-motor problems, learning disabilities, neurologic involvement, or mental retardation.

J. Evaluate the child's learning skills and other factors that affect language learning including independent learning and organization skills, attending behavior, ability to follow directions, parental involvement and acceptance of handicap, teacher-peer interactions, and the physical environment of classroom.

K. If the problems are more severe than hearing loss or educational history would predict, refer the child for psychologic or social services consultation or consult with the school administration.

L. Formulate a therapy plan based on all test results and identification of child's strengths as well as weaknesses if the problems are consistent with the degree of hearing loss and the educational history.

## References

Erber NP. Auditory Training. Washington, DC: AG Bell Association for the Deaf, 1982.

Ling D. Speech and the hearing impaired: theory and practice. Washington, DC: AG Bell Association for the Deaf, 1976.

Moeller MP, McConkey AJ, Osberger MJ. Assessing the communication skills of hearing-impaired children. Audio 1983; 8:113.

Osberger MJ, ed. The Language and Learning Skills of Hearing-Impaired Students. Washinton, DC: ASHA Monograph. No. 23 March, 1986.

Ross M. Hard of Hearing Children in Regular Schools. Englewood Cliffs, NJ: Prentice-Hall, 1982.

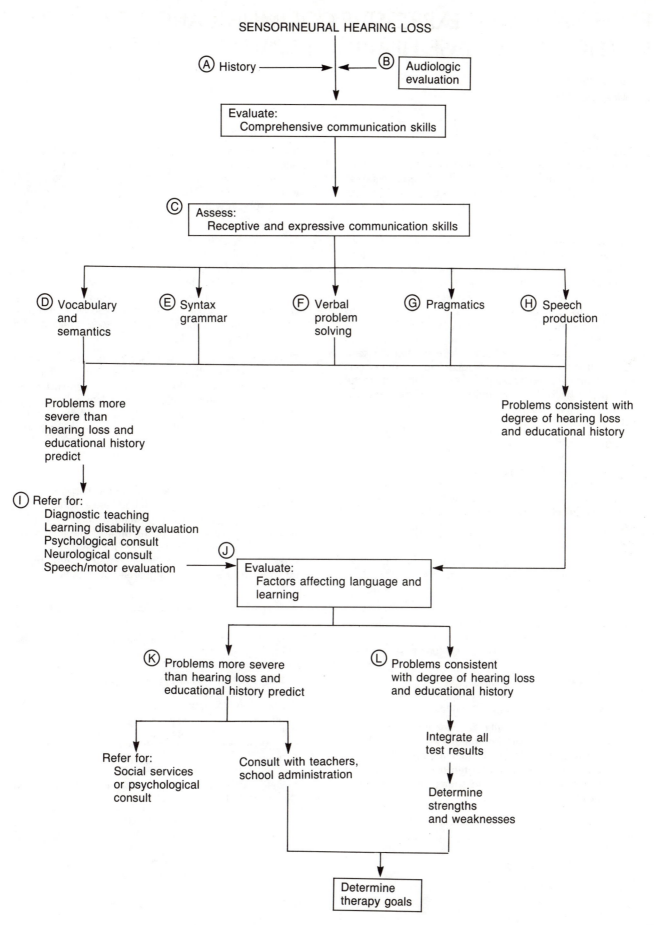

# REMEDIATION OF EXPRESSIVE COMMUNICATION PROBLEMS IN THE SCHOOL-AGE HEARING-IMPAIRED CHILD

*Mary Joe Osberger, Ph.D.*
*Mary Pat Moeller, M.S.*

A. Determine history of speech and language therapy and consistency of hearing aid use. Check functioning of hearing aid, and determine speech sound targets (segmental and/or suprasegmental). Suggested training sequence is appropriate for children using oral or total communication.

B. Begin with drills with the target in simple context (nonsense syllables or monosyllabic words) (Ling, 1976). Tasks should be imitative, having the child produce a target modeled by the clinician on the basis of auditory cues only. The clinician's model should be removed, and child should produce speech pattern on demand; the pattern can be elicited with pictures or orthographic representation. Auditory discrimination requires the child to identify a speech pattern from a closed set that is meant to develop the auditory-oral feedback loop. Emphasis is placed on the child learning to monitor and evaluate the quality of his or her own productions (Osberger et al, 1978).

C. The child may need cues through sensory channels in addition to the impaired auditory system (Calvert and Silverman, 1983). Tactile and visual cues may be added to facilitate production and discrimination of the target speech sound. When the child can perform the task, additional sensory cues should be withdrawn in order to facilitate development of auditory-oral skills.

D. Drills can be conducted using larger linguistic units (words, phrases, sentences). Initially, facilitative speech contexts (such as carrier phrases containing facilitative phonemic environments) should be used. Generalization to numerous phonemic environments should be incorporated.

E. Initially, target speech sounds can be embedded in familiar phrases and used in situations in which the listeners have abundant contextual cues to support the linguistic message. Listeners should be highly familiar with the speech of the child. Children who use total communication should practice producing and receiving speech without the support of signs.

F. If the child is not successful in functional communicative situations, the clinician should model repair and clarification strategies for the child. The child needs to be able to monitor and evaluate his or her own productions so he or she can determine the source of the listener's difficulty.

G. Increase the complexity of the task by putting the speech target in more novel linguistic contexts, and reduce the amount of environmental and contextual support available to the listener. The child should practice functional use of speech with persons not highly familiar with his or her speech.

H. The child must incorporate the speech target in utterances that he or she formulates. The structure of utterances should be varied and should include sentence-length requests, comments, or questions. Context sensitivity can be developed through role-playing activities. Speech skills should be developed in the context of contingent responding in order to formulate a solid base for discourse skills.

I. The utterance length is increased to conversation. Pragmatic language skills can be developed in parallel with speech production skills. The child is given structured practice in discourse skills including learning the rules of topic negotiation, turn-taking, and informativeness (Kretschmer and Kretschmer, 1978). The child should learn to formulate comments in conversation so that they follow a logical sequence. Speech targets can be embedded in these language activities.

J. The child produces the speech target in spontaneous conversations. He or she should be able to monitor and evaluate his or her own productions and self correct when necessary. If errors occur, appropriate repair and clarification strategies should be employed. The child should assume responsibility for communication repair by spontaneously applying learned strategies.

## References

Calvert DR, Silverman SR. Speech and deafness. Washinton, DC: AG Bell Association for the Deaf, 1983.

Kretschmer R, Kretschmer L. Pragmatics: development in normal-hearing and hearing-impaired children. In: Subtelny J, ed. Speech assessment and speech improvement for the hearing impaired. Washington, DC: AG Bell Association for the Deaf, 1980.

Ling D. Speech and the hearing-impaired child: theory and practice. Washington, DC: AG Bell Association for the Deaf, 1976.

Osberger MJ, Johnstone A, Levitt H, Swarts E. Evaluation of a model speech training program for the deaf. J Commun Disord 1978; 11:293.

SCHOOL-AGE HEARING-IMPAIRED CHILD

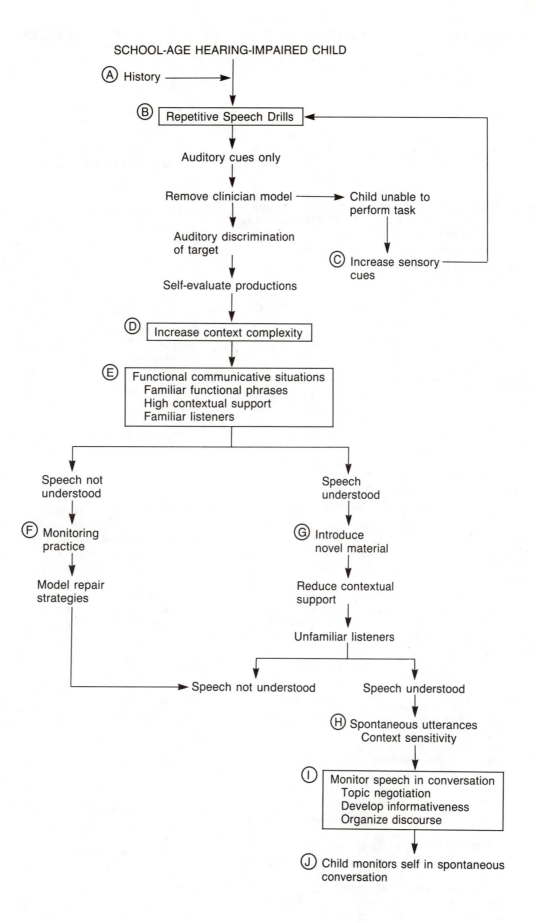

Ⓐ History

Ⓑ Repetitive Speech Drills

Auditory cues only

Remove clinician model ⟶ Child unable to
perform task

Auditory discrimination
of target

Ⓒ Increase sensory
cues

Self-evaluate productions

Ⓓ Increase context complexity

Ⓔ Functional communicative situations
Familiar functional phrases
High contextual support
Familiar listeners

Speech not
understood

Speech
understood

Ⓕ Monitoring
practice

Ⓖ Introduce
novel material

Model repair
strategies

Reduce contextual
support

Unfamiliar listeners

Speech not understood

Speech understood

Ⓗ Spontaneous utterances
Context sensitivity

Ⓘ Monitor speech in conversation
Topic negotiation
Develop informativeness
Organize discourse

Ⓙ Child monitors self in spontaneous
conversation

# ACQUIRED HEARING LOSS IN THE ADULT: ASSESSMENT

*Dean C. Garstecki, Ph.D.*

Common causes of hearing loss in the adult include conditions affecting the outer ear (collapsed canal, disease, deformity, accident, foreign body, cerumen, tympanic membrane perforation), middle ear (eustachian tube dysfunction, cholesteatoma, ossicular chain discontinuity, malleus fixation, otitis media, otosclerosis), inner ear (Meniere's disease, noise, skull trauma, ototoxicity, presbycusis, perilymph fistula), and the neural pathway to the brain (acoustic neuroma, intracranial tumors, multiple sclerosis, vascular disturbances).

A. Begin with identifying information, reason for referral (note mention of pending medical-legal action or compensation), and referral source. Note age, familial hearing loss, noise exposure, head trauma, vascular disorders, balance disorders, syndrome stigmata, and use of ototoxic medications. Indicate the reported cause, onset, and progression of hearing loss. Note possible influence of hearing loss on speech and voice. Fluctuations in hearing are often suggestive of mild to moderate loss. The patient with conductive loss will hear better in noise than the patient with sensorineural loss. A patient with bilateral, high-frequency, sensorineural hearing loss complains about being unable to understand others in noisy situations. Investigate reports of medical treatment for hearing loss, related conditions (tinnitus, dizziness), and general health problems. Review attempts to manage problems related to hearing loss (lipreading classes, hearing-aid use, aural rehabilitation [Martin, 1984]).

B. Inspect the ear canal and visualize the tympanic membrane, noting physical condition and possible signs of obstruction. Measure pure tone air and bone conduction thresholds bilaterally with appropriate masking. Obtain speech reception thresholds (SRT), suprathreshold speech discrimination scores, tympanograms, and acoustic reflex thresholds. If a hearing aid is worn, measure its electroacoustic characteristics and determine the benefit derived from the hearing aid through behavioral audiometry.

Results from this basic battery may suggest:

1. no loss (all results normal);
2. conductive lesion (air-bone gap, SRT approximates pure tone average [PTA], good to excellent speech discrimination, type B, C, A$_S$, or A$_D$ tympanogram, absent or elevated acoustic reflex thresholds);
3. cochlear pathology (air-bone thresholds approximate and demonstrate loss, SRT approximates PTA, fair to good speech discrimination, normal tympanograms, low or absent acoustic reflex thresholds);
4. retrocochlear pathology (normal thresholds, no air-bone gap, SRT generally agrees with PTA, poor speech discrimination, normal tympanograms, abnormal reflex decay)(Rosenberg, 1978); and,
5. malfunctioning and/or inappropriate hearing aid for loss (Jerger and Jerger, 1981).

C. Through interview and use of hearing handicap scales, note the impact of hearing loss of everyday communication, personal safety, and ability to earn a living.

D. Otologic evaluation should precede audiologic evaluation. Vestibular examination is warranted when a balance problem or dizziness is reported or when attempting to rule out retrocochlear lesion. Tomography enables the clinician to visualize structural abnormalities of the cochlea and locate acoustic tumors. Electroencephalography is critical for diagnosis of brain pathology that may impact on the auditory system. A psychological evaluation provides information relating to intellectual ability and personality that assists in management and rehabilitation.

E. Rule out a conductive lesion by adding a static compliance test to the otoadmittance battery. A low value suggests a stiff tympanic membrane and/or ossicular chain. A high value indicates disarticulation of the ossicular chain.

F. Rule out cochlear pathology by administering: (1) Performance intensity function for phonetically balanced words; PI-PB ratio is less than 0.40; (2) Monaural-Alternate Binaural Loudness Balance Tests (positive recruitment); (3) Tone Decay Test (slight decay); and, (4) Bekesy Audiometry (Type II tracing).

G. Rule out retrocochlear pathology by administering: (1) Performance intensity function for phonetically balanced words; PI-PB ratio is greater than 0.40; (2) Monaural-Alternate Binaural Loudness Balance Test (no recruitment or decruitment); (3) Tone Decay Test (marked decay); (4) Bekesy Audiometry (Type III or IV); and, (5) Auditory Brainstem Response (no response on side with lesion or significant difference in I-V interpeak latency on impaired side; abnormal tracings ipsilaterally and contralaterally found for posterior cranial fossa lesions)(Jerger and Jerger, 1981).

H. Rule out central auditory pathology by administering Synthetic Sentence Intelligibility task with ipsilateral (SSI-ICM) and contralateral (SSI-CCM) competing messages. Sentence intelligibility will be poorer than monosyllabic word discrimination scores in the the patient with neural involvement central to the cochlea. Dichotic listening task results demonstrate reduced auditory function for the ear contralateral to a temporal lobe lesion (Rintleman, 1979).

## References

Jerger S, Jerger J. Auditory disorders: a manual for clinical evaluation. Boston: Little, Brown, 1981.

Martin F. Principles of audiology: a study guide. Baltimore: University Park Press, 1984.

Rintleman WF. Hearing assessment. Baltimore: University Park Press, 1979.

Rosenberg PE. Differentiating cochlear and retro-cochlear dysfunction. In: Katz J, ed. Handbook of clinical audiology. 2nd ed. Baltimore: Williams & Wilkins, 1978:159.

# ACQUIRED HEARING LOSS IN THE ADULT: ASSESSMENT

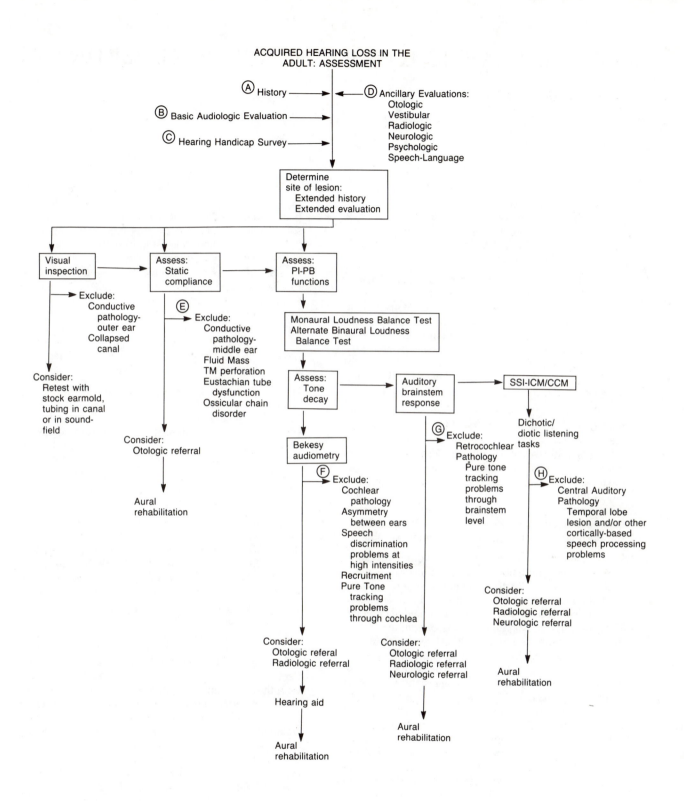

Ⓐ History

Ⓑ Basic Audiologic Evaluation

Ⓒ Hearing Handicap Survey

Ⓓ Ancillary Evaluations:
Otologic
Vestibular
Radiologic
Neurologic
Psychologic
Speech-Language

Determine
site of lesion:
Extended history
Extended evaluation

Visual
inspection

Assess:
Static
compliance

Assess:
PI-PB
functions

Exclude:
Conductive
pathology-
outer ear
Collapsed
canal

Ⓔ Exclude:
Conductive
pathology-
middle ear
Fluid Mass
TM perforation
Eustachian tube
dysfunction
Ossicular chain
disorder

Monaural Loudness Balance Test
Alternate Binaural Loudness
Balance Test

Consider:
Retest with
stock earmold,
tubing in canal
or in sound-
field

Consider:
Otologic referral

Aural
rehabilitation

Assess:
Tone
decay

Auditory
brainstem
response

SSI-ICM/CCM

Dichotic/
diotic listening tasks

Bekesy
audiometry

Ⓖ Exclude:
Retrocochlear
Pathology
Pure tone
tracking
problems
through
brainstem
level

Ⓗ Exclude:
Central Auditory
Pathology
Temporal lobe
lesion and/or other
cortically-based
speech processing
problems

Ⓕ Exclude:
Cochlear
pathology
Asymmetry
between ears
Speech
discrimination
problems at
high intensities
Recruitment
Pure Tone
tracking
problems
through cochlea

Consider:
Otologic referral
Radiologic referral
Neurologic referral

Consider:
Otologic referal
Radiologic referral

Consider:
Otologic referral
Radiologic referral
Neurologic referral

Aural
rehabilitation

Hearing aid

Aural
rehabilitation

Aural
rehabilitation

# ACQUIRED HEARING LOSS IN THE ADULT: REHABILITATION

*Dean C. Garstecki, Ph.D.*

A. Describe and provide rationale for each major program component. Present options for participation. Request joint participation of spouse, family member, or close friend. Elicit description of primary problem and offer plan to address it. Explain instructional format. Provide fee and schedule information.

B. Obtain further description of chief complaint and reason for seeking rehabilitative care at this time. Review history of hearing loss and success in its management. Note presence of medical conditions related (tinnitus, dizziness) and unrelated (visual impairment, neurologic disorders) to hearing loss and their prescribed treatment. Observe influence of hearing loss on interpersonal communication skills. Note adjustment problems and information deficits (Garstecki, 1982).

C. When suggested by the history and/or observation, referral should be made for otological evaluation and treatment. A vestibular examination is needed when balance/dizziness problems are reported. Tomograms are required to visualize the structure of the cochlea and/or the location of acoustic tumors. Electroencephalograms aid in the diagnosis of brain pathology. Psychological evaluation and treatment is helpful when an individual experiences an inability to accept hearing loss and responsibility for self-management of related problems.

D. Extend the audiologic test battery to include measures of speech discrimination in quiet and noise situations (multi-talker babble; 0 dB signal-to-noise ratio) in sound field at conversation level (60 dB sound pressure level) under the most usual listening mode, unaided or aided. This provides a reasonable estimate of communication difficulty experienced in difficult, yet commonly occurring, listening conditions. Self-report of hearing handicap and observations of others known by the hearing-impaired individual assists in gaining insight into specific communication conditions. Also, handicap scale results provide insight into the psychological impact of hearing loss. This information is useful for counseling and education purposes. An estimate of binocular visual acuity alerts the audiologist to the possible need for referral and it provides an indication of the hearing-impaired individual's ability to compensate for hearing loss through use of visual cues (speechreading). Snellen charts are used for screening visual acuity. Auditory-visual communication skills are assessed using word and sentence materials presented in the test conditions noted above. Auditory and auditory-visual speech discrimination scores constitute a baseline measure for auditory and auditory-visual training (Garstecki, 1984).

Earmold impressions should be made if consideration is to be given to selection of a hearing aid, a change in earmold configuration, or use of an earmold with an assistive listening device.

E. Objective measures that parallel those employed in behavioral evaluations of speech discrimination in hearing-aid selection, should be used to evaluate and select assistive listening devices (personal amplifiers, telephone amplifiers, television listening devices, portable loop induction systems). Other devices (telephone message decoders, vibrotactile aids, telephone signalers, TV captioners, home alerting or warning systems) should be selected on the basis of the hearing-impaired individual's interests, needs, and ability to use the device without assistance. Long-term satisfaction and use of assistive devices should be assessed by written questionnaire; user satisfaction is helpful when advising new device users (Kasten and McCroskey, 1982).

F. Hints for improving everyday communication are discussed and learned through role-playing activities. These include strategies for using speechreading and nonverbal and situational cues. Stagemanaging strategies are exercised. Hints for improving assertiveness in difficult communication conditions are provided. Information on ways to improve message understanding is also given to individuals with normal hearing who regularly interact with hearing-impaired individuals.

G. Communication strategies are applied to exercises designed to improve message understanding under conditions of decreasing redundancy of information. Materials vary in linguistic content from words (low) to stories (high). They are presented in varying competing noise conditions ranging from quiet to cafeteria noise/multi-talker babble at an unfavorable signal-to-noise ratio. Situational cues range from those that complement the message to message distractors. Each of these parameters is isolated and systematically recombined to create messages of graded redundancy. Initial use of highly redundant material acquaints the hearing-impaired individual with the communication task in a way that is motivating. As materials become less redundant, greater effort must be directed toward application of communication strategies. Ultimately, the intent is to optimize the hearing-impaired individual's ability to follow everyday conversation. Using these principles, exercises are designed to develop auditory communication skills (message perception through audition alone as in telephone conversation or when communicating with someone in another room) and auditory-visual communication skills (combined auditory and visual message perception as in face-to-face conversation or when watching a television program) (Garstecki, 1981).

H. The counseling process begins with the identification of problems related to the personal acceptance and/or management of hearing loss. Problems are evaluated in terms of the feasibility of their being resolved. An approach toward problem solving is developed. It may re-

# ACQUIRED HEARING LOSS IN THE ADULT: REHABILITATION

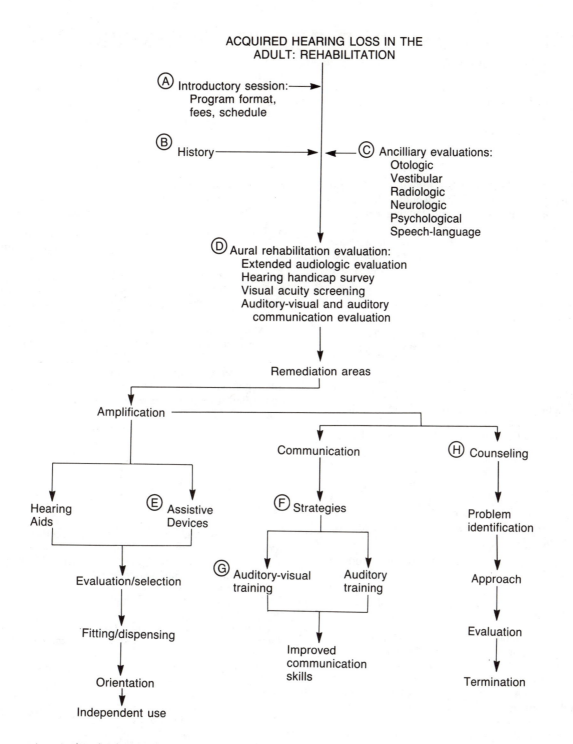

quire individual counseling or involve other hearing-impaired individuals, spouses, and family members in communication therapy, assertiveness training, and other counseling techniques. Success in resolving the remediable problem is evaluated. Decisions are made either to refer for additional care and/or to terminate the counseling relationship. An invitation is extended for the hearing-impaired individual to return to the program for future advice and assistance as needed (Wylde, 1982).

## References

Garstecki DC. Aural rehabilitation for the aging adult. In: Alpiner J, ed. Handbook of adult rehabilitative audiology. Baltimore: Williams & Wilkins, 1982.

Garstecki DC. Auditory-visual training paradigm for hearing-impaired adults. J Acad Rehab Aud 1981; 14:223.

Garstecki DC. Techniques for adult aural rehabilitation. In: Perkins WM, ed. Current therapy for communication disorders. New York: Thieme-Stratton, 1984.

Kasten RN, McCroskey R. The hearing aid as related to rehabilitation. In: Alpiner J, ed. Handbook of adult rehabilitative audiology. Baltimore: Williams & Wilkins, 1982.

Wylde M. The remediation process: Psychologic and counseling aspects. In: Alpiner J, ed. Handbook of adult rehabilitive audiology. Baltimore: Williams & Wilkins, 1982.

# AUDITORY PROCESSES IN THE ADULT OR GERIATRIC INDIVIDUAL: ASSESSMENT

Daniel J. Orchik, Ph.D.
David J. Wark, Ph.D.
Daniel S. Beasley, Ph.D.

Audiological assessment is approached from the perspective of a freestanding audiology facility. This would include a private practice, community speech and hearing center, or university-based clinic. It is assumed that the audiologic assessment entails not only the process of selecting an appropriate assessment battery, but also involves making otologic referrals where indicated and at the appropriate place in the assessment process.

A. The case history chronicles the onset and duration of hearing loss and possible contributing factors. In particular, suggestions of significant balance disorder, sudden hearing loss, ear pain, or drainage would necessitate direct medical referral (Rosenberg, 1978).

B. Otoscopic examination is completed prior to any testing to determine whether any obstruction exists, which would require medical referral before valid audiologic assessment could be completed. The most common obstruction is impacted cerumen, although other obstructions may be found.

C. The basic audiologic evaluation (BAE) includes immittance audiometry, pure-tone audiometry (air and bone conduction), and speech audiometry. The relationships among these tests determine in large part the processes to follow (Jerger, 1983; Jerger et al, 1974; Hayes and Jerger, 1980).

D. Patients reporting significant balance disorder, sudden onset of hearing loss, persistent ear pain, or drainage are referred for otologic evaluation. A direct medical referral is made following the basic audiologic evaluation irrespective of the outcome of the test battery.

E. Individuals presenting a significant conductive component to their hearing loss are referred for otologic examination and possible treatment. The basic audiologic evaluation should be repeated following completion of otologic management. If the hearing problem has been successfully corrected, no further evaluation is indicated. If the hearing loss could not be reversed medically, the patient is directed toward evaluation for communication management (Jerger et al, 1974).

F. An individual with normal hearing typically requires no further evaluation. However, an individual who presents normal hearing and yet reports hearing difficulty warrants further evaluation. The most appropriate measure at this point is evaluation of the auditory brainstem response (ABR). Assessment of central auditory function using measures such as the staggered-spondaic word test (SSW), synthetic sentence identification (SSI), or time-altered speech are also appropriate. Middle-latency auditory-evoked potentials (MLR) should be considered as well (Jerger et al, 1985; Jerger et al, 1980; Jerger and Jerger, 1975; Musiek and Guerkink, 1982).

G. A patient with sensorineural hearing loss (SNHL), in addition to a careful history, should be scrutinized for symmetry of hearing loss. With symmetrical pure-tone and speech audiometric data, the patient can be directed toward communication management. However, any asymmetry in either pure-tone thresholds or speech discrimination (WDS) warrants further study. Evaluations of the ABR should be done in all cases of asymmetry. Other speech audiometric measures, such as the SSI might also be utilized. Tests for acoustic reflex latency, amplitude growth, and reflex decay, would be diagnostically useful (Jerger et al, 1985; Jerger and Jerger, 1975; Mangham et al, 1980; Clemis and Samo, 1980; Hayes and Jerger, 1982).

# References

Clemis J, Samo C. The acoustic reflex latency test: clinical applications. Laryngoscope 1980; 90:601–611.

Hayes D, Jerger J. Effect of degree of hearing loss on diagnostic audiometric tests. Am J Otol 1980; 2:91–96.

Hayes D, Jerger J. Signal-averaging of the acoustic reflex: diagnostic applications of amplitude characteristics. Scan Audiol 17 (suppl) 1982;31–36.

Jerger J. Strategies for neuroaudiologic evaluation. Sem Hear 1983; 4:109–120.

Jerger J, Anthony L, Jerger S, Mauldin L. Studies in impedance audiometry III: middle ear disorders. Arch Otolaryngol 1974; 99:165–171.

Jerger J, Jerger S. Clinical validity of central auditory tests. Scand Audiol 1975; 4:147–163.

Jerger J, Neely J, Jerger S. Speech, impedance and auditory brainstem response audiometry in brainstem tumors. Arch Otolaryngol 1980; 106:218–223.

Jerger J, Oliver T, Stach B. Auditory brainstem response testing strategies. In: Jacobsen J, ed. The auditory brainstem response. San Diego: College-Hill Press, 1985.

Mangham C, Lindeman R, Dawson W. Stapedius reflex quantification in acoustic tumor patients. Laryngoscope 1980; 90:242–250.

Musiek F, Guerkink N. Auditory brainstem response and central auditory test findings for patients with brainstem lesions: a preliminary report. Laryngoscope 1982; 92:891–900.

Rosenberg P. Case history: the first test. In: Katz J, ed. Handbook of clinical audiology, 2nd ed. Baltimore: Williams & Wilkins, 1978.

PATIENT WITH HEARING LOSS

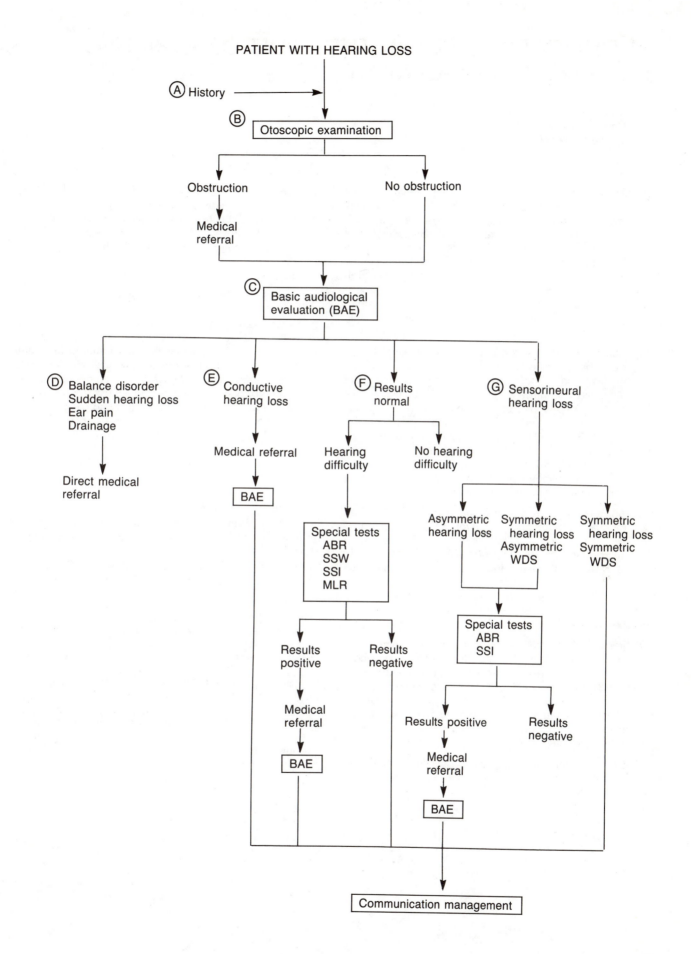

# AUDITORY PROCESSES IN THE ADULT OR GERIATRIC INDIVIDUAL: MANAGEMENT

David J. Wark, Ph.D.
Daniel J. Orchik, Ph.D.
Daniel S. Beasley, Ph.D.

A. Amplification assessment must first ensure that the client has a thorough understanding of the advantages and disadvantages of amplification in general. Secondly, various amplification systems must be selected and evaluated comparatively for each client; emphasis needs to be given to the evaluation of assistive listening devices for this population (Vaughn et al, 1983). Finally, the clinician needs to ensure that each client receives appropriate orientation in the use of his amplification system, including instruction in its use with other electronic media such as the telephone, radio, and television.

B. Communication assessment places primary emphasis on a current description of the client and the psychological, physical, and socioeconomic considerations that impact upon his or her present communication abilities (Loebel and Eisdorfer, 1984; Weinstein, 1984). Both informal assessment tools (interview and case history) and more formal ones (standardized tests and self assessment questionaires) should be used in the process (Weinstein, 1984; Giolas, 1982; Demorest and Erdman, 1987). Including family members or significant others in gathering appropriate information is a helpful strategy.

C. An individualized profile of the client's specific communication needs and skills is formulated. Again, input is solicited from both client and family members when appropriate. The profile provides a structure that facilitates decision making in determining an appropriate course(s) of action. The profile may suggest that the client's communication skills are adequate for his or her particular needs at this time. In this case the client would be dismissed.

D. Rehabilitation often consists of two general approaches. A client's profile may suggest the need for one or both of these approaches. Communication counseling is traditionally a didactic approach designed to develop specific communication skills. Communication therapy offers an alternative to more traditional approaches by assisting the client in the development of appropriate communication patterns.

E. Communication training provides specific instruction to enhance the client's skills in the use of auditory and visual cues in communication. It is particularly important to use situation based therapy materials that are geared to the client's specific communication needs. Manual communication instruction should be available for those clients who might benefit from the use of these skills.

F. Communication counseling provides an opportunity for clients to develop an awareness of communication problem areas and to identify their present interaction patterns. This can best be accomplished through an interactive group structure that includes both clients and family members. The therapist serves primarily as a catalyst who provides direction to group discussion. The group not only serves as a "laboratory" for describing alternative interaction patterns, but also provides a setting in which to develop the skills necessary to use these patterns (Fleming-Haspiel and Clement, 1980).

## References

Demorest ME, Erdman SA. Development of the communication profile for the hearing impaired. J Speech Hear Disord 1987; 52(2):129.

Fleming-Haspiel M, Clement JR. The communication workshop; an alternative approach to hearing therapy for adults. Communication Disorders: An Audio Journal for Continuing Education. 1980; 5(3).

Giolas TG. Assessment of hearing handicap: self-report procedure (Chapter 4). In: Giolas TG. Hearing handicapped adults. Englewood Cliffs, NJ: Prentice-Hall, 1982.

Loebel JP, Eisdorfer C. Psychological and psychiatric factors in the rehabilitation of the elderly. In: Williams TF, ed. Rehabilitation in the aging. New York: Raven Press, 1984.

Vaughn GR, Lightfoot RK, Gibbs SD. Assistive listening devices: SPACE ASHA 1983; 25(3):33.

Weinstein BE. Management of the hearing impaired elderly. In: Jacobs-Condit L, ed. Gerontology and communication disorders. Rockville, MD: American Speech-Language-Hearing Association, 1984.

PATIENT WITH COMMUNICATION IMPAIRMENT

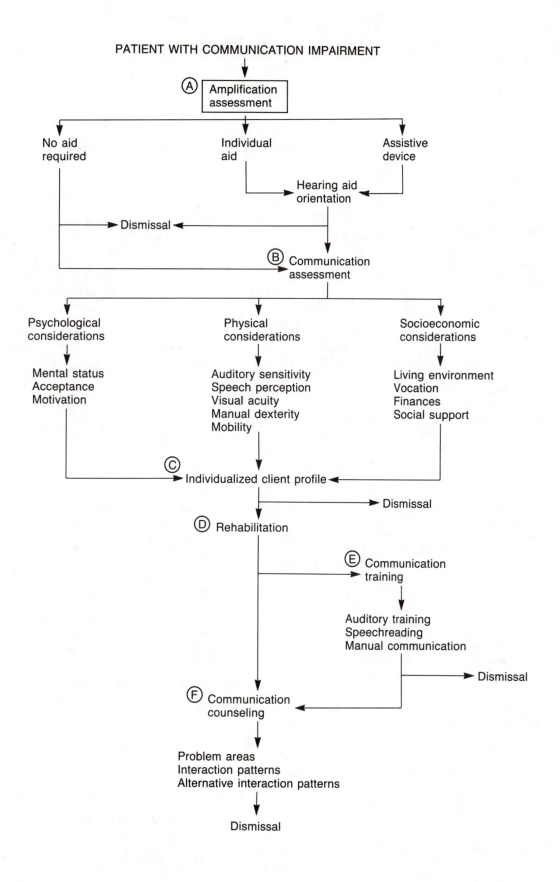

Ⓐ Amplification
assessment

No aid
required

Individual
aid

Assistive
device

Hearing aid
orientation

Dismissal

Ⓑ Communication
assessment

Psychological
considerations

Physical
considerations

Socioeconomic
considerations

Mental status
Acceptance
Motivation

Auditory sensitivity
Speech perception
Visual acuity
Manual dexterity
Mobility

Living environment
Vocation
Finances
Social support

Ⓒ Individualized client profile

Dismissal

Ⓓ Rehabilitation

Ⓔ Communication
training

Auditory training
Speechreading
Manual communication

Dismissal

Ⓕ Communication
counseling

Problem areas
Interaction patterns
Alternative interaction patterns

Dismissal

# AUDITORY PROCESSING DIFFICULTIES

*Christine Sloan, Ph.D.*

A. Auditory processing difficulties (APD) often present as more general speech, language, or learning problems (Sloan, 1980a; Tallal, 1980). The clinician must assess a range of speech, language, and learning behaviors in order to ascertain whether deficits in these areas could be attributed fully or in part to problems in auditory processing (Sloan, 1980b).

B. History information is used to help differentiate APD from other disorders. Several findings suggest APD may be present: (1) inconsistent response to speech; (2) parental concern about hearing; (3) difficulties listening to or comprehending speech, particularly when noise or other distractions are present; (4) frequent need for repetition of what is said; (5) difficulties remembering what is said. Obtain school records and achievement test results. Classroom behavior such as poor listening, misunderstanding, and difficulties following directions suggest APD. Analyze achievement test results for poor word attack skills, low reading recognition, poor phonetic analysis of words, and poor spelling. Reading and spelling errors show confusion among phonetically and auditorily similar sounds (Sloan, 1986).

C. The outcomes of a general speech and language assessment may be quite variable depending on the child's age, environment, experience, language background, level of development, abilities, and motivation in testing. Generally the assessment yields a scattered profile of abilities such that an overall speech and language delay can be ruled out. Be aware of how language tests or test items increase the demand for auditory processing and specific phonetic retrieval (e.g., by providing no other cues, by reducing redundancy, by presenting stimuli of short duration, by having increased phonetic complexity, by containing phonetically/auditorily confusing elements) (Lasky and Cox, 1983; Sloan 1980b; Sloan 1986). Usually, test results for phoneme identification/discrimination, auditory memory, sentence repetition, and general information (elicited by the auditory modality alone) are low (Sloan, 1980b).

D. Reasons other than APD that cause a child to "tune out" or respond inappropriately or inconsistently to speech must be ruled out. However, it is also possible that an APD is a concomitant problem.

E. Tests of auditory perception might include commercially available tests or the clinician's own assessment. Phoneme discrimination/identification should be tested using sound pairs that are phonetically or auditorily similar (e.g., t-d, b-d, s-sh, m-n) (Sloan, 1980b; Sloan, 1986).

F. Central auditory tests can contribute to the diagnosis of APD. Currently there is no single test that is conclusive. A central auditory assessment should include a battery of tests (Pinheiro and Musilk, 1985).

G. Analyze assessment data for evidence of APD. Evidence should be available from several sources. With older children or very bright children, test to the ceiling of their abilities rather than an average level, so that more subtle deficits in auditory processing are identified (Sloan, 1980a).

H. The performance of some children often reflects a general weakness of auditory skills rather than a clear auditory processing deficit. Sometimes these children have a history of illness, middle-ear disease, or prolonged absences from school. They seem to have missed some critical experiences for developing good listening and auditory discrimination skills. They need short-term intervention to facilitate the development of these skills, such as a program of training in auditory discrimination of speech sound contrasts, and general listening strategies. Include generalization of these skills to reading, spelling, and classroom behavior. If short-term intervention does not result in a good response, treatment should be more extensive, as for APD (Sloan, 1986).

I. Treatment should include direct therapy for APD, including training in discrimination and identification of speech-sound contrasts, and extension to reading and spelling skills (if school-aged) (Sloan 1986). Inform the family and teachers about the effect of APD on the child's behavior and learning. Suggest: (1) repeating directions to the child; (2) encouraging the child to repeat to himself; (3) using a slower speaking rate; (4) being aware of the detrimental effects of a noisy environment; (5) preferential seating; (6) individualized programming when appropriate (Lasky and Cox, 1983). Integrate treatment for APD with other therapy programs the child is receiving, e.g., for language disorder. Be sure that the purpose of each is clear to the child. APD may be either part of a learning disability or a primary cause of problems in reading and spelling. Integrate therapy for APD with the teaching of reading and spelling if possible. Early intervention, before too much failure and frustration develop, is very important. A team approach in management is best.

J. APD can affect learning and especially the development of reading and spelling. Young children should be followed through the early school years to prevent these problems (Sloan, 1980a).

## References

Lasky EZ, Cox LC. Auditory processing and language interaction: evaluation and intervention strategies. In: Lasky EZ, Katz J, eds. Central auditory processing disorders. Baltimore: University Park Press, 1983.

Pinheiro ML, Musiek FE. Assessment of central auditory dysfunction: foundations and clinical correlates. Baltimore: Williams & Wilkins, 1985.

Sloan C. Auditory processing disorders and language development. In: Levinson P, Sloan C, eds. Auditory processing and language: clinical and research perspectives. New York: Grune & Stratton, 1980a:101.

Sloan C. Auditory processing disorders in children: diagnosis and

UNDIFFERENTIATED SPEECH, LANGUAGE OR
LEARNING PROBLEM

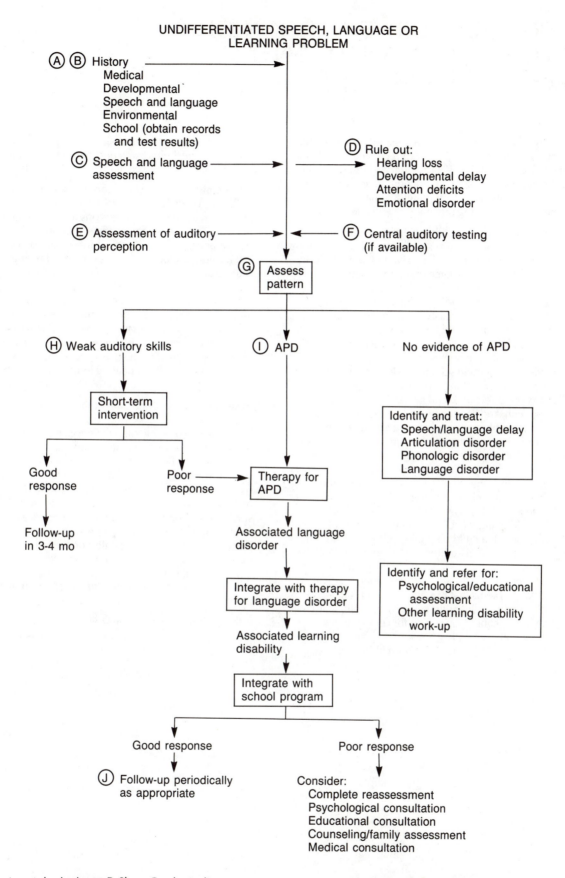

treatment. In: Levinson P, Sloan C, eds. Auditory processing and language: clinical and research perspectives. New York: Grune & Stratton, 1980b:117.

Sloan C. Treating auditory processing difficulties in children. San Diego: College-Hill Press, 1986.

Tallal P. Auditory processing disorders children. In: Levinson P, Sloan C, eds. Auditory processing and language: clinical and research perspectives. New York: Grune & Stratton, 1980:81.

# CENTRAL AUDITORY EVALUATION OF THE LEARNING DISABLED CHILD

*Frank E. Musiek, Ph.D.*

The decision making process in the assessment of central auditory function in the learning disabled (LD) child is difficult due to many factors, including individual and test variability and a lack of knowledge of the neurocommunicative process. This commentary attempts to highlight some of the major steps in the decision making process in this challenging area.

A. Not all school-age LD children have central auditory problems. Therefore, the first step in screening is to question the referral source as to observation of an auditory problem. If the referral source can substantiate instances of auditory difficulty, further information must be obtained to determine candidacy for central testing. Psychological and educational evaluations are necessary to determine (1) that the child has an overall normal IQ, (2) that his academic achievement significantly lags his potential, and (3) differences in performance on verbal vs. nonverbal subjects in school. Developmental, speech, and hearing history-taking are necessary to identify any delays in communication and/or neuromotor systems. A recent speech and language evaluation including the Token test, can provide insight into a potential problem. Medical history or a report of a thorough medical examination can provide information about neurologic, otolaryngologic, or pediatric problems that could affect test results and the diagnosis of a central auditory problem. At our facility, children must achieve at a second grade level or higher and have a mental age of at least 7 years to allow accurate evaluation of central auditory function. If a child meets the aforementioned clinical criteria for central auditory test candidacy, then one can proceed. Strict criteria for candidacy identifies the child who has psychological, achievement, medical, or intellectual problems that may interfere with valid assessment of central auditory function by audiological means. Obviously, candidacy criteria for central testing vary; however, the above are key areas from which to gather information to aid in the decision making process.

B. The basic audiological evaluation should include at least pure tone thresholds by air and bone conduction, spondee thresholds, and speech recognition testing.

C. If the child reveals a significant hearing loss in one or both ears, we do not complete the central auditory evaluation. There are two main reasons for not pursuing central tests: (1) the basis for a child's auditory difficulty may be the peripheral loss, and (2) interpretation of central test results is contaminated by peripheral hearing deficits. If there is a conductive loss, medical treatment and audiological follow-up are recommended. If the hearing loss is sensorineural, then medical evaluation, possible amplification, aural rehabilitation, and educational considerations must be pursued. Special educational planning may also be required for the child with conductive hearing loss, but this is also dependent on many factors. If there is no peripheral hearing impairment, central testing can be initiated.

D. In central auditory evaluation of the LD child, some type of dichotic speech task should be included in the test battery. Also, some measure of temporal sequencing ability is a valuable tool in assessment (e.g., pitch patterns and two-tone ordering). Monaural distorted speech tasks, such as filtered, compressed, interrupted or competing speech, can be valuable in assessment. In our experience, however, distorted speech tests are not as sensitive as dichotic or temporal sequencing tasks. It is important to have at least one test to assess low brainstem integrity to rule out or alert one to acoustic neuroma or, more commonly, a brainstem lesion in the LD child. Although these lesions seldom occur in children, it is important not to overlook the possibility. If the child passes the test battery, he is dismissed.

E. If the central test results are below the norm, the findings should be analyzed. There should be some quantification of the deficit (i.e., severe, moderate, or mild).

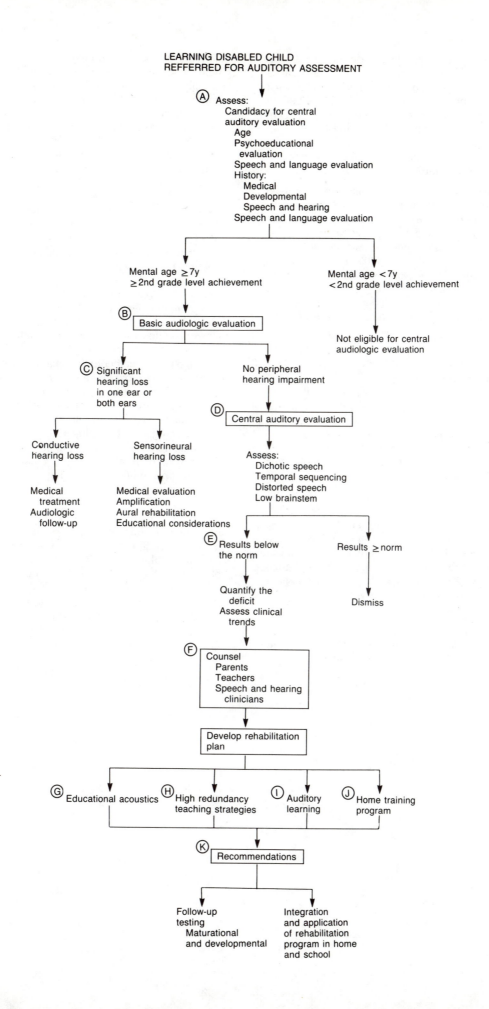

LEARNING DISABLED CHILD
REFFERED FOR AUDITORY ASSESSMENT

(A) Assess:
    Candidacy for central
    auditory evaluation
       Age
       Psychoeducational
       evaluation
    Speech and language evaluation
    History:
       Medical
       Developmental
       Speech and hearing
    Speech and language evaluation

Mental age ≥ 7y
≥ 2nd grade level achievement

Mental age < 7y
< 2nd grade level achievement

(B) Basic audiologic evaluation

Not eligible for central
audiologic evaluation

(C) Significant
hearing loss
in one ear or
both ears

No peripheral
hearing impairment

(D) Central auditory evaluation

Conductive
hearing loss

Sensorineural
hearing loss

Assess:
    Dichotic speech
    Temporal sequencing
    Distorted speech
    Low brainstem

Medical
treatment
Audiologic
follow-up

Medical evaluation
Amplification
Aural rehabilitation
Educational considerations

(E) Results below
the norm

Results ≥ norm

Quantify the
deficit
Assess clinical
trends

Dismiss

(F) Counsel
    Parents
    Teachers
    Speech and hearing
    clinicians

Develop rehabilitation
plan

(G) Educational acoustics

(H) High redundancy
teaching strategies

(I) Auditory
learning

(J) Home training
program

(K) Recommendations

Follow-up
testing
    Maturational
    and developmental

Integration
and application
of rehabilitation
program in home
and school

Any trends, such as left ear deficits on most tests, normal performance on one type of test, and severe deficits on another task should be used for interpretation. Test analyses should be used to obtain information about the type of auditory processes that are problematic. It is important to realize that abnormal central test results can indicate an active neurological problem that should be ruled out or managed by appropriate medical consultation (Musiek et al, 1986).

F.  After findings are analyzed, parents and teachers need to be counseled about the implications of the test results. A rehabilitation plan must be delineated at a separate meeting with parents and all professionals involved in the child's education. The plan is designed around the central auditory test results, the child's current academic program, and input from the parents. Many of the children we see for evaluation travel a great distance to get to our facility; therefore, we depend on parents and school professionals to follow through on the recommendations.

G.  One of the first items in the rehabilitation scheme is educational acoustics. This involves determining, either directly or indirectly, the noise level of the educational environment. If noise seems to be a problem, the concepts of signal-to-noise ratio and academic performance are discussed. A handout is given (usually to the classroom teacher) on how to reduce ambient noise levels and reverberation times at minimal cost. If noise levels cannot be reduced, the use of assistive listening devices (e.g., auditory trainers) is discussed.

H.  High redundancy teaching strategies are important to the child's academic performance. Handouts are made available to the classroom teacher outlining these approaches. The suggested guidelines include ways to use multisensory approaches for relaying information, classroom placement and seating arrangements, ways to emphasize inflection and gestures when speaking, and ways to gain attention. The key point is to make the presentation of educational material as redundant as possible.

I.  Auditory training can be done at home or school. Our auditory training paradigms are quite different from the classical approaches. Though much is dependent on the type of deficit and the child's own inclinations toward therapy, some approaches seem to work well with most children. For example, a primary exercise teaches and trains the child to listen for and distinguish among various subtle types of inflections that affect the meaning of a phrase or sentence. Use of the Language Master in this therapy has proven valuable in making immediate comparisons of stressed versus nonstressed words or phrases. Transferring auditory input to a motor activity and then to a verbal output is not only a good therapy concept, but can often be developed as a strategy to help in the integration and retention of auditory information. Most of these training techniques are of low redundancy and challenge the child. This approach is appropriate for training, but must not be used in the educational setting.

J.  The home training program is an important part of the rehabilitation plan. We believe that the child must work daily at developing listening skills and strategies, a consistency which often cannot be established in school. Parents and teachers must be aware of each other's efforts and work together in the rehabilitation process. The home training program can be a continuation of what has been started at school or it may be a simplified version of the school plans. Vocabulary building, electronic listening games, reading aloud emphasizing inflection, and listening games developed around bedtime stories are some therapies easily adapted for home use. The key factor in home training is that it is daily, short, and intense activity, unless the listening activity is incorporated into something leisurely such as a bedtime story.

K.  Additional recommendations for follow-up testing may be critical to long-range therapy plans. That is, some deficits in central auditory function may be related to lack of neural maturation while others may not (Musiek et al, 1984; Musiek et al, 1986). If maturational factors have affected auditory abilities, the therapy plan will differ from that for a static condition. Finally, it is important that the recommendations for management of the LD child with a central auditory problem be integrated into the school and home environment. Follow-up meetings with teachers and parents and some type of ongoing evaluation of the child's auditory and academic behavior are necessary in order to monitor the effectiveness of the program and the child's progress.

# References

Bornstein S, Musiek F. Implications of temporal processing for children with learning and language problems. In: Beasley D, ed. Contemporary issues in audition. San Diego: College Hill Press, 1984.

Musiek F, Geurkink N. Auditory imperception in children: considerations for the otolaryngologist and audiologist. Laryngoscope 1980; 90:962.

Musiek F, Gollegly K, Baran J. Myelination of the corpus callosum and auditory processing problems in children: Theoretical and clinical correlates. Semin Hear 1984; 5:231.

Musiek F, Gollegly K, Ross M. Profiles of types of auditory processing deficits in children with learning disabilities. J Child Commun Disord (in press).

# REFERRAL FOR AUDIOLOGY

*David E. Palm, Ph.D.*

A. The audiologic evaluation consists of pure tone and speech audiometry. Pure tone audiometry assesses sensitivity to air- and bone-conducted pure tone signals and defines the type (sensorineural, conductive) and degree of loss (mild, moderate, severe, profound). Speech audiometry measures sensitivity for speech and also the ability to discriminate words. It provides information about the impact of the loss on communication ability. Additional testing may be considered to provide information about the status of the middle ear (impedance audiometry), 8th nerve (electronystagmography and evoked potential audiometry), or central pathways (evoked potential audiometry, sensitized speech tests). In the case of neonates and children who cannot be tested using adult techniques, both subjective (orienting response and observation audiometry) and objective techniques (evoked potential audiometry) are used to estimate hearing levels (Keith, 1976).

B. Normal hearing is conventionally defined in terms of the ability to hear pure tones in relation to a specified standard. Pure tones are used because they are a standardized signal that can be easily measured on relatively inexpensive equipment. Because pure tones represent only one parameter of auditory experience, the ability to hear them within a specified range is not necessarily synonymous with normal hearing ability. The ability to understand speech in the presence of noise or auditory competition may require skills that are not measured using conventional pure tone and speech audiometric techniques. It is, therefore, not unusual to find individuals who have "normal audiometric results" and still have significant complaints about their ability to hear in less than ideal listening situations.

C. Listening behavior is complex, and difficulty in listening can result from many causes. Children with attention deficit disorders, auditory processing problems, language and behavior problems, and certain medical conditions may all show similar patterns of behavior in the classroom. Proper education and medical management depends upon the ability to distinguish among these alternatives. The evaluation of central auditory processing problems involves the use of dichotic and/or distorted speech tests to assess processing abilities. The results of this testing can provide some indication of how a child can be expected to function in less than ideal listening conditions, such as those that exist in classrooms. While auditory processing disorders are rarely the sole reason for failure to learn, they can contribute to school problems and are a valuable part of a comprehensive medical/educational evaluation of children (Kinsbourne, 1983).

D. Hearing loss may be due to lesions involving the outer or middle ear (conductive), inner ear (sensorineural), 8th cranial nerve (retrocochlear), or central nervous system pathways and centers subserving audition (central). Conductive hearing losses are most commonly caused by fluid or changes in middle ear structures, resulting from chronic ear disease. Sensorineural hearing loss is associated with aging, Meniere's disease, noise exposure, and congenital or hereditary factors. Retrocochlear lesions usually involve tumors affecting the 8th cranial nerve. Central hearing loss is associated with cerebral vascular problems, congenital factors, infectious processes, and demyelinating or degenerative disease (Balloh, 1984). The vast majority of conductive hearing losses are correctable either by medication or surgery. Hearing losses due to lesions involving inner ear, 8th nerve or central nervous system, are generally not correctable, although treatment of the cause or associated symptoms may be required.

E. When medical or surgical treatment cannot improve the hearing to adequate levels, the possibility of amplification or other rehabilitative measures should be considered. Most individuals can benefit to some degree from amplification, but require counseling and periodic follow-up to maximize their hearing abilities. Some people cannot or will not use hearing aids and may require specialized devices to improve communication. Such things as telephone amplifiers, infrared systems, FM auditory trainers, teletypewriters, and listening devices are often recommended to improve communication skills and hearing abilities (Smaldino and Traynor, 1982).

## References

Balloh RW. The essentials of neurotology. Philadelphia: FA Davis, 1984.

Keith RW. The audiologic evaluation. In: Northern JL, ed. Hearing disorders. Boston: Little, Brown 1976: 10.

Kinsbourne M. Pediatric aspects of learning disorders. In: Lasky E, Katz J, eds. Central auditory processing disorders. Baltimore: University Park Press, 1983: 49.

Smaldino J, Traynor R. Comprehensive evaluation of the older adult for audiological reconditioning. Ear Hear 1982; 3:148.

PATIENT WITH SUSPECTED HEARING LOSS

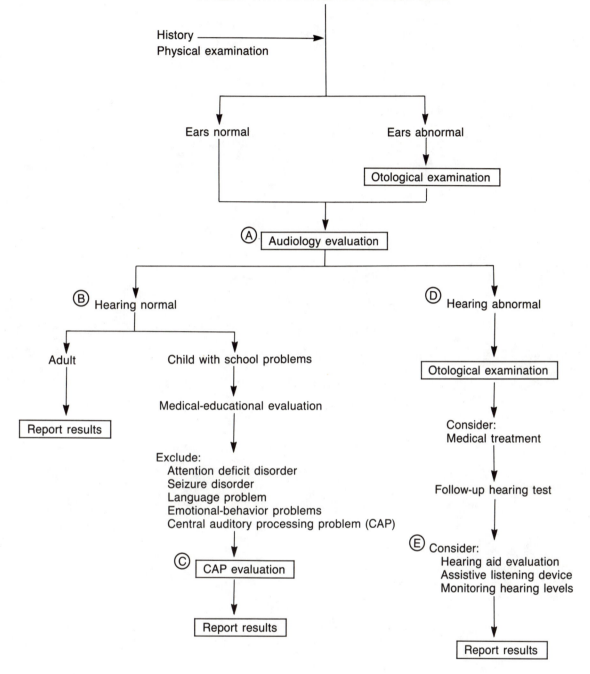

History
Physical examination

Ears normal

Ears abnormal

Otological examination

Ⓐ Audiology evaluation

Ⓑ Hearing normal

Adult

Child with school problems

Report results

Medical-educational evaluation

Exclude:
    Attention deficit disorder
    Seizure disorder
    Language problem
    Emotional-behavior problems
    Central auditory processing problem (CAP)

Ⓒ CAP evaluation

Report results

Ⓓ Hearing abnormal

Otological examination

Consider:
Medical treatment

Follow-up hearing test

Ⓔ Consider:
    Hearing aid evaluation
    Assistive listening device
    Monitoring hearing levels

Report results

# II: Language, Cognition, and Communication Systems

The chapters in this section cover a wide range of topics related to language learning, use, and disorders across the life span. The role of cognition in learning and using language is well recognized and has become such an integral part of the decision process in assessing and managing language behaviors that it begins this section. The decisions related to learning and using a first language ($L_1$) are different from those for second-language learners ($L_2$), and the difficulties encountered by children and adults of $L_1$ and $L_2$ who have accompanying language disorders present yet different decision processes. For the individual who has the cognitive and language comprehension ability but a severe production system deficit, alternative and augmentative communication system decisions must be provided. For those individuals who have limited cognitive, language, and motor behavior as a result of congenital or acquired disorders, there are special program decisions to be made. The length of the chapters in this section vary in scope and detail. This is due partly to the problem under consideration and partly to the perspective of individual authors. The chapters in this section do not necessarily build on each other; however, the reader will find interrelated notions in many of them, thus providing a frame of reference for the larger clinical picture.

# COGNITIVE FUNCTION: ASSESSMENT

*Margaret M. Rosin, M.S.*
*Gary D. Gill, Ph.D.*

A. Cognition is a general term that encompasses all forms of knowing. Cognitive processes include such constructs as sensation, perception, discrimination, memory, conceptualization, mental operations, thought, and judgment. These systems or processes are complex, dynamic, and interrelated and are influenced by environmental input (Muma, 1978). Cognitive assessment protocols are designed to sample various aspects of these processes. These assessment instruments can focus on the product of cognitive systems, knowledge, or they can explore more directly the individual's ability to manipulate and interrelate observations to create knowledge.

B. There are at least three major sets of assessment variables that must be considered in selecting methods of cognitive assessment. These include: (1) situation (environment), (2) child (what the child brings to the task), and (3) task (what the task demands of the child). Aspects of the situation that may have an impact on the method of evaluation are: where (setting), when (time of day), and who (familiarity with evaluator). The child variables are of crucial consideration in determining the best fit between the child and the assessment protocol. The child's age, estimated developmental level, sensory and motor abilities (e.g., hearing, vision, perceptual motor, fine motor), communication skills, behavior, and motivation all contribute to the decision making process when selecting the assessment format. The task variables (e.g., input to child, child's mode of response, memory constraints, length of test) must be appropriate, so that the child has the best chance of demonstrating his ability level (McCormick and Schiefelbush, 1984).

C. With all variables being considered, the clinician must then choose the specific protocol that best allows the child to demonstrate his cognitive abilities. The tests selected can be formal and standardized, informal and nonstandardized, or a combination of both methods. We advocate a systems approach to assessment rather than simply a psychometric or intelligence quotient (IQ) testing approach; therefore, a combination of procedures is generally recommended. A test is said to be standardized if validity and reliability data are available. Conversely a test is nonstandardized if those data are not available. The formality of the standardized test requires that the child meet certain test restrictions or requirements. In an informal approach the task demands can be varied and redesigned with a specific child in mind. Informal measures are based on a combination of criterion-referenced items, developmental theory, and careful observations of learning strategies and styles. A formal test utilizes a built-in scoring format to organize and summarize the data; with an informal measure the examiners must organize and interpret the data based on their knowledge of developmental theory and assessment strategies.

D. A test outcome should ideally yield a cognitive profile detailing the child's current abilities and level of functioning. With this information described, the clinician knows how the evaluated child compares with his peers and how the child best learns (i.e., strengths and weaknesses or learning style) and can decide whether treatment is necessary. Three test outcomes are possible, including normal, delayed, and deviant profiles. If significant delays exist, the child may be mentally retarded. The American Association on Mental Deficiency defines retardation as "significantly subaverage general intellectual functioning existing concurrently with deficits in adaptive behavior and manifested during the developmental period." IQs below 68 or 70 are considered in the mentally retarded range (Owens 1984). A test outcome categorized as deviant is one in which delays may or may not be present across the cognitive profiles, but one or more processes are significantly disordered. For example, children with learning disabilities have normal IQs but can exhibit significant difficulty in the acquisition and development of any or all of the following area: listening, speaking, reading, writing, or mathematical abilities. Autistic children provide another example of deviant cognitive profiles.

## References

McCormick L, Schiefelbush R. Early language intervention. Columbus: Charles E. Merrill, 1984.

Muma JR. Language handbook. Englewood Cliffs: Prentice-Hall, 1978.

Owens RE. Language development: an introduction. Columbus: Charles E. Merrill, 1984.

ASSESSMENT OF COGNITIVE FUNCTION

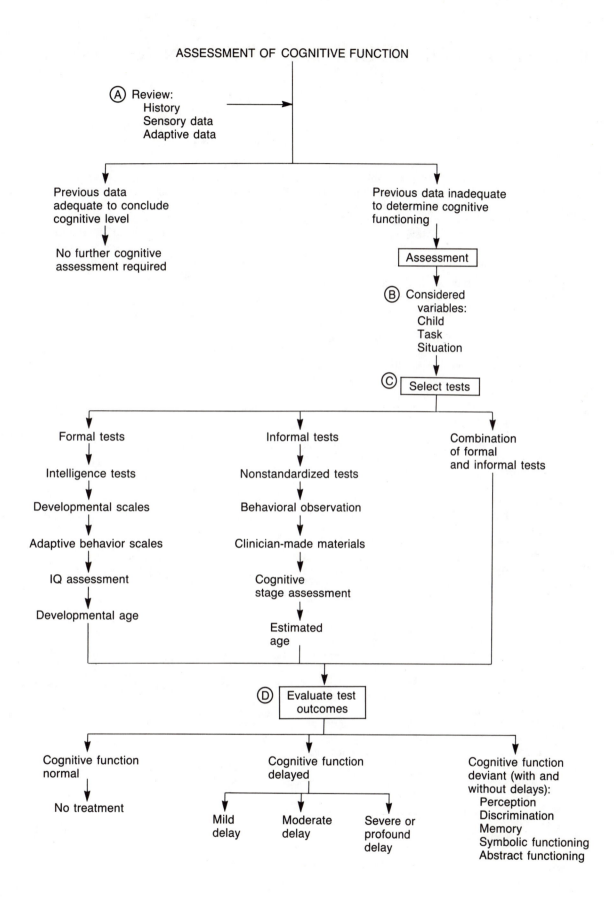

# IMPLICATIONS OF COGNITIVE FUNCTION ASSESSMENT

Gary D. Gill, Ph.D.
Margaret M. Rosin, M.S.

A. Child variables (McCormick and Schiefelbush, 1984) (e.g., chronological age [CA], sensory abilities, motor skills, behavior) must be considered in addition to cognitive profile in determining the optimum type of communication treatment. A successful intervention depends on the degree to which the treatment program matches the child variables and stimulates the child within his level of cognitive functioning.

B. The precise relationship between language and the cognitive processes is not well understood (Owens, 1984). Most cognitive theorists agree that language and cognitive development correlate in the normal child. We can say that in a general sense language does not significantly exceed a child's cognitive level. Given a child's level of cognitive functioning, this principle allows us to: (1) identify realistic communication goals for the child, (2) develop better statements of prognosis, (3) determine appropriate entry points for programming, and (4) better estimate the rate of learning.

C. Decalage literally means unwedging or uncoupling. Horizontal decalage is a phenomenon that occurs within a developmental period; it is the ability to uncouple an idea from the context in which it was first learned and to apply it across a set of appropriate contexts. Vertical decalage is a phenomenon that occurs across developmental periods; it is the restructuring of basic cognitive strategies, the unwedging of interrelated ideas, and their reformulation into structures typical of the next level of development (Rosen, 1977). When a child is expected to continue making developmental changes, it is important to intervene developmentally, to teach functional linguistic concepts and communicative behaviors that broaden the horizontal decalage. When the horizontal decalage is broad, when skills and abilities are spontaneously used with a variety of people and in many appropriate contexts that demonstrate proficiency at a developmental level, only then should the clinician focus the therapy on moving vertically to the next developmental level. With some people it is not reasonable to expect developmental changes. With such individuals we advocate switching from a developmentally based approach to a functionally based approach, which may strive to teach behaviors beyond an individual's cognitive level of functioning. Regardless of the developmen-

tal level, teach the behaviors that the person needs to communicate effectively (McCormick and Schiefelbush, 1984). In such situations we do not expect the behavior learned out of developmental sequence to be generalizible or to be used by the individual outside the context in which it is learned. With either approach, the clinician should never lose sight of the fact that people learn best when they have a reason to learn, when the skill or ability is functional. Likewise people in a functionally based program learn best if the skills and abilities that they need to acquire are expressed in a form as close to their developmental level as possible.

D. Treatment is the planning, organizing, and manipulating of environmental conditions to promote learning. By learning we mean some change in the internal structures that govern a child's communication system, i.e., the use of abilities generatively across contexts. If the implication of comparing the cognitive evaluation with the communication evaluation reveals that they are equal but delayed in regard to chronological age, the clinician may use either direct or indirect therapy, but usually chooses indirect therapy. If comparing cognitive and communication evaluations reveals that communication skills are significantly delayed in comparison to cognitive abilities, either direct or indirect therapy may be used; in this instance, direct therapy is usually preferred. In direct therapy the clinician personally delivers the service; in indirect therapy the service is provided by an intermediary. In both cases it is the responsibility of the speech and language pathologist to design and manage the intervention program.

## References

McCormick L, Schiefelbush R. Early language intervention. Columbus: Charles E. Merrill, 1984.

Muma JR. Language handbook. Englewood Cliffs: Prentice-Hall, 1978.

Owens RE. Language development: an introduction. Columbus: Charles E. Merrill, 1984.

Pyle DW. Intelligence: an introduction. London: Routledge and Kegan Paul, 1979.

Rosen H. Pathway to Piaget. Cherry Hill: Post-graduate International, 1977.

COGNITIVE FUNCTION ASSESSMENT

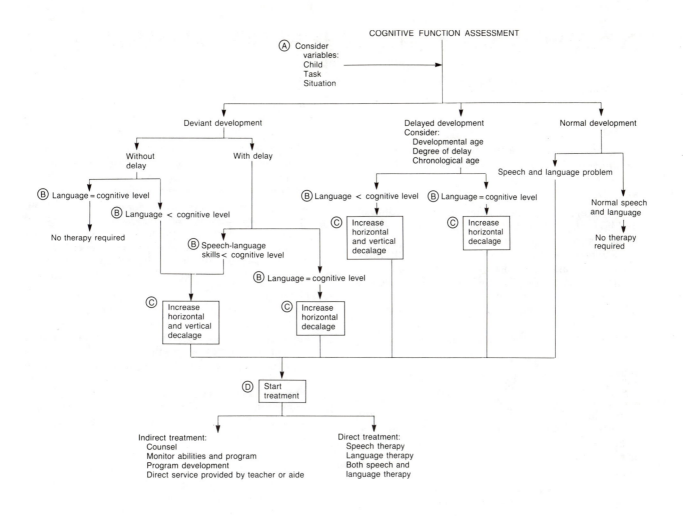

Indirect treatment:
  Counsel
  Monitor abilities and program
  Program development
  Direct service provided by teacher or aide

Direct treatment:
  Speech therapy
  Language therapy
  Both speech and
  language therapy

# COGNITIVE IMPAIRMENT IN THE ADULT

*Kathryn A. Bayles, B.S., M.S., Ph.D.*

Adult cognitive impairment can vary in severity and result from a variety of causes many of which are associated with speech or communication problems.

A. The assessment process necessarily involves obtaining information about medical, educational, occupational, and linguistic history and neurological status in order to distinguish patients with focal brain damage from those with diffuse (Cummings and Benson, 1983). Historical information assists in determining disease course and estimating premorbid intelligence. Further, because depression, sensory impairment, and drug effects can all adversely affect cognitive and communicative functioning, it is necessary to rule out their presence or quantify their contribution to the patient's test performance.

B. The speech-language pathologist will be concerned primarily with those cognitively impaired patients with irreversible conditions, but may routinely evaluate patients with treatable conditions such as adverse drug reactions, long-term alcohol abuse, infections, and neoplasms. Although these patients may be responsive to treatment, residual cognitive or communicative deficits may remain and therapy may be appropriate.

C. Patients with diffuse brain damage due to a degenerative irreversible process should have comprehensive neuropsychological evaluation of orientation, memory, perception, attention, visuo-spatial function, reasoning, and associative ability. Further, the possibility of depression or affective disorder should be explored (Lezak, 1983). In addition to information about intellectual capacity, information about functional abilities is valuable for planning patient care. Periodic reevaluation by a neuropsychologist is recommended to monitor change in the patient's abilities and the disease course.

D. Diffuse brain damage associated with degenerative cognitive impairment and fluctuating course is most likely to be associated with vascular disease. Dementia and communication disorders in these individuals result from the cumulative damage of repeated strokes (Burst, 1983). The nature of the observed behavioral deficits depends on the number and distribution of infarcts. For example, speech and language disorders are more probable with middle cerebral artery disease in the language dominant hemisphere than with disease in the posterior cerebral artery. Neuropsychological and language-speech evaluations should be given to define the pattern of deficits as a prelude to judgments about therapy. Some patients will be able to compensate for certain of their disorders and information about the patient's behavioral deficits is essential to caregivers. Patients with vascular dementia typically have a history of hypertension, abrupt onset of intellectual deficits, stair-step progression of illness, and focal neurologic signs and symptoms. Periodic reevaluation of these patients is recommended.

E. An important condition that differentiates among patients with degenerative brain disease is the presence of mo-

tor dysfunction (Cummings and Benson, 1983). Diseases associated with motor dysfunction, as well as dementia, in which the locus of primary damage is subcortical, often are referred to as subcortical dementing diseases. The most notable subcortical dementias are Huntington's disease, Parkinson's disease (PD), and progressive supranuclear palsy. Patients with Alzheimer's disease in the early and moderate stages typically have normal motor function with the exception of a small subgroup in whom extrapyramidal symptoms are present.

F. Huntington's disease, an inherited degenerative brain disease, is always associated with dementia and a movement disorder. Thus, patients have language, communication, and speech problems. Disease onset is typically in middle age and the first sign may be a motor, cognitive, or personality problem, or combination of the three. In addition to dysarthria, patients may exhibit impairment in communicative functioning, for example, display deficits in vocabulary, descriptive linguistic ability, verbal associative reasoning, and naming.

G. Although speech disorders traditionally have been recognized as a common clinical feature of Parkinson's disease (due to basal ganglia pathology), language and communication deficits have not (Bayles and Kaszniak, 1986). It recently has been recognized that many PD patients have select intellectual deficits, and in some cases a global dementia. On the average, the prevalence of dementia is estimated at 7 to 15 percent. Those PD patients with dementia, and many with select intellectual deficits, have language and communication disorders. Because of the marked variability in the Parkinson patient population, a comprehensive evaluation of intellectual, communicative, and speech functions is recommended. Then too, care must be taken to account for drug effects and depression. Results of speech-language evaluation may be valuable for helping the patient and family compensate for deficits. Periodic reevaluation is recommended and caregiver counseling is important.

H. The dementia of progressive supranuclear palsy is typified by forgetfulness, changes in affect, slowness in thinking, and impairment in the manipulation of acquired knowledge. Pathology of many subcortical structures is present with nerve cell loss, gliosis, formation of neurofibrillary tangles, and granulovacuolar changes.

I. Patients with abnormal motor function may have speech problems in addition to dementia-associated communication disorders. Although patients with Huntington's disease, in whom dementia is always present, will have communication disorders, patients with Parkinson's disease may not. The presence and degree of intellectual and communicative impairment in patients with Parkinson's disease is highly variable. Among patients with progressive supranuclear palsy, speech problems are most common.

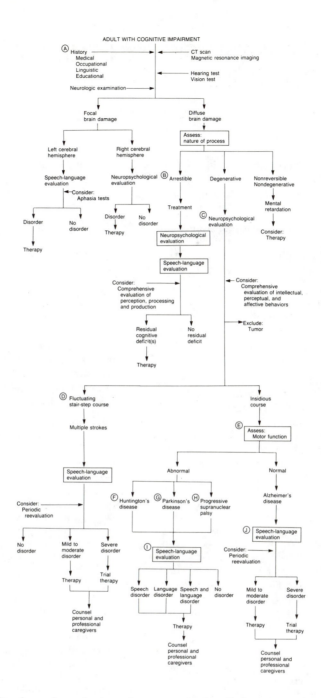

ADULT WITH COGNITIVE IMPAIRMENT

J. Because communicative ability depends on the integrity of the perceptual, memory/learning, attentional, and reasoning capabilities of an individual, it is necessarily diminished in Alzheimer's disease, a disease in which all cognitive abilities insidiously deteriorate. To detect impairment in the early stages of this disease, communication measures must be generative, active, creative, and involve reasoning. Generative naming tests, verbal description tasks, and tests of verbal memory have been found particularly sensitive to early stage deficits. Communicative functions have been found suitable for monitoring the disease course. Results of recent studies suggest the existence of subgroups within the Alzheimer's population defined by: presence of extrapyramidal signs, familial history, age at onset, rate of disease progression, history of head trauma, and handedness. Therapy is recommended for patients in the mild and moderate stages to give clinicans an opportunity to de-

termine if alterations of situational and linguistic variables will improve the patient's ability to process information and communicate. Periodic reevaluation is recommended to document the disease course and provide caregivers with information about the patient's strengths and weaknesses.

## References

Bayles KA, Kaszniak AW. Communication and cognition in dementia. San Diego: College-Hill Press, 1986.

Burst JCM. Dementia and cerebrovascular disease. In: Mayeaux R, Rosen WG, eds. The dementias. New York: Raven Press, 1983:131.

Cummings JL, Benson DF. Dementia: a clinical approach. Boston: Butterworths, 1983.

Lezak MD. Neuropsychological assessment. New York: Oxford University Press, 1983.

# LANGUAGE COMPREHENSION IN THE INFANT AND PRESCHOOL CHILD

*Robin S. Chapman, Ph.D.*

Assess comprehension whenever cognitive, hearing, or language production status is queried or when child is reported to be noncompliant. Parental report (or anecdotal observation) of linguistic comprehension is unreliable.

A . Cognitive delay, autistic behaviors, unresponsiveness to sound, seizures, hearing loss, or history of ear infections, head injuries, meningitis, encephalitis are all medical factors associated with comprehension problems.

B . Check language(s) spoken in the home; history of developmental milestones for comprehension; amount and times of language interaction with child; and the communicative situations in which child seems to understand best, has problems, or encounters most frequently.

C . Try to determine developmental level and problems of comprehension in pragmatics, semantics, and syntax. Outcomes in these three areas can be different. Assess pragmatics from birth onward through items on developmental inventories; observation of child in best, most frequent, and problem listening situations (Gallagher and Prutting, 1983; Lund and Duchan, 1983); and identification of comprehension strategies (Chapman, 1978). No standardized tests exist. Assess semantics and comprehension from 9 months informally (e.g., Miller et al, 1980) or from 2 to 3 years on, through tests (Darley, 1979).

D . For 0- to 3-year-old language levels, evaluate input in play and daily activities for developmental appropriateness in length, purpose, amount, topic, conversational routines, content, lexical choice, and prosody; is the child attentive, cooperative, able to take speaker's meaning from words and situation (Chapman, 1981)? For 3- to 6-year-old language levels, add samples of adult input about remote times and places, storytelling, and peer play input.

E . Embed functional, developmentally appropriate language input in social and cognitive enrichment programs. Introduce new language forms for familiar functions and content in situations that allow the child to figure out their meanings. Use language the child already understands to talk about new experiences and concepts. Adjust environmental expectations and input to the child's level.

F . For 0- to 3-year-old language levels, increase the time spent in mother-child and clinician-child interaction (following the principles of F) in play contexts where child determines the activity and topic; the adult comments on the child's activity. For 3- to 6-year-old language levels, add peer play in cooperative and sociodramatic contexts. Consider augmentative systems (pp 72–75) for input if there is no progress. Consider single word input for autistic children.

G . Create or increase the frequency of daily and play routines that make the communicative intent clear. Make the initial input formulaic and simple for developmentally appropriate demands.

H . Using the principles outlined in F, focus on increasing the frequency of lexical input for objects and actions that the child already appreciates. Choose words that correspond to the child's categories. When the child's attention is already focused on referent, increase the variety of exemplars and situations of concept. Use the same word consistently until it appears in use.

I . Again following the principles of F for 0- to 3-year-old language levels, focus on expansions of the child's utterances and extensions of the child's topic. For 3- to 6-year-old language levels, model new constructions in contexts that clarify the meaning; model old constructions in activities that increase reliance on language (stories, conversations about past and future events, imaginary play).

## References

Chapman RS. Comprehension strategies in children. In: Kavanagh JF, Strange W, eds. Speech and language in the laboratory, school, and clinic. Boston: MIT Press, 1978:308.

Chapman RS. Mother-child interaction in the second year of life: its role in language development. In: Schiefelbusch R, Bricker D, eds. Early language: acquisition and intervention. Baltimore: University Park Press, 1981:178.

Darley F, ed. Evaluation of appraisal techniques in speech and language pathology. New York: Addison-Wesley, 1979.

Gallagher T, Prutting C. Pragmatic assessment and intervention issues in language. San Diego: College Hill Press, 1983.

Lund NJ, Duchan JF. Assessing children's language in naturalistic contexts. Englewood Cliffs, NJ: Prentice-Hall, 1983.

Miller JF, Chapman RS, Branston MB, Reichle J. Language comprehension in sensorimotor stages V and VI. J Speech Hear Res 1980; 23:384.

COMPREHENSION QUERIED

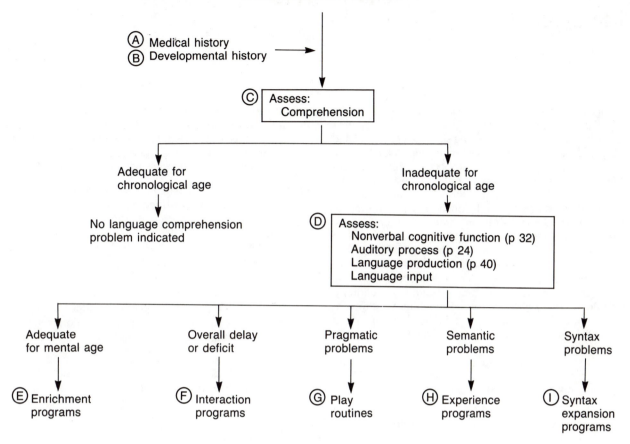

# LANGUAGE PRODUCTION IN THE PRESCHOOL CHILD

*Jon F. Miller, Ph.D.*

Language disorders in the preschool years are associated with a variety of etiologies that affect cognitive processes, perceptual integrity, information processing skills, physiological and motor performance, and environmental support for communication. Identification of children suspected of having deficits in language production can be done in two ways: (1) in the first year of life through the identification of an associated condition such as mental retardation, and (2) through recognizing a failure to establish basic communication skills using words or word approximations at 10 to 12 months. Where language behavior is the source for identification, medical, perceptual, and cognitive evaluations should follow to identify primary etiology that can often be treated, e.g., hearing loss caused by middle ear infection. Regardless of etiology, since frequently no etiology can be identified, the evaluation of productive language must proceed to confirm a productive language problem. The first step is to review the child's developmental, environmental, and medical histories to determine the child's general level of development and any special problems. Second, given the child's level of development, select appropriate procedures to evaluate language and related behaviors.

A. The primary method to evaluate language production skills is recording (video or audio) a free speech sample. Initial samples should reflect a variety of communication situations: free play with toys, routines and verbal games for younger children, and story telling for older children. This first sample should be a mother-child interaction with the examiner observing and taking notes (Lund and Duchan, 1983).

B. General analysis of the speech sample begins with transcription following Systematic Analysis of Language Transcripts (SALT) (Miller and Chapman, 1986) conventions, entering the transcript into a computer file, and analyzing using SALT, a computer program designed to analyze free speech samples. General analyses will include the following measures for both the child and mother: mean length of utterance (MLU); number of different words; number of utterances and words per minute; percent complete and intelligible utterances; distribution of utterances by utterance length; number of utterances containing false starts, repetitions, and reformulations; and number of utterances per speaking turn. These measures provide a general index of the child's knowledge of syntax, lexical semantics, and discourse requirements. The outcomes of this analysis can be three: no problem identified, questionable performance requiring periodic monitoring of developmental change, and the identification of a production problem.

C. The identification of a production problem at this level of assessment leads to three broad areas of classification: (1) fluency and rate problems associated with stuttering and cluttering, (2) intelligibility deficits resulting from phonetic or phonological problems (p 118), (3) productive language deficit that is symbolic in nature. Further characterization of all three areas is necessary to describe performance in detail to (1) differentiate fluency disorders from word finding and sentence formulation problems and limitations in language production owing to physiological constraints (e.g., speech motor deficits), and (2) to initiate the appropriate intervention program.

D. Detailed analysis of language production requires additional speech samples directed toward eliciting specific language characteristics (e.g., question asking and answering). Word, morpheme, utterance, and discourse levels of analysis are performed to characterize the deficit areas and the conditions under which the deficits occur, as well as the conditions that facilitate performance, e.g., topics or pragmatic conditions (Miller, 1981).

E. Evaluate language comprehension abilities for the content areas of suspected deficit in conjunction with measures of general language comprehension ability (p 38).

F. When questions regarding the child's cognitive status emerge and other performance data cannot be used to infer cognitive ability, assessment of nonverbal cognitive ability is necessary. Using such tests as the Leiter International Performance Scale, the Columbia Test of Mental Abilities, or the Wechsler Intelligence Scale for Children (WISC), a mental age can be established to determine expectations for language performance. In general, language performance should be equal to general mental abilities.

G. Characterizing the language production problem involves determining if the child's language is best described as a general delay in acquiring linguistic knowledge or as a deficit in a specific linguistic domain, in expression of particular meanings, or in communicating in certain situations. Some children evidence delays or deficits in language production only and some in both comprehension and production. The degree of deficit in vocabulary, syntax, semantics, and pragmatics must be determined for both comprehension and production skills. Decisions include: delay versus deficit, comprehension versus production, and severity of problem.

H. Intervention programs aimed at facilitating language production in young children with language delays are aimed at providing the child's parents with strategies for communicating with their child. The goal of these strategies is to incorporate intervention into everyday activities, where children naturally learn language. Techniques for improving language deficits require direct language intervention for the child provided by a certified speech-language pathologist.

## References

Lund NJ, Duchan JF. Assessing children's language in naturalistic contexts. Englewood Cliffs, NJ: Prentice-Hall, 1988.

Miller JF. Assessing language production in children. Austin, TX: Pro-Ed, 1981.

Miller JF, Chapman R. SALT: systematic analysis of language transcripts. Madison, WI: University of Wisconsin, 1986.

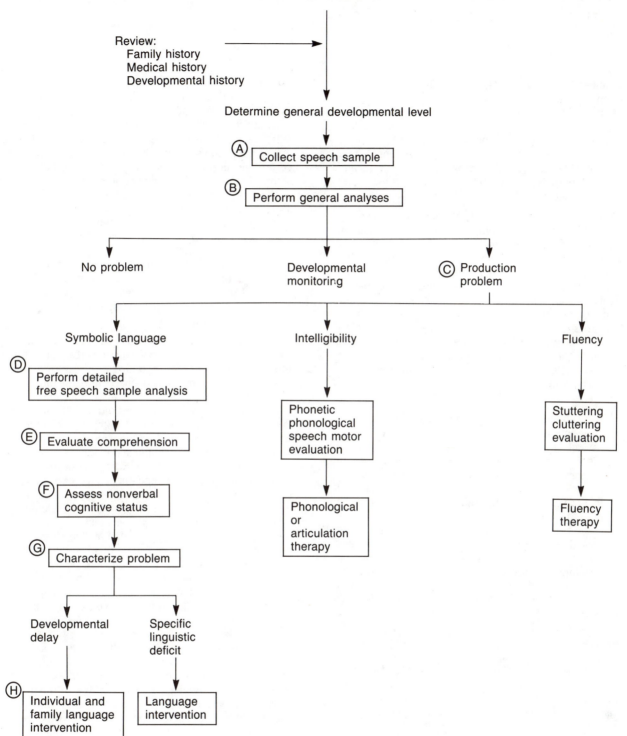

# SPECIFIC LANGUAGE LEARNING PROBLEMS

*Susan Ellis Weismer, Ph.D.*

The treatment approach discussed in this chapter is primarily designed for young children with specific language deficits (as described by Stark and Tallal, 1981 and Leonard, in press). That is, this intervention framework reflects the assumption that management programs should be geared to the particular type of child being served. Although the present chapter focuses on direct intervention involving the clinician and child, the importance of indirect intervention in managing specific language disorders is recognized.

A.  The areas of focus and entry levels of intervention goals should be based on a comprehensive communication profile including assessment across language domains (content, form, function) and processes (comprehension and expression), as well as an evaluation of cognitive and social skills. Consideration of case history information is also crucial in establishing intervention goals. For children who exhibit linguistic deficits in a number of different areas, decisions must be made about which area(s) to address first in therapy. As a general guideline, early stages of training should focus on the functions language serves and its content, with emphasis on the form of the message coming later.

B.  Since it is clear that language disordered children have failed to identify the rules governing language in the normal way, intervention strategies must include special considerations in terms of the type of linguistic input provided. The likelihood that linguistic patterns will be discovered can be maximized by imposing a certain structure upon the language sample presented to the child. One way of accomplishing this is through the use of focused repetition in which a particular linguistic rule is isolated and numerous clear examples of this rule are presented using a range of different models. Another means of structuring the linguistic input is to ensure that it is appropriately timed such that meaning relations are clarified through the co-occurrence of the target form and its referent. Timing considerations also entail capitalizing upon children's attentional predispositions by labeling objects or describing events in which they demonstrate interest. The saliency of a particular linguistic form can be increased by the manner in which it is presented. Positioning a target form at the beginning or end of an utterance when feasible (rather than in the middle) may heighten its perceptual saliency. The use of vocal stress can also serve to call attention to a given construction and may increase the probability that it will be produced by the child. Presenting linguistic stimuli at slower than normal rates may be useful in reducing processing demands and allowing children to focus attention on target forms. For certain children, it may be beneficial to provide a stable, visual representation of auditory input during the initial stages of training. For example, a picture or symbol corresponding to each word or grammatical morpheme in a sentence could be presented. The effectiveness of these linguistic input modification techniques is likely to depend upon the specific target form and/or the child's learning style and needs to be established for each case individually.

C.  In addition to modifying and structuring linguistic input, it is necessary to manipulate the intervention context so that it is maximally facilitating for language learning. To accomplish this, the therapy milieu should consist of interactive situations that are functional in nature. Functional significance implies that a legitimate reason for communication underlies therapy activities. The interactive character of the intervention context refers both to the child's interaction with people and with objects. Ideally, language intervention should be conducted within small groups or preschool classrooms, since these contexts offer greater flexibility in creating situations that promote social interchanges (e.g., through the use of uninformed listeners or requests to convey information to another person). Materials used in training should consist of real objects associated with ongoing events such that interaction with the physical enviroment is encouraged.

D.  A variety of training techniques have been found to be effective in promoting language learning (Leonard, 1981; in press). These include modeling procedures, modeling accompanied by evoked productions of the target (which do not simply involve imitation of the clinician's utterance), and direct imitation procedures. The majority of training studies have centered on improving children's productive syntactic skills. One can conjecture that imitation procedures are better suited for this focus than for training of semantic or pragmatic abilities; whereas modeling techniques and modeling plus evoked production techniques may be more widely applicable than imitation procedures. Several important considerations that relate to the selection of training techniques include the use of reinforcement, instructional feedback and generalization. Natural or "functional" reinforcement that is directly tied to the communication event should be employed when possible (e.g., giving the child an object following an appropriate request). With respect to the issue of feedback, it is critical to remember that the objective of intervention is to train, not test, the child. It is particularly important to provide as many cues as possible and to give immediate, informative feedback regarding the child's performance during the initial phases of training in order to facilitate discovery of linguistic rules. Generalization is promoted in this intervention approach by employing activities that involve the use of language in social, communicative contexts. In addition, various means of systematically engineering generalization can be employed throughout the course of intervention (e.g., input cues and structure can be reduced as training progresses to aid the child in moving toward generalized use of the target through gradual increases in task demands).

E.  Measurement of clinical change is essential to determining the effectiveness of a language intervention program. Pre- and post-testing procedures can be utilized to ascertain if the amount of gain in linguistic skills exceeds that expected on the basis of maturation alone. Combined series or multiple baseline single-case design methodol-

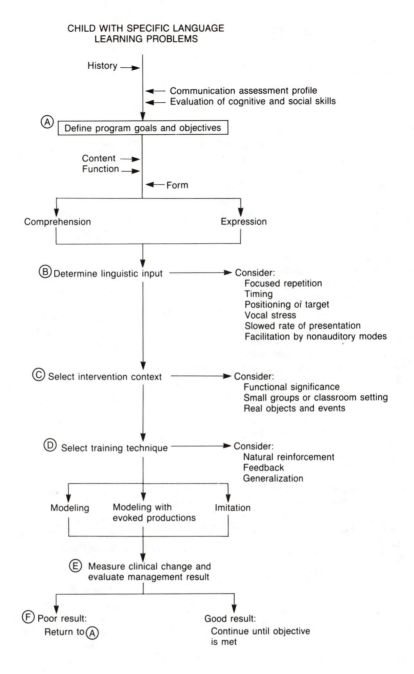

CHILD WITH SPECIFIC LANGUAGE
LEARNING PROBLEMS

History →

← Communication assessment profile
← Evaluation of cognitive and social skills

(A) Define program goals and objectives

Content →
Function →
← Form

Comprehension          Expression

(B) Determine linguistic input → Consider:
    Focused repetition
    Timing
    Positioning of target
    Vocal stress
    Slowed rate of presentation
    Facilitation by nonauditory modes

(C) Select intervention context → Consider:
    Functional significance
    Small groups or classroom setting
    Real objects and events

(D) Select training technique → Consider:
    Natural reinforcement
    Feedback
    Generalization

Modeling    Modeling with        Imitation
            evoked productions

(E) Measure clinical change and
    evaluate management result

(F) Poor result:                Good result:
    Return to (A)               Continue until objective
                                is met

ogy might also be employed to evaluate the effects of treatment across a variety of linguistic targets for an individual child. In addition to making quantitative measurements, it is important to assess qualitative changes (particularly error patterns) that may signal progress toward acquisition of the target.

F.  If the evaluation of management results is poor, a re-examination of program goals and objectives is indicated (i.e., return to A). However, if good results are obtained, intervention should continue until objectives are met for each area of focus.

## References

Leonard LB. Children with specific language impairment. In: Brookhouser P, Rubin A, Netsell R, eds. Communication disorders in children. Philadelphia: Praeger, in press.

Leonard LB. Facilitating linguistic skills in children with specific language impairment. Appl Psycholing 1981; 2:89.

Stark R, Tallal P. Selection of children with specific language deficits. J Speech Hear Disord 1981; 46:114.

# LANGUAGE DISORDERS IN THE SCHOOL-AGE CHILD

*Mary Lovey Wood, Ph.D.*

A. When the clinician has determined that intervention is to be pursued, a precursor to beginning is to establish which facets of direct and indirect intervention are indicated. Direct intervention encompasses direct clinician-child interaction designed to minimize deficiencies and to expand the child's use of learning strengths to compensate for language weaknesses. Indirect intervention, which may be in conjunction with direct intervention, usually incorporates consultation with—and referral to—others who are intrinsic to the child and to remedial endeavors. The prioritizing of targets within both direct and indirect intervention programs reflects the relative importance of various dimensions of the language disorder to the child's functioning. Top priority usually is given to those features that most seriously interfere with the child's realization of potential, as well as to features that are most offensive to the child and the family. Some early priority may be given to certain compensatory devices that make an immediate difference to the child and his or her environment, thereby helping to bind the child and family to long-term intervention efforts.

B. Three major categories of direct intervention include: (a) focus on language deficits, (b) teaching devices to facilitate functioning in language-related areas, and (c) consultation with the child and family regarding their responsibilities in the intervention program. Intervention targets focused on specific language deficits may encompass aspects of all subsystems of structure, content, and use or may be specialized within a single subsystem, depending on the child's disorder. Clinicians frequently emphasize both processing and production at each phase of intervention; an increasingly common practice is to include both spoken and written components of language remediation. Devices to facilitate functioning in language-related areas include use of cognitive strengths to imbed newly learned language skills and to enhance learning in difficult situations.

C. Family consultation in direct intervention involves attempts to help the child and family understand the child's proficiencies and deficiencies, and to obtain family assistance and commitment to intervention plans. The family often needs the clinician's direction in making changes in the home while not sacrificing all the family's resources for one child. The child gradually can learn to take responsibility for applying newly acquired proficiencies to daily life.

D. Indirect intervention is the coordinated effort to provide the child with other services that are deemed important for his changing needs and proficiencies. The targets of indirect intervention change with the child just as the targets of direct intervention. For example, many children with language-learning deficiencies experience adjustment problems in social and family life and in self-perception. However, many children cannot profit from psychotherapy until their language skills are sufficiently intact to allow communicative interaction and participation in abstraction and self-growth.

E. Tutoring frequently is indicated for language impaired children and may involve supervised study or repetition, review, and restatement of academic work. Supervised study involves the overseeing of homework tasks, completion of assignments, and verification of assignments with the teacher. Teacher contact by the clinician may consist of explanation of the child's disorder in terms that relate the disorder to the child's functioning in the classroom and that provide the teacher with specific ways of managing the child. The school may also offer special services appropriate for the child that can be coordinated and facilitated by the clinician. Occasionally some intervention goals can be attained through a clinician directed home program; in some situations, illness or vacation necessitates a home program. Clinicians sometimes find that a family intends to "do something" whether the clinician advocates it or not; in these instances, some direction from the clinician can turn a potentially harmful force into a constructive one.

F. Integral to an intervention program is frequent reassessment of the child's functioning and the redesign of intervention. A slightly abbreviated version of the original assessment, sometimes including assessment tools that could not be used with the child in the initial evaluation process, is useful in modifying the priorities and targets of intervention. The alteration of intervention plans also takes into account the changing expectations of the child's social, academic, and family environments. In relatively few instances is the permanent termination of intervention indicated for the seriously language deficient child. Although a respite or vacation may be integrated into an intervention program, the clinician must consider the complexities of language and language-related behaviors at each level of achievement. Each level of achievement involves companion expectations for the child. The clinician should not ignore the continuing possibilities of discrepancies between the child's performance and appropriate expectations.

## References

Laughton J, Hasenstab MS. The language learning process: implications for management of disorders. Rockville, MD: Aspen Publications, 1986.

Masters LF, Mori AA. Teaching secondary students with mild learning and behavior problems: methods, materials, strategies. Rockville, MD: Aspen Publications, 1986.

Wallach GP, Butler KG, eds. Language learning disabilities in school-age children. Baltimore: Williams & Wilkins, 1984.

Westby C. Learning to talk—talking to learn: oral/literate language differences. In: Simon CS, ed. Communication skills and classroom success: therapy methodologies for language-learning disabled students. San Diego: College-Hill Press, 1985.

# REMEDIATION OF LANGUAGE DISORDERS

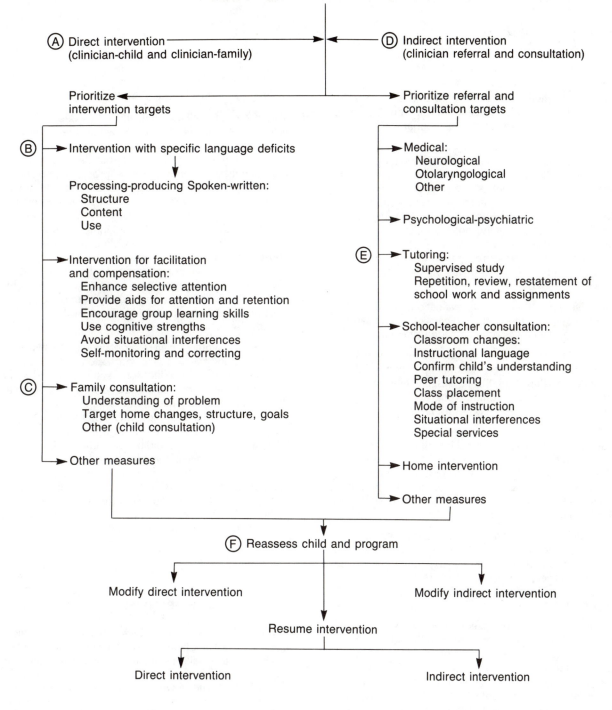

(A) Direct intervention
(clinician-child and clinician-family)

(D) Indirect intervention
(clinician referral and consultation)

Prioritize
intervention targets

Prioritize referral and
consultation targets

(B) → Intervention with specific language deficits

Processing-producing Spoken-written:
   Structure
   Content
   Use

→ Intervention for facilitation
and compensation:
   Enhance selective attention
   Provide aids for attention and retention
   Encourage group learning skills
   Use cognitive strengths
   Avoid situational interferences
   Self-monitoring and correcting

(C) → Family consultation:
   Understanding of problem
   Target home changes, structure, goals
   Other (child consultation)

→ Other measures

→ Medical:
   Neurological
   Otolaryngological
   Other

→ Psychological-psychiatric

(E) → Tutoring:
   Supervised study
   Repetition, review, restatement of
   school work and assignments

→ School-teacher consultation:
   Classroom changes:
   Instructional language
   Confirm child's understanding
   Peer tutoring
   Class placement
   Mode of instruction
   Situational interferences
   Special services

→ Home intervention

→ Other measures

(F) Reassess child and program

Modify direct intervention

Modify indirect intervention

Resume intervention

Direct intervention

Indirect intervention

# LANGUAGE DISORDERS IN THE ADOLESCENT: ASSESSMENT

*Vicki Lord Larson, Ph.D.*
*Nancy L. McKinley, M.S.*

A. Determine whether the adolescent is in an early, middle, or late stage of adolescent development (Mitchell, 1979) in order to select the appropriate assessment procedures.

B. Language comprehension-listening evaluation should include: auditory comprehension of linguistic features (syntax and semantics), informational listening (following oral directions, selecting main ideas and relevant details in spoken language, understanding lecture format, and applying effective notetaking skills) and critical listening (engaging in inductive and deductive reasoning, recognizing propaganda devices, detecting false reasoning) (Boyce and Larson, 1983; Larson and McKinley, 1987).

C. Language production-speaking evaluation should emphasize the assessment of phonology, syntax, and semantics as they relate to communication pragmatics.

D. Obtain IQ test data from the psychologist, assess the adolescent's concrete versus formal operational abilities (Inhelder and Piaget, 1958), and observe potential for improved cognitive functioning (Feuerstein, 1980). Compare and contrast these data points. Determine matches and mismatches.

E. Testing should consist of formal instruments (norm- and criterion-referenced tests) and informal procedures (directed tasks and discourse samples). The discourse samples, both narrations and conversations, should be obtained from two or more communication situations (Larson and McKinley, 1987).

F. Consider all formal and informal assessment data in regard to the stage of the adolescent's development. Data will be interpreted differently dependent upon the adolescent's need to reach academic (Ac), personal-social (P-S), and vocational (Voc) goals. Different goals are more important at different stages of development.

G. The educational system needs to be assessed to determine whether the problem is within the adolescent or the educational system. If the problem is within the educational system (e.g., a teacher's language that is too complex, a curriculum that is disorganized), it would preclude labeling the adolescent as being language disordered. A number of aspects of the educational system need to be evaluated (Larson and McKinley, 1987): (1) the actual educational structure of the secondary-level schools, using a specified checklist; (2) the teacher's language, using a self-evaluation procedure; (3) the teachers' and administrators' attitudes toward adolescents with communication disorders, using an attitudinal scale; and (4) the curriculum, using a curriculum analysis form.

H. The environmental system needs to be evaluated to determine whether the problem is within the adolescent or the environmental system. If the problem is within the environmental system (e.g., parents denying that the adolescent has a communication problem, peers teasing adolescents about their problem), the environmental system needs to be modified. To determine where the problem rests, the speech-language pathologist should investigate the following: (1) the family members' perceptions of the adolescent's problem and the possible consequences, (2) the feelings and attitudes of environmental system members toward the adolescent, and (3) the communication styles of environmental system members to isolate whether a language disorder or difference exists. Each of these dimensions can be evaluated using either observations or interviews.

I. Analyze and synthesize all data obtained up to this point to determine matches and mismatches among the adolescent's language, educational system demands, and environmental system to decide whether no service, direct service, or indirect service is warranted. If, for example, the language of the educational system is adequate and it matches the adolescent's language (i.e., adequate), no service would be recommended. If, for example, the language of the educational system is inadequate and it mismatches the adolescent's language (i.e., adequate), indirect service to the educational system would be recommended (i.e., the speech-language pathologist would consult with other professionals who are working directly with the adolescent).

## References

Boyce N, Larson VL. Adolescents' communication: development and disorders. Eau Claire, WI: Thinking Publications, 1983.

Feuerstein R. Instrumental enrichment. Baltimore: University Park Press, 1980.

Inhelder B, Piaget J. The growth of logical thinking from childhood to adolescence—an essay on the construction of formal operational structures. New York: Basic Books, 1958.

Larson VL, McKinley N. Communication assessment and intervention strategies for adolescents. Eau Claire, WI: Thinking Publications, 1987.

Mitchell J. Adolescent psychology. Toronto: Holt, Rinehart & Winston, 1979.

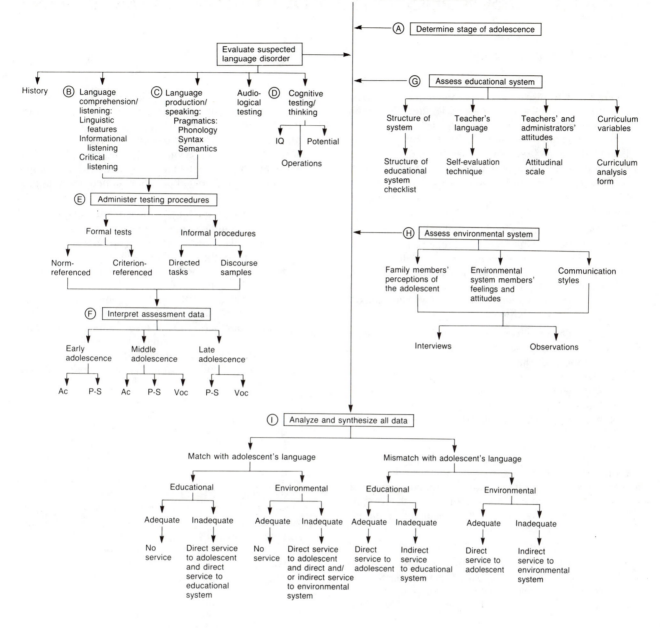

# LANGUAGE DISORDERS IN THE ADOLESCENT: INTERVENTION

*Vicki Lord Larson, Ph.D.*
*Nancy L. McKinley, M.S.*

A. Using a match-mismatch model, determine if the locus of service is with the adolescent and/or the educational and environmental systems. If a mismatch occurs, the intervention is delivered to the area found to be inadequate. If a match occurs (e.g., both the language of the adolescent and the educational system are inadequate), the intervention is delivered to both areas. If a match occurs in which both systems are adequate, no intervention is warranted.

B. Direct service provides individual or group language intervention to the adolescent utilizing a variety of delivery models (e.g., itinerant, resource room, self-contained language classroom, and outpatient) whereas, indirect service provides intervention to the adolescent's educational and/or environmental systems (Boyce and Larson, 1983; Larson and McKinley, 1987).

C. Collaborative planning of goals and objectives is essential to the adolescent's assuming responsibility for the modification of the language disorder. Additional incentives may be necessary to motivate the adolescent, such as offering language intervention as a course for credit, assisting in the procurement of a general education degree, reaching predetermined vocational goals, and contracting for improved communication performance. Counseling adolescents about their language disorder is an integral part of providing direct services. This counseling consists of giving information about the impact of the language disorder on academic progress, personal-social growth, and vocational aspirations; securing information about the adolescent's perspective of the impact of the language disorder; and providing release and support for the adolescent's feelings.

D. The stage of adolescence (early, middle, late) affects the selection of goals and objectives to be emphasized. In general, goals for early adolescents focus on developing the language necessary for academic progress and personal-social growth. In late adolescence, goals focus on developing the language necessary for enhancing personal-social growth and vocational aspirations. In middle adolescence, any or all of the three areas might be emphasized.

E. Thinking, listening, and speaking behaviors (terms selected because of their familiarity to adolescents) are taught within an interactive communication context as they relate to academic, personal-social, and vocational objectives. Thinking behaviors include three phases: input, the gathering of the data; elaboration, the manipulating of the data; and output, the communicating of the results of the data processing (Feuerstein, 1980). Listening behaviors have been described on page 12. Within speaking behaviors, communication pragmatics serves as the all-encompassing parameter under which phonology, syntax, and semantics are assumed and taught.

F. Depending upon the adolescent's needs and objectives, one of several intervention approaches can be selected. The basic skills remediation model emphasizes skills not acquired during the elementary years. The survival skills approach emphasizes language needed for daily communication situations, by teaching either prerequisites (e.g., addition and subtraction) or compensatory strategies (e.g., using the calculator). The communication strategies approach emphasizes how to learn to apply thinking, listening, and speaking behaviors across a variety of communication settings and situations. The communication strategies approach is the one selected most frequently by the authors to enhance the adolescent's communication behaviors.

G. Dismissal may be precipitated by a variety of factors: adequate language for academic and/or personal-social and/or vocational potential, lack of motivation, or insufficient progress over time.

H. Within indirect service to the adolescent, intervention to the educational and environmental system may be direct or indirect. Direct service to these systems involves contact among the speech-language pathologist and the adolescent's teachers and/or family and/or peers. Indirect service to these systems involves contact with persons or agencies outside of the adolescent's immediate life space in order to affect constructive modifications.

## References

Boyce N, Lord Larson V. Adolescents' communication: development and disorders. Eau Claire, WI: Thinking Publications, 1983.

Feuerstein R. Instrumental enrichment. Baltimore: University Park Press, 1980.

Larson VL, McKinley N. Communication assessment and intervention strategies for adolescents. Eau Claire, WI: Thinking Publications, 1987.

# LANGUAGE DISORDERS IN THE ADOLESCENT: INTERVENTION

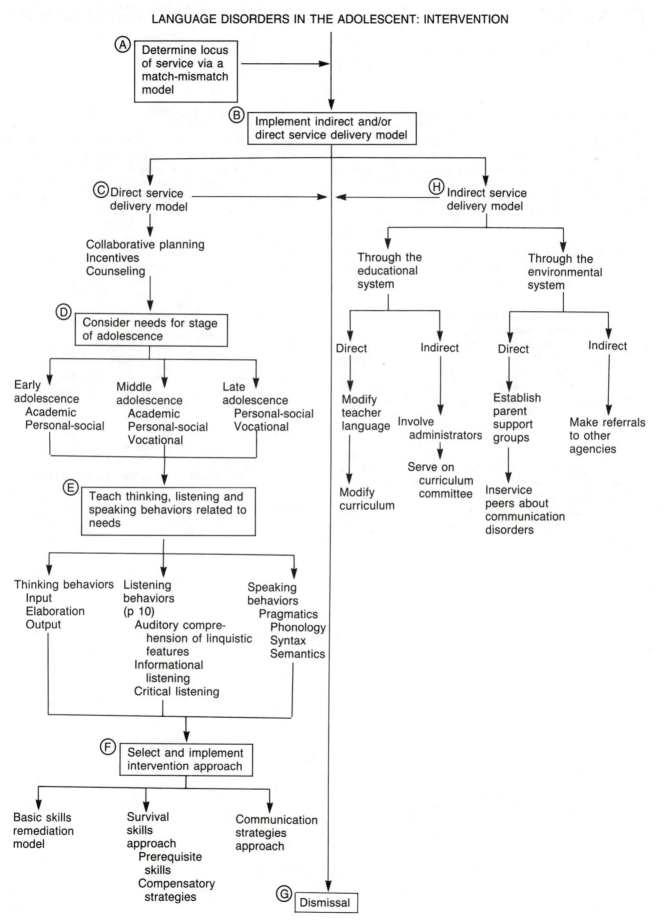

# DISMISSAL CRITERIA FOR THE LANGUAGE-IMPAIRED CHILD

*Marc E. Fey, Ph.D.*

This chapter represents an initial attempt to develop a systematic and principled means for determining when an intervention program for a language impaired child should be discontinued. Temporal criteria that are proposed should be taken only as suggestions, because there are no data to suggest that these criteria are better than a set derived by the clinician for a particular child. It is assumed that the decision to dismiss a client is not irrevocable. Rather, the dismissal decision constitues a hypothesis that further intervention at the present time is either no longer necessary or serves no significant benefit to the child and/or the child's family and significant others. This hypothesis must be carefully evaluated so that the decision to dismiss can either be further justified or reversed.

A.  Dismissal from intervention must be a consideration from the beginning of intervention planning (i.e., conditions for dismissal should be determined before therapy is begun [Kemp, 1983]). It is important to note that each specific goal behavior reflects a step toward the most basic goal: *improved performance in communication and/or communication-related processes* (e.g., problem-solving, reading, establishing positive peer relations). Potential goal behaviors for a child that cannot serve these functions would not be selected as specific goals (Fey, 1986, Chapter 4). The type of plan for program evaluation that is developed depends to a large extent on the types of goals that are selected and the intervention approach that is adopted for reaching those goals. For example, a plan that involves the facilitation of a set of language forms using a fairly traditional trainer-oriented approach could probably be evaluated using a multiple-baseline experimental design (Fey, 1986, Chapters 7 and 8). This design may be inadequate, however, to evaluate a program designed to facilitate the systemic development of a number of unspecified language structures, using a child-oriented intervention approach (Fey, 1986, Chapter 9). At the very least, the clinician should observe the child's production of potential target behaviors on several occasions before intervening to establish the reliability of the pretherapy measures and the stability of the child's performance under nontherapy conditions. The plan should also contain a set of statements that reflects the amount of progress toward stated goals that is expected at the end of a monthly period. These statements generally take the form of subgoals, which can be assessed routinely in fairly structured contexts. For example, progress toward subgoals often reflects improved performance on probes, including sentence imitation tests, spontaneous responses to sets of nontrained picture stimuli, and increased conversational responsiveness to the intervention agent but not others. Some improvements in these limited contexts may occur prior to generalized gains made in naturally-occurring, social-communicative situations. Therefore, they may serve as valuable indices of progress toward specific goals even before new developments appear in discourse contexts.

B.  The child's progress on targeted behaviors should be evaluated approximately once a month. Ideally, perfor-

LANGUAGE-IMPAIRED CHILD

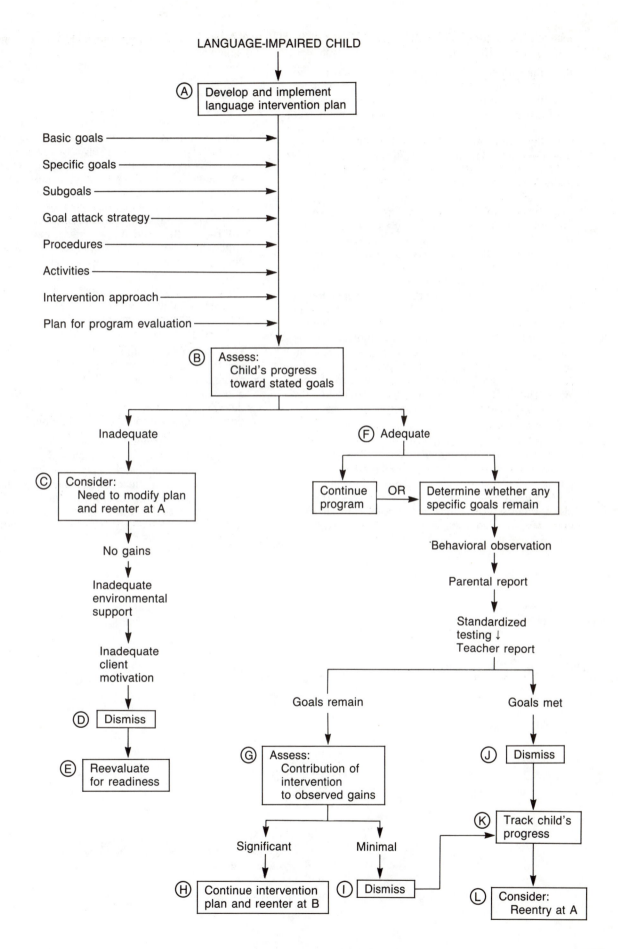

mance on structured probes and in more naturalistic, social-communicative conditions should be evaluated.

C. If, at the end of a 1-month period, the child has not reached at least one subgoal, the clinician must reexamine the program as a whole and consider the need to modify it in some way to foster the facilitation of targeted behaviors. Any individual component of the plan may be manipulated. After a period of 1 month of intervention, it is likely that only minor adjustments in the program will be needed. For example, the set of goals and intervention approach may remain constant, but new activities reflecting greater or lesser degrees of naturalness may be called for. Some adjustments in the procedures utilized within these activities may also be necessary. If these minor adjustments have not resulted in adequate improvements after 3 months, more dramatic changes in the intervention plan must be considered. These might include changes in specific goals, changes in the intervention approach, and a change of the primary intervention agent. Changing intervention agents should be carefully considered if the clinician has been the primary agent up to this point. In this way, the clinician can begin to train other individuals close to the child in the development of activities and use of procedures expected to facilitate target behaviors. Some valid form of intervention could then be continued, even if the child is dismissed from the clinician's active caseload.

D. If the child has not met stated goals after a period of 6 months, the clinician should strongly consider dismissal. This decision would reflect the clinician's hypothesis that continued intervention efforts on the clinician's part *at the present time* are not likely to bring about the desired gains in communicative performance. This decision is never a pleasant one, but every clinician must come to grips with its necessity. Indeed, one must con-

sider the ethics of continuing an expensive program that is unlikely to have a positive outcome, especially if other needy children and their families are waiting for services. The dismissal decision is fully justifiable when a comprehensive intervention plan has been developed and implemented with essentially no progress or a prolonged plateau in performance and when repeated attempts to modify the child's intervention plan also have been unsuccessful. This decision receives further justification in two other instances. In many cases, the success of the intervention plan may depend on at least some degree of participation by the child's family, caretakers, and/or school personnel. When this environmental support is not provided, the likelihood that continued intervention will benefit the child significantly is minimized. Similarly, with older children, significant improvement depends to a large extent on the child's level of motivation and extent of cooperation. Taking steps to increase a child's motivation and to ensure cooperation should be considered a part of every clinician's role. In many cases, however, these efforts are not successful. Under these circumstances, dismissal is warranted.

E. The clinician's hypothesis that continued intervention would not result in significant gains should be evaluated approximately 6 months following dismissal (Olswang and Bain, 1986, for some important considerations for determining readiness for intervention). For some children, readmission to therapy is warranted at this time.

F. If the child meets monthly subgoals, the program should be continued. After approximately 3 months of such progress, however, the clinician must answer the questions, ''Has the child reached all planned specific goals?'' and ''Do any valid specific goals remain?'' A thorough reassessment of the child's communicative functioning should be performed to answer these questions.

G. It is important to estimate the extent to which observed gains are due to the intervention program rather than influences external to intervention, such as maturation. Multiple baseline experimental designs are especially useful in evaluating the efficacy of intervention (Fey, 1986, Chapter 7). When such a design has not been implemented, the clinician should study as carefully as possible the child's performance on targeted and nontargeted behaviors.

H. If the child's gains are restricted to targeted behaviors and behaviors closely related to therapy targets, the hypothesis that the intervention program is responsible for the child's gains is reasonable. Continuation of the intervention plan is well justified under these circumstances.

I. If the child's progress over the intervention period has been relatively general and not treatment-specific, it is reasonable to assume either that the gains were due to factors other than intervention or that the intervention program has successfully stimulated the child's language-learning mechanisms to function more adequately on their own. Under either assumption, the decision to dismiss the child from treatment is appropriate. This decision reflects the clinician's hypothesis that the child will continue to exhibit significant improvements in language functioning without intervention.

J. In some cases, reassessment enables the clinician to determine that the child is no longer language impaired. In other cases, especially with older children who have severely impaired communication and cognitive systems, it can be determined that, despite the child's restricted functioning, new, potentially attainable skills would not add significantly to the child's communicative potential. No valid specific goals remain under either of these conditions and a decision to dismiss is appropriate.

K. The dismissal hypothesis can be tested by tracking the child's performance at 3-month intervals (see McDermott, 1985, for more information on the concept of tracking). An assessment of behaviors relevant to the child's original basic goals, including targeted and nontargeted specific goal behaviors, should be performed, and the child's growth curves should be analyzed. If the dismissal hypothesis is confirmed at the 3- and 6-month follow-ups (i.e., growth following dismissal is as great as during intervention), subsequent follow-ups could be made less formally through phone conversations with the parents, teachers, and child, or through the review of audio tapes and diary information prepared by the parents or other caregivers.

L. If the dismissal hypothesis is refuted based on a plateau in development or regression from previous levels of performance, a new intervention program should be begun immediately or tracking should continue for 6 more months.

# References

Fey ME. Language intervention with young children. San Diego: College Hill Press, 1986.

Kemp J. The timing of language intervention for the pediatric population. In: Miller J, Yoder D, Schiefelbusch R, eds. Contemporary issues in language intervention. Rockville, MD: American Speech-Language-Hearing Association, 1983:183.

McDermott L. Service alternatives. In: Snope T, ed. Caseload issues in schools: how to make better decisions. Rockville, MD: American Speech-Language-Hearing Association, 1985:18.

Olswang LB, Bain BA, Rosendahl PD, Oblak SB, Smith AE. Language learning: moving performance from a context-dependent to independent state. Child Lang Teach Ther 1986; 2:180.

# APHASIA: ASSESSMENT

Malcolm R. McNeil, Ph.D.
Edythe Strand, Ph.D.

A. The fundamental assumptions about the nature of aphasia (which lead to decisions regarding purposes and methods of assessment) are embodied in the following definition: "Aphasia is a physiologically based inefficiency with verbal symbolic functions. It is caused by damage to the cortical and subcortical structures in the hemispheres dominant for such verbal symbolic behavior." (McNeil, 1984).

B. If signs or symptoms are persistent (i.e., if long time post onset and patient is medically stable), there may be no need for a medical evaluation and focus of assessment is on the aphasia.

C. The presence of any signs or symptoms consistent with the stated or implied definition of aphasia provided above are sufficient reason for referral to a speech-language pathologist.

D. The speech pathologist may proceed from a number of potential purposes for assessment. These include differential diagnosis of presenting deficits, detection or confirmation of an existing aphasia, classification of type of aphasia, detection of site of lesion, determination of severity, determination of treatment candidacy and prognosis, and determination of treatment approach and measurement of change (McNeil, 1984).

E. A complete medical, social, and speech and language history is important in interpreting the data obtained for each of the purposes for assessment (Wertz, 1985).

$F_1$. Patients frequently present with a variety of sensory, perceptual, motor, or cognitive deficits that either can be confused with aphasia or can complicate the assessment. Detection of acuity or perceptual deficits is important early in the assessment process. Auditory or visual perceptual defects may be detected through observation (e.g., observation of failure to manipulate objects in one field; leaving food on one-half of the plate, and ignoring the presence of a person on one side as indications of the presence of a hemianopsia). Motor speech disorders such as apraxia of speech (AOS) and dysarthria may be present with or without concomitant aphasia. This differentiation is essential, as the underlying mechanisms and the eventual treatments take very different forms.

$F_2$. The symptomatology of higher cognitive disorders such as dementia, psychoses, or language of confusion may include abnormalities in verbal behavior even though aphasia is not the presenting disorder. Dementia is a disorder that crosses domains, affecting language less than other cognitive functions. Symptoms include impaired memory, attention, and learning; disturbance in emotional affect (often depressed); personality changes; and difficulty with abstract thinking. The disorder may present with an acute onset but is more commonly progressive. The primary symptoms of schizophrenia—disruption in thinking, mood, and behavior—are not always exhibited in language behaviors. Tasks to appraise language in schizophrenic patients should include those that tap relevance in communication, such as conversation and open-ended questions. The language of confusion is comprised of irrelevance and confabulations. The patient exhibits no word finding deficits and uses good syntax. The disorder often follows bilateral brain injury, is often of acute onset, and may improve rapidly and markedly (Wertz, 1984).

G. In order to be consistent with the diagnosis of aphasia, one needs to demonstrate that the deficits are exhibited across the oral, written, and gestural modalities ($G_1$); that the deficits are performance rather than competence based ($G_2$); and that the deficits are exhibited in language behaviors ($G_3$) (McNeil, 1984). Standardized tests such as the Porch Index of Communicative Ability (PICA) (Porch, 1967), the Boston Diagnostic Aphasia Examination (BDAE) (Goodglass and Kaplan, 1983), and the Western Aphasia Battery (WAB) (Kertesz, 1982) illustrate modalities in which deficits are demonstrated (Linebaugh, 1979). Examination of variability within each subtest provides information about the level of performance on a particular task the patient is able to achieve, even if that performance is not typical ($G_4$) (Linebaugh, 1979; McNeil, 1984). Detection involves the process of probing to determine whether problems exist that may not be apparent. The process of confirmation involves probing for an ambiguous sign or symptom in order to identify it.

H. Inherent in aphasia diagnosis and treatment is a long history of the process of classifying patients into particular groupings. Most commonly, one approaches this process with basic assumptions that lead one to identify particular patient types according to neurolinguistic models (e.g., Broca, Wernicke, Conduction) ($H_1$) or according to language behaviors (e.g., type I to VII Schuell) (Schuell, 1965) ($H_2$). The BDAE and the PICA systems differentially classify (or label the patient unclassified) while the WAB forces a classification.

I. Assessment of severity can be accomplished through the use of any of a number of standardized tests. There is no one measure of severity. One examines the overall severity of the aphasia in general, the severity of involvement in each of the verbal, written, reading, and gestural modalities, and the degree to which the patient is hampered in his ability to convey and receive messages (Darley, 1979). The best measures are those that attempt to quantify—e.g., PICA for overall severity and Revised Token Test (RTT) (McNeil and Prescott, 1978) for auditory-receptive modality.

J. The presence and nature of the symptomatology may at times have predictable neuropathological substrates. At present, the direct correlates are made primarily by aphasic classifications.

K. A patient's prognosis needs to be determined either with or without treatment. If the patient chooses no treatment,

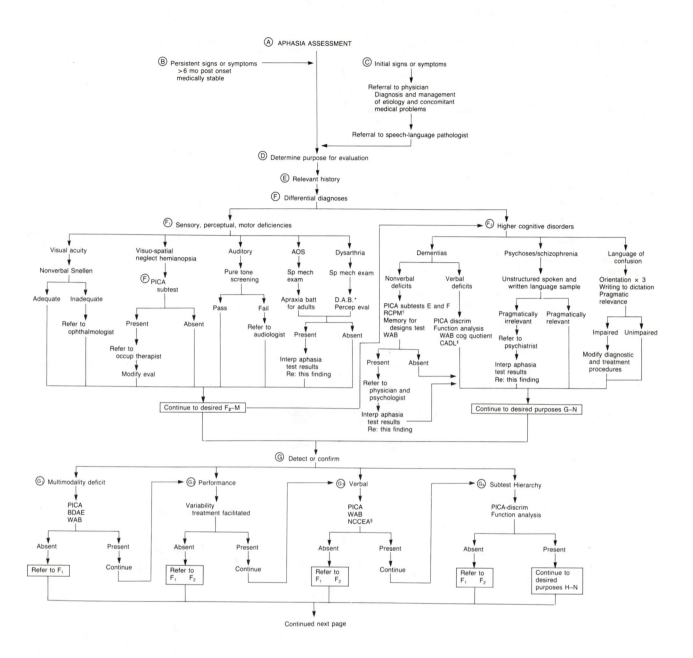

* D.A.B. – Darley, Aronson, and Brown
† RCPM – Raven Coloured Progressive Matrix
‡ CADL – Communicative Abilities in Daily Living
§ NCCEA – Neurosensory Center Comprehensive Examination for Aphasia

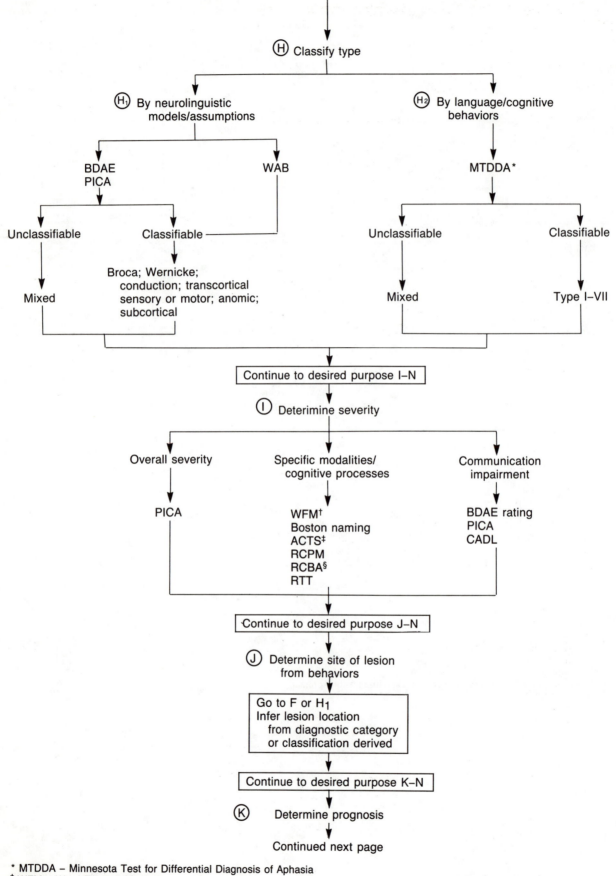

* MTDDA – Minnesota Test for Differential Diagnosis of Aphasia
† WFM – Word Fluency Measure
‡ ACTS – Auditory Comprehension Test for Sentences
§ RCBA – Reading Comprehension Battery for Aphasia

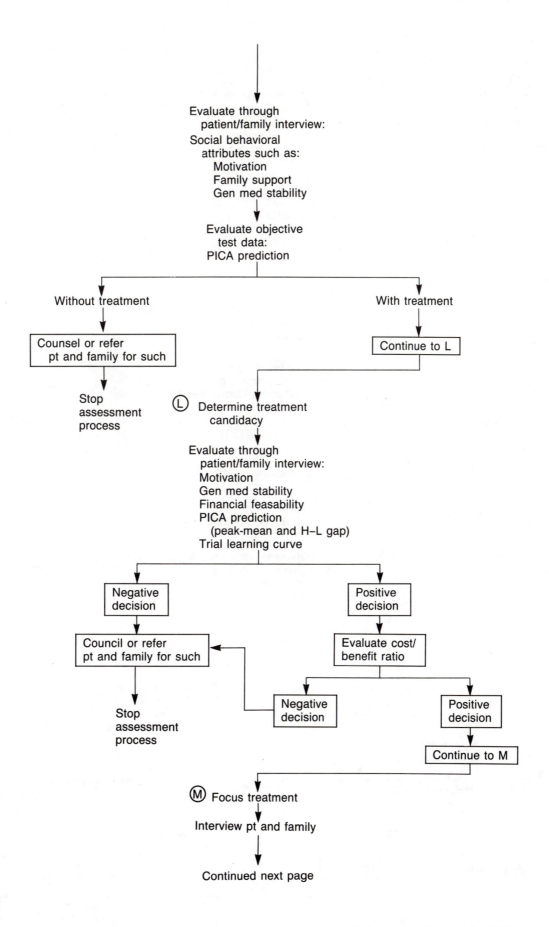

Evaluate through
  patient/family interview:
Social behavioral
  attributes such as:
    Motivation
    Family support
    Gen med stability

Evaluate objective
  test data:
  PICA prediction

Without treatment

With treatment

Counsel or refer
pt and family for such

Continue to L

Stop
assessment
process

Ⓛ Determine treatment
candidacy

Evaluate through
  patient/family interview:
  Motivation
  Gen med stability
  Financial feasability
  PICA prediction
    (peak-mean and H–L gap)
  Trial learning curve

Negative
decision

Positive
decision

Council or refer
pt and family for such

Evaluate cost/
benefit ratio

Stop
assessment
process

Negative
decision

Positive
decision

Continue to M

Ⓜ Focus treatment

Interview pt and family

Continued next page

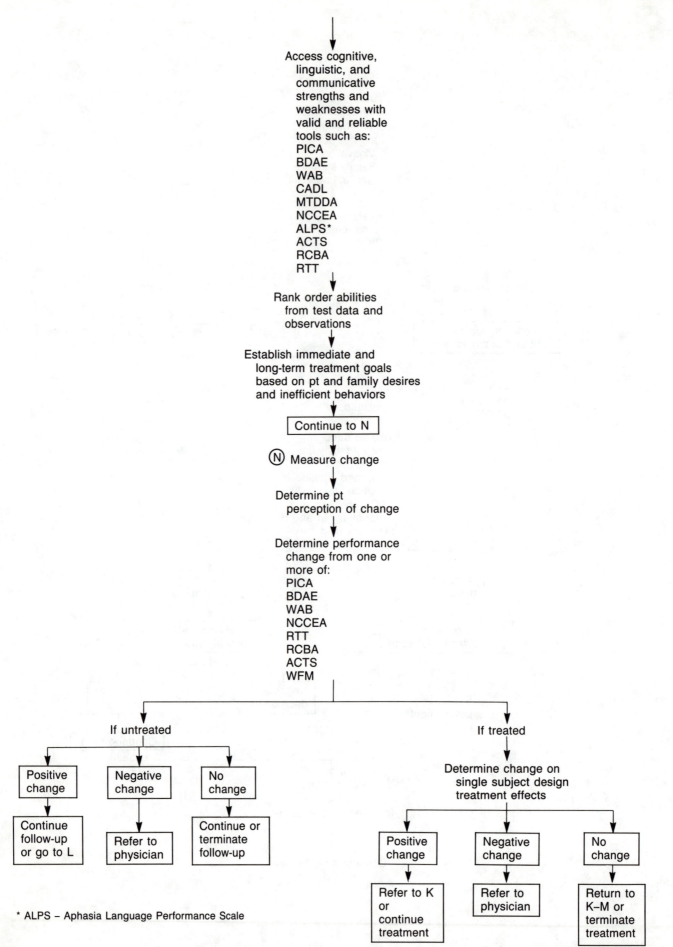

Access cognitive, linguistic, and communicative strengths and weaknesses with valid and reliable tools such as:
PICA
BDAE
WAB
CADL
MTDDA
NCCEA
ALPS*
ACTS
RCBA
RTT

Rank order abilities from test data and observations

Establish immediate and long-term treatment goals based on pt and family desires and inefficient behaviors

Continue to N

Ⓝ Measure change

Determine pt perception of change

Determine performance change from one or more of:
PICA
BDAE
WAB
NCCEA
RTT
RCBA
ACTS
WFM

If untreated

| Positive change | Negative change | No change |
| --- | --- | --- |
| Continue follow-up or go to L | Refer to physician | Continue or terminate follow-up |

If treated

Determine change on single subject design treatment effects

| Positive change | Negative change | No change |
| --- | --- | --- |
| Refer to K or continue treatment | Refer to physician | Return to K–M or terminate treatment |

* ALPS – Aphasia Language Performance Scale

the patient or family needs to be informed of the potential for improvement with and without treatment. Counseling or referral to appropriate professional may be necessary. If treatment is desired, the same information should be given, and additional measures to determine treatment candidacy should be initiated.

L.  The diagnosis of aphasia or the desire for treatment does not automatically indicate that the patient is a candidate for treatment. If the patient is not medically stable or is negative in attitude regarding intervention, postponement of treatment may be indicated. Financial considerations or living arrangements of the patient may necessitate counseling with the family regarding how to effectively enhance the patient's ability to communicate in lieu of treatment. The prognosis for improvement must be weighed against the financial and emotional costs of intervention.

M.  The focus of treatment is motivated by patient-family need and desire and the patient's specific strengths and weaknesses; the clinician's philosophy of intervention may also yield specific treatment approaches. For example, those who believe intervention should yield increased interpersonal communication would choose approaches such as PACE (Davis and Wilcox, 1981), while those favoring a more linguistic approach might choose to manipulate linguistic variables.

N.  It is sometimes important to measure change when the patient is not receiving intervention, including: determining a suspected new onset or progression of lesion, potential physiological changes, and whether treatment is now indicated for a patient for whom treatment had been deferred. Measurement of change for patients undergoing treatment may be obtained through perceptual, acoustic, or physiological methods. The patient's opinion, as well as objective measures, is taken into account in order to make decisions regarding changing the therapeutic approach, continuing treatment, or terminating the intervention. Single subject time series designs are appropriate methods to use to determine the efficacy of the intervention.

# References

## General

Darley FL. The differential diagnosis of aphasia. In: Brookshire RH, ed. Clinical aphasiology. Minneapolis: BRK Publishers, 1979a:23.

Darley FL. Evaluation of appraisal techniques in speech and language pathology. Philadelphia: Addison-Wesley, 1979b.

Davis GA, Wilcox MJ. Incorporating parameters of natural conversation in aphasia treatment. In: Chapey R, ed. Language intervention strategies in adult aphasic. Baltimore: Williams & Wilkins, 1981.

Goodglass H, Kaplan E. Boston diagnostic aphasia examination. 2nd ed. Philadelphia: Lea & Febiger, 1983.

Kertesz A. The western aphasia battery. Orlando: Grune & Stratton, 1982.

Linebaugh CW. Assessing the assessments: the adequacy of standardized tests of aphasia. In: Brookshire RH, ed. Clinical aphasiology. Minneapolis: BRK Publishers, 1979:8.

McNeil MR. Current concepts in adult aphasia. Internat Rehab Med, 1984; 6:128.

McNeil MR, Prescott TE. Revised token test. Baltimore: University Park Press, 1978.

Porch BE. Porch index of communicative ability. Palo Alto, CA: Consulting Psychologists Press. 1967.

Schuell H. The Minnesota test for differential diagnosis of aphasia. Minneapolis: University of Minnesota Press, 1965.

Wertz RT. Language disorders in adults: state of the clinical art. In: Holland L, ed. Language disorders in adults. San Diego: College-Hill Press, 1984:1.

Wertz RT. Neuropathologies of speech and language: an introduction to patient management. In: Johns DF, ed. Clinical management of neurogenic communicative disorders. Boston: Little, Brown, 1985:1.

## Specific to Decision Tree

Borkowski JG, Benton AL, Spreen O. Word fluency and aphasia. Neuropsychologia 1967; 5, 135.

Dabul B. Apraxia battery for adults. Tigard, OR: CC Publishers, 1979.

Darley FL, Aronson AE, Brown JE. Motor speech disorders. Philadelphia: WB Saunders, 1975.

Deal JL, Deal L, Wertz RT, Kitselman K, Dwyer C. Right hemisphere PICA percentiles: some speculations about aphasia. In: Brookshire RH, ed. Clinical aphasiology. Minneapolis: BRK Publishers, 1979.

Graham FK, Kendall BS. Memory-for-designs test. Missoula: Psychological Test Specialists, 1960.

Holland AL, Communicative assessment in daily living. Baltimore: University Park Press, 1980.

Keenan JS, Brassell EG. Aphasia language performance scales (ALPS). Murfreesboro: Pinnacle Press, 1975.

LaPointe LL, Horner J. Reading comprehension battery for aphasia. Tigard, OR: CC Publications, 1979.

Porch BE, Collins MJ, Wertz RT, Friden TP. Statistical prediction of change in aphasia. J Speech Hear Res 1980; 23, 312.

Porch BE, Friden T, Porec J. Objective differentiation of aphasic versus nonorganic patients. Paper presented to the International Neuropsychological Society. Santa Fe, NM, 1977.

Raven JC. Coloured progressive matrices. London: HK Lewis, 1962.

Shewan CM. Auditory comprehension test for sentences. Chicago: Biolinguistics, Clinical Institutes, 1979.

Speen O, Benton AL. Neurosensory center comprehensive examination for aphasia. Victoria, BC: University of Victoria, 1969.

# APHASIA: TREATMENT

*Malcolm R. McNeil, Ph.D.*

A. Following the assessment decision making process, a decision is made about the patient's potential for improvement with and without treatment and the timing of that treatment. From an efficacy perspective, there is no reason to delay treatment, but neither is there a threat to the treatment's efficacy in delaying its implementation (Darley, 1982; McNeil, 1988). If treatment potential is judged positive, the desire for treatment is evaluated in step C.

B. If the potential for improvement with treatment is judged to be negative, the patient should be scheduled for a follow-up evaluation in order to assess any changes in medical, cognitive, linguistic, or psychosocial status that mitigated treatment at the present time.

C. If the desire for treatment from the patient or the patient's guardian is present, an evaluation of the cost-benefit is made in D. If the patient or guardian is uninterested in receiving treatment at the present, a follow-up evaluation should be offered to reassess the motivation for treatment at a later date. The timing of this reevaluation depends on the perceived causes for the lack of motivation.

D. The cost-benefit ratio is evaluated by the financial expenditure involved from the financially responsible party and the personal expenditure of the patient and the patient's family or caretakers, relative to the personal and financial resources available. The resources available relative to the financial and personal expenditures are evaluated against the predicted benefits of the treatment. If the cost-benefit ratio is judged by the clinican and the patient or the guardian or family to be unfavorable for the initiation of treatment, a follow-up evaluation should be offered (B). If the ratio is judged favorable for treatment, the treatment regimen should be initiated with the establishment of the methods for evaluating the efficacy of the treatment employed (E).

E. The precise methods for determining the efficacy of the treatment regimen adopted should be clearly specified (Chapey, 1986). This specification should include a clear statement of the stimuli used, the method of treatment, the criteria for patient change or treatment termination, the method of data collection, and the experimental design in which the patient and treatment will be evaluated. This establishment of method is necessary because there is currently insufficient evidence to predict that any one treatment procedure or method will be efficacious for any individual. Therefore, the efficacy of each procedure needs validation with each patient until a high degree of confidence can be given, a priori, that the treatment will be efficacious.

F. There is sufficient evidence to suggest that some input or output channels are typically stronger than others for carrying language information in individual subjects. Some treatment techniques have been devised to capitalize on this fact, such as "deblocking." Stronger and weaker language carrying channels (modalities) should be arranged in hierarchical orders to optimize the facilitation of language and communication.

G. While there is little evidence for complete dissociations among linguistic domains (e.g., syntax, semantics, phonology, morphology), there is evidence that the domains can be impaired to varying degrees for individual subjects (Davis, 1983). The degree to which there are rela-

APHASIA TREATMENT

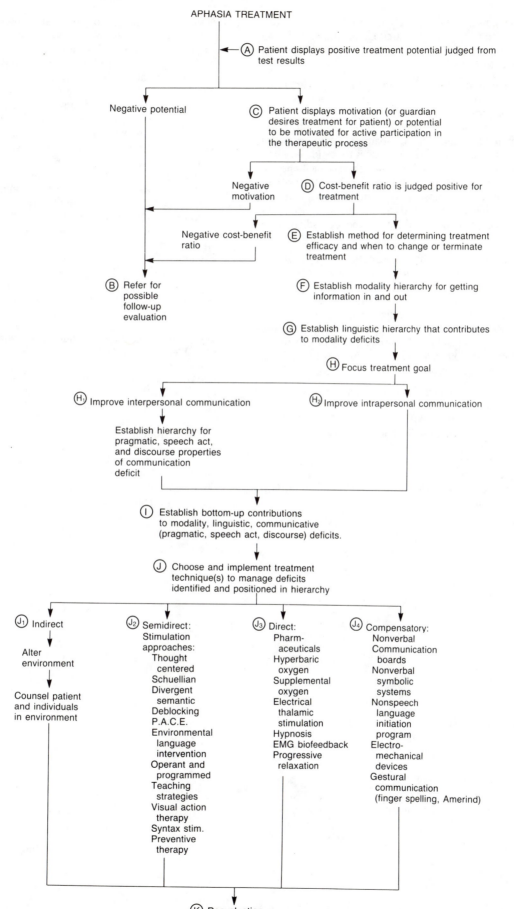

Ⓐ Patient displays positive treatment potential judged from test results

Negative potential

Ⓒ Patient displays motivation (or guardian desires treatment for patient) or potential to be motivated for active participation in the therapeutic process

Negative motivation

Ⓓ Cost-benefit ratio is judged positive for treatment

Negative cost-benefit ratio

Ⓔ Establish method for determining treatment efficacy and when to change or terminate treatment

Ⓑ Refer for possible follow-up evaluation

Ⓕ Establish modality hierarchy for getting information in and out

Ⓖ Establish linguistic hierarchy that contributes to modality deficits

Ⓗ Focus treatment goal

Ⓗ₁ Improve interpersonal communication

Ⓗ₂ Improve intrapersonal communication

Establish hierarchy for pragmatic, speech act, and discourse properties of communication deficit

Ⓘ Establish bottom-up contributions to modality, linguistic, communicative (pragmatic, speech act, discourse) deficits.

Ⓙ Choose and implement treatment technique(s) to manage deficits identified and positioned in hierarchy

Ⓙ₁ Indirect

Alter environment

Counsel patient and individuals in environment

Ⓙ₂ Semidirect:
Stimulation approaches:
Thought centered
Schuellian
Divergent semantic
Deblocking
P.A.C.E.
Environmental language intervention
Operant and programmed
Teaching strategies
Visual action therapy
Syntax stim.
Preventive therapy

Ⓙ₃ Direct:
Pharm-aceuticals
Hyperbaric oxygen
Supplemental oxygen
Electrical thalamic stimulation
Hypnosis
EMG biofeedback
Progressive relaxation

Ⓙ₄ Compensatory:
Nonverbal Communication boards
Nonverbal symbolic systems
Nonspeech language initiation program
Electro-mechanical devices
Gestural communication (finger spelling, Amerind)

Ⓚ Reevaluation (implement Ⓔ)

tive strengths and weaknesses across linguistic domains needs to be arranged in hierarchies to comply with one of the basic principles of treatment (working from strengths to weaknesses).

H.  With the establishment of specific modality and linguistic strengths and weaknesses, the specific targets of treatment need to be established to further refine and focus the treatment goals (Darley, 1982). See La Point (1983) for a more elaborate menu of treatment techniques. The first decision that needs to be made is to decide whether the initial treatment goal is to strengthen or facilitate the cognitive and linguistic operations used in interpersonal communication or those used in intrapersonal communication. This decision needs to be made because these two goals often require different treatment paradigms and techniques.

H$_1$. If the improvement of interpersonal communication is the goal of treatment, the hierarchies for those constructs that have been developed for the description of interpersonal communication and its impairments (e.g., pragmatics, speech acts, and properties of discourse such as coherence and cohesion) need to be established for the individual patient. As with other aspects of treatment, a primary principle is to work from sources of strengths to improve areas of weakness.

H$_2$. If the goal is to indirectly improve intrapersonal communication, such as the cognitive and linguistic processes involved in reading or writing or the linguistic abilities that actually structure intellect and much of behavior the clinician is likely to be less concerned with such communication variables as speech acts or discourse. In this case, the clinician moves to I for an evaluation of the bottom-up contributions to the intrapersonal communication deficits that exist.

I.  A systematic analysis of any basic sensory and motor deficits and any information processing (e.g., memory, attention, resource allocation, automaticity) deficits (bottom-up) that contribute to the modality, linguistic, or communicative deficits will be made and organized into hierarchies along with a specific plan of remediation for them (McNeil and Kimelman, 1986). In this way, the goal of therapy is to strengthen an inefficient cognitive system to effect change in the language and its use for interpersonal communication. It would be rare for a clinician to direct his therapeutic efforts to only one of these goals in an individual patient. It is probably more common to work on both interpersonal and intrapersonal communication in each patient. Most often this occurs simultaneously because the facilitation and manipulation of inefficient cognitive systems that support language and communication cannot be accomplished without having an indirect effect on those systems that they support. The opposite is also true. That is, direct remediation of speech acts or discourse necessarily involves and possibly changes the cognitive and linguistic apparatus that it uses to accomplish its goals.

J.  The most appropriate treatment technique or combination of techniques are selected for addressing the specific treatment goals and linguistic and modality strengths and weaknesses. One way to categorize the treatment approaches and techniques currently available to the clinical aphasiologist is to focus on the directness with which the technique affects the physiology of the patient (McNeil, 1988).

J$_1$. Indirect treatment techniques do not attempt to alter anything about the patient. Instead they attempt to alter the physical environment or individuals in the patient's environment. The counseling might include not only a realistic assessment of the patient's capabilities, but also strategies for persons in the patient's environment for enhancing the communicative or information processing abilities of the patient.

J₂. Semidirect techniques are those that generally fall within techniques that are called "stimulation approaches." They provide a semidirect impact on the physiology of the system as any sensory or motor stimulus does. These approaches represent the majority of the techniques used by the majority of clinical aphasiologists. Those studies that have demonstrated efficacious treatment for aphasia have used one or more semidirect stimulation approaches.

J₃. Direct techniques are those that provide a direct electrical or chemical impact on the physiology of the system. This electrical or chemical stimulation is focal in nature and is designed to stimulate those neural substrates that are believed to be most directly involved in the linguistic and cognitive behaviors associated with aphasia. Biofeedback and progressive relaxation might be classified better as semidirect techniques, but in the current classification schema they are classified as direct because they often use a sensitivity to physiological functions as a stimulus to change a particular physiological function.

J₄. Compensatory treatment techniques are those that use augmentative or alternative devices to circumvent the impaired communication processes. They do not attempt to alter the patient's environment or those individuals within that environment, the ways that language is processed in the patient, or the physiology of the patient. Compensatory techniques are frequently recommended clinically, and they usually appear within the clinical ar-

mamentarium of the clinical aphasiologist, but there is little evidence for their efficacy with aphasic persons.

K. Consistent with the schedule for reassessment established in E, the patient should be periodically reassessed with standardized, valid, and reliable measures that will reflect any changes that need to be made in the focus of the treatment (H) or in the decision to terminate treatment. The duration of time between assessments depends on a number of patient variables, including, but not limited to, the time after onset, motivation, complicating medical, social, or psychological illnesses, and frequency or quality of treatment.

# References

Chapey R. Language intervention strategies in adult aphasia. 2nd ed. Baltimore: Williams & Wilkins, 1986.

Darley FL. Aphasia. Philadelphia: WB Saunders, 1982.

Davis GA. A survey of adult aphasia. Englewood Cliffs, NJ: Prentice-Hall, 1983.

LaPointe LL. Aphasia intervention with adults: historical, present and future approaches. In: Miller J, Yoder DE, Shiefelbusch R, eds. Contemporary issues in language intervention. ASHA Reports 12. Rockville, MD: American Speech-Language-Hearing Association, 1983.

McNeil MR. Aphasia in the adult. In: Lass NJ, McReynolds LV, Northern JL, Yoder DE, eds. Handbook of speech-language pathology and audiology. Toronto: BC Decker, 1988: (in press).

McNeil MR, Kimelman MDZ. Toward an integrative information-processing structure of auditory comprehension and processing in adult aphasia. Sem Speech Lang 1986; 7:123.

# SOCIOCOMMUNICATIVE COMPETENCE IN THE SEVERELY/ PROFOUNDLY HANDICAPPED CHILD: ASSESSMENT

*Lee Snyder-McLean, Ph.D.*
*James E. McLean, Ph.D.*

A. The assessment and clinical management (see p 68) of sociocommunicative competencies in children with severe or profound handicaps require the clinician to view the "whole child" and to work closely with caregivers and other professionals in an interdisciplinary or transdisciplinary framework. Before beginning any assessment activities, the clinician will want to obtain several types of background information from these individuals and from client records. Information regarding the client's functional vision and hearing, as well as his or her neuromotor status and capabilities, is necessary in designing appropriate assessment activities and in meaningful interpretation of that assessment. It is also important to know what types of communication responses have been targeted in previous communication therapy with this client and with what results. Finally, the clinician should interview people who know the client to identify those individuals (including parents) who constitute this client's "significant others," or SOs (MacDonald and Gillette, 1984) and to identify materials or activities that are known to be motivating for this client.

B. The three-phase assessment process begins with an in-depth interview conducted with one (or more) of the client's SOs. The clinician should evoke descriptive information relative to the client's status on each of the major assessment variables identified in the lower sections of the decision chart. It is also important to determine the SO's major concerns and expectations regarding this client's current and future communicative abilities. Following this interview, the clinician should arrange to observe the client in one or two activities identified by the SO as times when the client communicates most consistently and successfully. If possible, have the SO participate in this observation and comment upon the representativeness of the communicative performance observed. On the basis of the interview and observation data collected up to this point, the clinician will probably be able to make many of the more global judgments called for in the decision chart. The final phase of assessment consists of structured evaluation activities designed to evoke specific types of expressive communication and dyadic interaction identified as areas of concern for this client. These activities generally involve the client's participation in one or more carefully scripted interaction sequences with the clinician. In planning these assessment sequences, the clinician can increase the probability of observing targeted response(s) by incorporating the types of materials and activities identified as motivating for this client and manipulating the interactive context in ways that invite or require client's communicative acts. While there are no published, standardized instruments for this purpose, several examples can be found in the literature (Cirrin and Rowland, 1985; Snyder, 1975; Wetherby and Prutting, 1984).

C. Perlocutionary communication is that which has an effect on some receiver, but does not seem to be clearly intended by the client to function as communication; whereas illocutionary communication is clearly directed toward a receiver and is produced with some expectation on the part of the client that he or she can have some effect on a receiver (Bates, 1976; McLean and Snyder-McLean, 1984). Of course, mature speakers communicate with both perlocutionary (e.g., "body language") and illocutionary acts. In clinical assessment, the client should be characterized as using perlocutionary communication only if there is little or no evidence that this client ever intends to communicate. If at least some communication acts can be classified as illocutionary, the clinician should select the "illocutionary communication" decision path.

D. The functions of perlocutionary communication acts are those ascribed to the client's behaviors by the SOs in his or her environment. Common perlocutionary functions include: obtaining a desired object or event; indicating

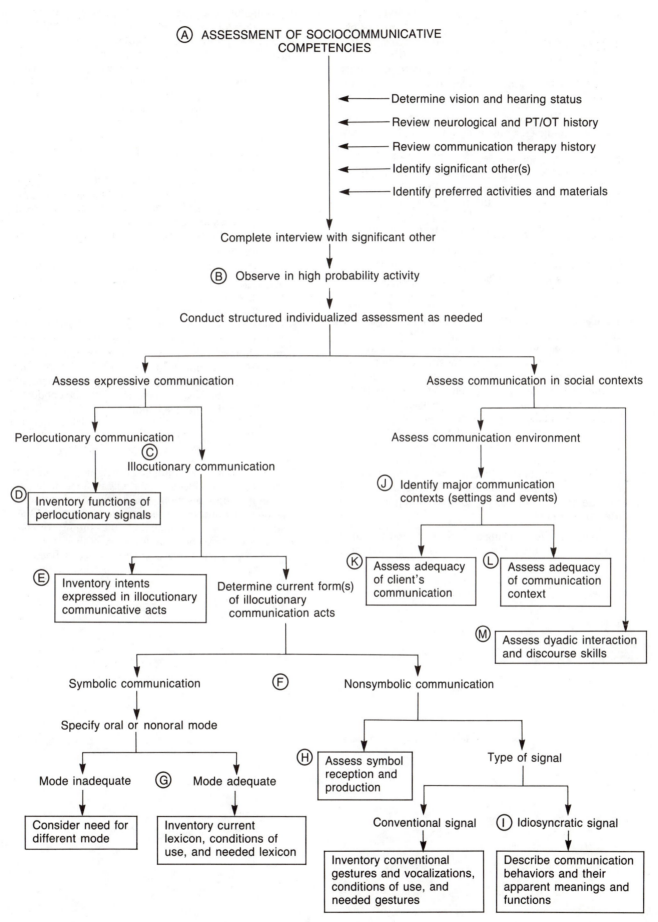

(A) ASSESSMENT OF SOCIOCOMMUNICATIVE COMPETENCIES

→ Determine vision and hearing status
→ Review neurological and PT/OT history
→ Review communication therapy history
→ Identify significant other(s)
→ Identify preferred activities and materials

Complete interview with significant other

(B) Observe in high probability activity

Conduct structured individualized assessment as needed

Assess expressive communication

Assess communication in social contexts

Perlocutionary communication

(C)
Illocutionary communication

(D) Inventory functions of perlocutionary signals

(E) Inventory intents expressed in illocutionary communicative acts

Determine current form(s) of illocutionary communication acts

Assess communication environment

(J) Identify major communication contexts (settings and events)

(K) Assess adequacy of client's communication

(L) Assess adequacy of communication context

(M) Assess dyadic interaction and discourse skills

Symbolic communication

(F) Nonsymbolic communication

Specify oral or nonoral mode

Mode inadequate

(G) Mode adequate

Consider need for different mode

Inventory current lexicon, conditions of use, and needed lexicon

(H) Assess symbol reception and production

Type of signal

Conventional signal

(I) Idiosyncratic signal

Inventory conventional gestures and vocalizations, conditions of use, and needed gestures

Describe communication behaviors and their apparent meanings and functions

**65**

notice of some interesting object or event; and indicating pleasure or displeasure about some internal or external state of affairs (McLean and Snyder-McLean, 1984). In assessing children with severe to profound handicaps, it is helpful to indicate whether the objects and events that evoke perlocutionary acts are food related or non-food related.

E.   The most common communicative intents included in inventories designed for use with severely and profoundly handicapped children are (a) to request an object or action, (b) to comment on or draw attention to an object or event, (c) to request information or permission, (d) to express an affective-emotional reaction to some state of affairs, (e) to greet, and (f) to answer or reply (Cirrin and Rowland, 1985; Wetherby and Prutting, 1984). Again, it is helpful to note whether these acts involve food.

F.   For the client who is producing at least some illocutionary (intentional) communication, the clinician will want to determine the particular form(s) used by that client to express his or her communicative intents. The first judgment that must be made is whether the client's communicative acts are symbolic or nonsymbolic. In this context, the term symbolic refers only to systems that allow their users to specifically represent or depict a variety of referent objects, events, and concepts. Common forms of symbolic communication include speech; manual sign language; traditional orthography; and various pictographic symbol systems, including Rebus and Bliss symbols. More broadly denotative communication systems, including both conventional and idiosyncratic gestures, are classified here as nonsymbolic forms of communication. In assessing this aspect of the client's communication, the clinician should identify the client's predominant or modal form of communicative act and also identify any other forms observed or reported to be used by the client.

G.   For the client who is using an oral or nonoral symbolic mode of communication, the clinician should next determine whether that mode is adequate to meet the client's current communications needs (see p 72). An adequate system is one that is both effective—i.e., that allows the client to clearly specify the range of referent meanings that he or she has to convey—and relatively efficient. A particular mode may be inadquate for a client because of internal limitations in the symbol system itself (e.g., photographs may be inadequate for a client who has many abstract meanings to convey); the client's inability to produce the symbols clearly or efficiently, or a lack of knowledge or acceptance of the symbol system in the client's communication environment. If the current mode is adequate, an inventory of the client's current lexicon should include the conditions in which words and symbols are produced (when and to whom) and those obligatory communication contexts in which the client produces no word or symbol or uses an inappropriate word or symbol.

H.   If the client's predominant form of communication is nonsymbolic, his potential for symbol use should be assessed. Receptive symbolization can be assessed using a match-to-sample procedure in which the client is presented with an array of referent objects and asked to select the one that is represented by a symbol presented by the clinician. This procedure can be used to assess receptive responding to spoken words, pictures, and manual signs. Stimulability testing (the ability to imitate a model presented by the clinician) should be conducted to determine the client's potential for productive use of different symbol systems. It is not unusual to find that severely handicapped clients can respond to symbols in modes that they themselves can not produce.

I.   The SO can assist in compiling a "dictionary" of idiosyncratic signals produced by the client. This dictionary should include a description of the client's communicative behavior and how it is interpreted by the SO. An inventory of any conventional gestures produced by the client should also be completed, including any use of a point; open palm request, wave, show, or head nod or shake. Further, it should be noted whether the client uses any intonated vocalizations, either alone or with gestures, to convey the illocutionary force of his or her communication acts.

J. Major communication contexts include those settings or activities in which the client spends a significant amount of time on a regular basis. These should be contexts that potentially offer the client both the need and the opportunity to communicate with others.

K. The adequacy of the client's current communication performance in each context should be assessed in terms of two criteria: (a) Is the client's communication effective and efficient enough to meet his or her needs in this context? (b) Are timing, duration, content, and forms of client's communication perceived as appropriate and acceptable by SOs in this context?

L. An assessment of the adequacy of each communication context should consider the following questions: (a) Do SOs in this context recognize and respond to the client's communication acts? (b) Is there both opportunity and expectation for client communication in this context? (c) Do SOs in this context encourage and expect client to use the highest, most efficient form of communication he or her can? (d) Do others in this context provide models of a broad range of communication meanings and intents? (e) Is the level of communication addressed to the client in this context appropriate to his or her comprehension abilities?

M. Dyadic interaction and early discourse skills should be assessed under optimal conditions—i.e., when the client is engaged one-on-one with the clinician or another adult in a simple game or activity that encourages joint attention and turn-taking. Care should be taken to avoid activities that are extremely motivating to the client, as these decrease the probability of his or her interacting with the examiner. Specific dyadic and early discourse skills to be assessed include the following: (a) attends to other person (not necessarily "eye contact"), (b) attends to the focus of activity, (c) pauses and allows other person to take turn, (d) fills own turn when appropriate, (e) successfully introduces topic(s) for communication, (f) maintains an established topic when responding to other's communication, and (g) demonstrates specific types of communication that serve to maintain conversation (answers questions, replies to statements, complies with requests for clarification or repetition, and requests clarification or repetition when needed).

## References

Bates E. Language and context. New York: Academic Press, 1976.

Cirrin FM, Rowland CM. Communicative assessment of nonverbal youths with severe/profound mental retardation. Ment Retard 1985; 23:52-62.

MacDonald JD, Gillette Y. Conversation engineering: a pragmatic approach to early social competence. Semin Speech Lang, 1984; 5(3).

McLean J, Snyder-McLean L. Recent developments in pragmatics: remedial implications. In: Muller DJ, ed. Remediating children's language: behavioural and naturalistic approaches. San Diego, CA: College-Hill Press, 1984.

Snyder L. Pragmatics in language disabled children: their prelinguistic and early verbal performatives and presuppositions. Unpublished doctoral dissertation, University of Colorado, 1975.

Wetherby AM, Prutting CA. Profiles of communicative and cognitive-social abilities in autistic children. J Speech Hear Res 1984; 27:364-377.

# SOCIOCOMMUNICATIVE COMPETENCE IN THE SEVERELY/ PROFOUNDLY HANDICAPPED CHILD: MANAGEMENT

*Lee Snyder-McLean, Ph.D.*
*James E. McLean, Ph.D.*

A. The previous chapter describes the types of assessment and historical data that should be obtained prior to planning a treatment program in the area of sociocommunicative skills for children with severe and profound handicaps. In implementing therapy, just as in assessment, input from the client's significant others (SOs) and all members of the interdisciplinary team is essential to success.

B. Client goals in the areas of expressive communication and dyadic interaction skills are derived on the basis of assessment procedures described in the previous chapter. Short-term objectives that will lead to the attainment of each of these goals are developed on the basis of the clinician's knowledge of the process and sequence of early communication development in general; as well as this client's unique needs and current abilities. (For reviews of early communication development see Bernstein and Tiegerman, 1985; Owens, 1984.) These objectives should be measurable and achievable within approximately 6 months. Initial objectives should focus on contexts, people, and stimulus events identified in the assessment process as having high probability for this client.

C. Vertical extension refers to the development of skills at a higher level than those currently displayed by client; horizontal expansion refers to increasing the range of client's communication at his or her current skill level (e.g., increasing the number of different gestures produced; the number of situations in which gestures are used). Generally a program for a severely/profoundly handicapped client includes both vertical extension and horizontal expansion objectives. An important principle in setting these objectives is to target new (higher) forms first to express existing meanings or functions and to target new meanings and functions using already established forms. The clinician should avoid targeting both a horizontal extension and a vertical expansion in the same objective.

D. A response development objective targets a response that was never produced spontaneously during assessment and that could not be readily evoked using imitative, verbal, or minimal physical prompts. If the target response is available under these conditions but is targeted for therapy because it is not used spontaneously or consistently, the objective is one of attaining appropriate stimulus control of that response.

E. For response development objectives, traditional massed trial procedures are generally most effective and efficient. Specific therapy methods may include modeling, shaping, chaining, fading, or the use of successive levels of prompting. Concurrent with such massed trial training, the client should be experiencing situations in which the new response will be functional. Once a response is available and is targeted in a stimulus control objective, more naturalistic, in situ procedures are used to bring the response under control of the natural stimuli that must evoke and maintain the response. (For a review of naturalistic procedures, see Warren and Kaiser, 1986.)

F. Direct recording of client responding on all trials is usually the preferred mode of data collection in massed trial therapy. For naturalistic, in situ programming, it is generally more practical to use a probe procedure, fol-

# MANAGEMENT OF SOCIOCOMMUNICATIVE THERAPY

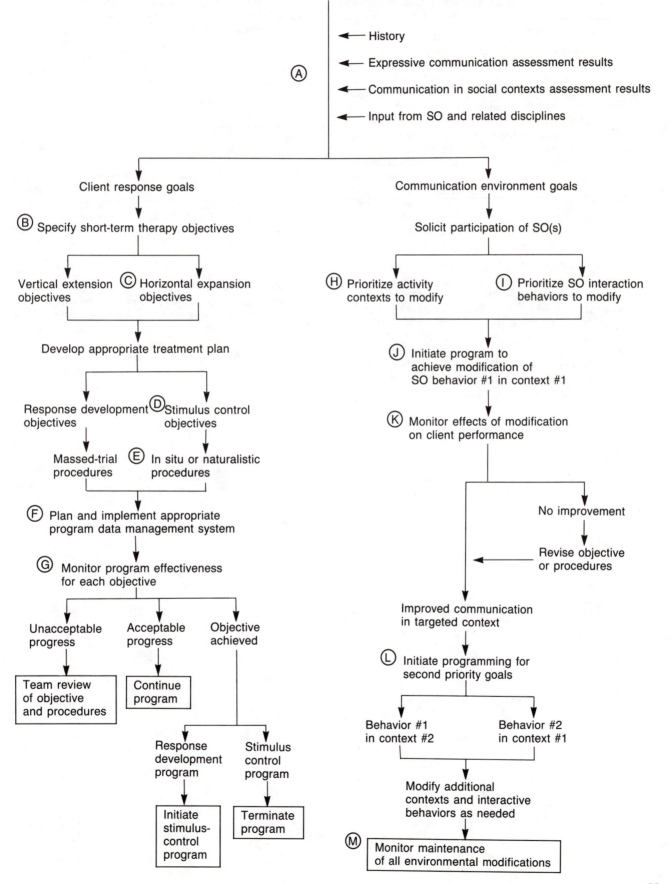

(A) ← History
← Expressive communication assessment results
← Communication in social contexts assessment results
← Input from SO and related disciplines

Client response goals

(B) Specify short-term therapy objectives

Vertical extension objectives (C) Horizontal expansion objectives

Develop appropriate treatment plan

Response development objectives (D) Stimulus control objectives

Massed-trial procedures (E) In situ or naturalistic procedures

(F) Plan and implement appropriate program data management system

(G) Monitor program effectiveness for each objective

Unacceptable progress | Acceptable progress | Objective achieved

Team review of objective and procedures | Continue program

Response development program | Stimulus control program

Initiate stimulus-control program | Terminate program

Communication environment goals

Solicit participation of SO(s)

(H) Prioritize activity contexts to modify | (I) Prioritize SO interaction behaviors to modify

(J) Initiate program to achieve modification of SO behavior #1 in context #1

(K) Monitor effects of modification on client performance

No improvement

Revise objective or procedures

Improved communication in targeted context

(L) Initiate programming for second priority goals

Behavior #1 in context #2 | Behavior #2 in context #1

Modify additional contexts and interactive behaviors as needed

(M) Monitor maintenance of all environmental modifications

lowing a predetermined schedule, to monitor client progress. For the severely or profoundly handicapped client, data usually do not need to be recorded daily but probably should be recorded at least once a week on each treatment objective.

G. Judgments about the adequacy of progress on any one program by a severely or profoundly handicapped client reflect some consideration of that client's characteristic rate of progress in previous therapy programs. In the event that progress falls to an unacceptable rate, the original interdisciplinary team may be consulted to determine whether adjustments are needed in the objective itself or in one or more aspects of the treatment procedure. If criterion performance is achieved on a response development objective, it is generally appropriate to target that new response in a stimulus control objective. Once the criterion performance level is reached on a stimulus control objective, formal programming can be terminated, but ongoing probes are advisable to promote and monitor skill maintenance.

H. Assessment data on the adequacy of different major communication contexts are reviewed to determine whether modifications should be sought in one or more of these contexts (see p 64). If more than one context is targeted for modification, these are prioritized so that modifications are introduced first into the context that offers the highest probability of success. Factors considered are the motivation of SOs in each context, the current activity structure in each context, and the client's motivation to participate in activities in each context.

I. If assessment results indicate that SOs in the client's communication environment do not demonstrate certain interaction strategies that support client communication development, these specific strategies may be targeted for modification. Initially just one of these strategies is selected by the clinician and SO to be targeted. Factors to consider in prioritizing these strategies include the perceived ease or difficulty of each for a particular SO, with priority given to those that can be acquired most easily and successfully; and the degree to which different strategies might be expected to contribute to an improved communication environment for the client and SO, with priority given to strategies that offer the greatest immediate improvement.

J. Generally modification of communication contexts is achieved through modification of SO interaction patterns in those contexts. Specific guidelines for modifying caregiver interaction behaviors, using videotape analysis and feedback, are provided by McDade and Simpson (1984). For some SOs, the "ECO" procedures developed by MacDonald and Gillette (1984) are useful in developing the basic elements of dyadic interaction between the SO and child. In addition, there are several procedures that can be used to modify the overall level of expectation and opportunity for client communication in any context. These include the "joint action routine" (Snyder-McLean, Solomonson, et al, 1984), the "mand-model" procedure (Rogers-Warren and Warren, 1980), and the interrupted sequence or delay procedure (Halle, Marshall et al, 1979).

K. The decision to modify any aspect of a client's communication environment, including the interaction patterns of SOs in that environment, represents a disruption of an established ecology. It is important to closely monitor the effects of such modifications for both expected and unexpected outcomes. This is typically accomplished through an informal process of observation and ongoing dialogue with the SO(s) involved in intervention, supplemented by careful monitoring of client program performance data. Environmental modification objectives or procedures may need to be changed if there is any indication that these procedures are either ineffective or are associated with undesired changes in the quality of client-SO interactions.

L. After the SO has mastered the first priority interaction strategy in the first priority context, the environmental intervention can be expanded to include additional interaction strategies and additional contexts. If a second interaction strategy is targeted for the SO, this is most effectively introduced in an already modified context. Similarly, modifications introduced into a second context should require only those interaction strategies already mastered by the SO. This process of introducing new strategies in established contexts and using established strategies in new contexts is continued until all targeted interaction strategies are used consistently by the SO in all major communication contexts.

M. It is common for SOs to revert to earlier interaction patterns after the period of formal intervention is over. Periodic monitoring by the clinician is important until these newly learned interaction strategies are habituated by the SO.

# References

Bernstein J, Tiegerman E. Language and communication disorders in children. Columbus: Charles E. Merrill, 1985.

Halle JW, Marshall AM, Spradlin JE. Time delay: a technique to increase language use and facilitate generalization in retarded children. J Appl Behav Anal, 1979; 12:431-439.

MacDonald JD, Gillette Y. Conversation engineering: a pragmatic approach to early social competence. Semin Speech Lang, 1984; 5(3).

McDade HL, Simpson MA. Use of instruction, modeling, and videotape feedback to modify parent behavior: a strategy for facilitating language development in the home. Semin Speech Lang, 1984; 5(3).

Owens R. Language Development: an introduction. Columbus: Charles E. Merrill, 1984.

Rogers-Warren AK, Warren SF. Mands for verbalization: facilitating the generalization of newly trained language in children. Behav Modif 1980; 4:230-245.

Snyder-McLean L, Solomonson B, McLean J, Sack S. Structuring joint action routines: a strategy for facilitating communication and language development in the classroom. Semin Speech Lang, 1984; 5:(3).

Warren SF, Kaiser AP. Incidental language teaching: a critical review. J Speech Hear Disord, 1986; 51:291.

# AUGMENTATIVE COMMUNICATION SYSTEMS FOR THE CHILD AND ADOLESCENT

*David E. Yoder, Ph.D.*
*Donna J. DePape, M.S.*

A. Table I illustrates the three areas to consider in the communication needs assessment: (1) *the communication situation*: Communication needs are assessed with respect to the internal and external environments in which communication takes place. External environment also includes the person's own unique physical position which is influenced by their disability; (2) *the manner of the interaction*: The manner in which communication takes place considers the needs for conversation and writing. Within this area we are mainly concerned about the way in which the augmentative communication system is or will be used; and (3) *communicative events and/or functions*: It is important to assess the communication needs relative to the user's success in conveying the intended message. One assesses the usual communication functions used by normal speakers to determine which ones are also available and/or used by the nonspeaking individual. One examines the extent of participation in conversation, turn taking, topic initiation, communication breakdown, and strategies for repair (Beukelman et al, 1984; Bottorf and De Pape, 1982).

B. Table 2 outlines the assessment process necessary to describe whether the individual with severe speech impairment has an adequate or inadequate communication system. There are three integral components to a communication system: person, tools, and environment. The interaction of these components with the six features listed in the left column of Table 2 constitutes the framework for assessing the communication system. The information listed in the left column of Table 2 relates to components of the communication system being examined. Across the top we have listed three integral aspects of the system that effect the factors of the system (Owens and House, 1984; Shane, 1981; Shane and Bashir, 1980).

C. Acceptance of the system and the interactional process are considered the overriding factors when addressing issues in user skill, the system, and the environment.

D. User skill, system, and environment are areas for specific change within the total system for interaction. Listed below those headings are particular activities or areas that may need to be addressed as part of an ongoing evaluation to move to a more sophisticated communication system in the future (Goossens and Crain, 1986).

E. The intradisciplinary team including the family and potential user participate in the discussion. As a result of this discussion the system is specified including the user's skills, the tools, and the environment (Bottorf and De Pape, 1982).

F. Fitting and training are considered integral parts of the assessment process as well as part of the follow-up. It is important to consider the amount of time and effort involved in the actual fitting and training of a user for effective use of their tools. This time factor may also be important in considering funding options.

G. The communication system's success depends upon following the user and the program development, reassessing the system's adequacy, and developing procedures to provide long-term support, equipment, maintenance, and troubleshooting.

## References

Beukelman DR, Yorkston KM, Dowden PA. Communication augmentation: a casebook of clinical management. San Diego: College Hill Press, 1984.

Bottorf L, DePape D. Initiating communication systems for severely speech-impaired persons. Topics in Language Disorders, 1982; 2:55.

Goossens C, Crain S. Augmentative communication: assessment resources. Lake Zurich, IL: Don Johnson Developmental Equipment, 1986.

Owens RE, House LJ. Decision-making processes in augmentative communication. JSHD 1984; 49:18.

Shane H. Early decision making in augmentative communication use. In: Schiefelbusch RL, Bricker DD, eds. Early language: acquisition and intervention. Baltimore: University Park Press, 1981.

Shane HC, Bashir AS. Election criteria for the adoption of an augmentative communication system: preliminary considerations. JSHD 1980; 45:408.

PATIENT WITH COMMUNICATION NEEDS

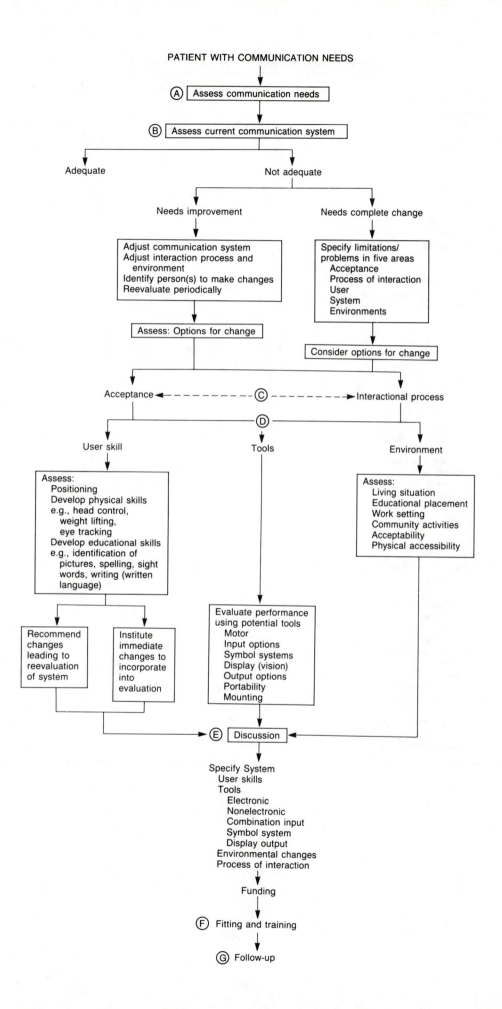

## TABLE 1  Communication Needs: Current and Future

| Situation | Manner | Event/Function |
|---|---|---|
| External | Conversation | Primary communication |
|   People |   Private |   function |
|     Family |   Public |     Requesting action |
|     Strangers |   Group |     Calling |
|     Peers |     Small |     Protesting |
|     Teachers |     Large |     Greeting |
|     Allied health |   Formal presentation |     Labeling |
|       service providers |     Private |     Requesting answer |
|     Colleagues |     Public |     Repeating |
|   Personal Restrictions | |     Answering |
|     Vision | |     Practicing |
|     Hearing | |     Teasing (humor) |
|     Familiarity with | | |
|       system | | |
|     Patience | | |
|     Reading skills | | |
|   Place/activity | Writing | User success in |
|     Home |   Personal |   conveying |
|       Bed |   Note writing |   Intention |
|       Wheelchair |   Math manipulation |   Communication function |
|       Walker |   Drawing, plotting, | |
|     School |     graphing | |
|     Work |   Homework | |
|     Hospital |   Editing/correcting | |
|     Community |   Computer | |
|     Recreation |   Lists | |
|     Church |   Prepared printed | |
|     Car |   Prepared auditory | |
|     Moving from | | |
|       place to place | | |
|     Primary position | | User role in |
|     for communication | | conversation |
|       prone | |   Initiation |
|       supine | |   Turn taking |
|       sitting upright | |   Repairing |
|       standing | |   Correction |
|       sidelying | | |
| Internal | | |
|   Physical needs | | |
|     Hunger | | |
|     Pain | | |
|     Change | | |
|     Position | | |
|     Safety | | |
|     Security | | |
|   Psychosocial affective | | |
|   needs | | |
|     Feelings | | |
|     Social contact | | |
|   Creative needs | | |
|     Arts | | |
|     Playing with ideas | | |
|     Daydreaming | | |
|     Role playing | | |

## TABLE 2  Assessment of Current Communication System

| Features | Person | Tools | | Environment |
|---|---|---|---|---|
| Means to indicate | Physical status:<br>  Motor facility<br>  Positioning<br>  Movement<br>Sensory skills<br>Cognitive abilities<br>Health and disease<br>  process<br>Acceptance/motivation | Indicators:<br>  Vocalizations/speech<br>  Natural nonverbal<br>  behavior<br>  Gesture<br>  Sign<br>  Encoding<br>  Combination of above | | Social:<br>  Receiver's acceptance<br>  Receiver's ability<br>  Receiver's<br>  knowledge/cognition<br>Physical:<br>  User's positioning<br>  User's adaptative ability<br>  Receiver's sensory status |
| Natural nonsymbolic interaction | Physical Status:<br>  Motor facility<br>  Positioning<br>  Movement<br>Sensory skills<br>Cognitive abilities<br>Language intentions<br>Health and disease<br>  process<br>Acceptance/motivation | Behavioral reactions<br>  Body states (vegetative)<br>  Protest and pleasure<br>Signals<br>  Early communicative intents<br>*Intent*<br>Negation<br><br><br><br><br>Attention/interest<br>choice, request<br><br>Questioning<br><br>Yes/no | *Possible body signals*<br>Avert head<br>Raise hand<br>Close eyes<br>Facial expression<br><br>Vocalization<br>Gaze<br>Reaching<br>Raise eyebrows<br>Quizzical look<br>Vocal<br>Head movement<br>Eye gaze<br>Body shifting | Social:<br>  Receiver's acceptance<br>  Receiver's ability<br>  Receiver's knowledge/<br>  cognition<br>Physical:<br>  User's positioning<br>  User's adaptation to<br>  other equipment<br>  Receiver's sensory status |
| Symbol system | Physical status:<br>  Motor facility<br>  Positioning<br>  Movement<br>Sensory skills<br>Cognitive abilities<br>Health and disease<br>  process<br>Acceptance/motivation<br>Language knowledge | *Technique*<br>Gesture<br>Sign<br><br><br>Visual graphic | *Ideographic Form*<br>Amer-Ind<br>American sign<br>language (ASL)<br><br>Photo<br>Line drawing<br>Symbol collections<br>Symbol systems<br>Traditional<br>orthography | Social:<br>  Receiver's acceptance<br>  Receiver's ability<br>  Receiver's knowledge/<br>  cognition<br>Physical:<br>  User's positioning<br>  User's adaptative ability<br>  Other equipment<br>  Receiver's sensory status<br>  Situations<br>  Expectations |
| Vocabulary | Motor facility (sign)<br>Cognitive abilities<br>Sensory skills<br>Experiences<br>Language knowledge<br>Interests<br>Experiences<br>Acceptance/motivation<br>Intentions<br>Situations<br>Health and disease<br>  process | Vocabulary selection:<br>  Do not limit vocabulary because<br>  of symbol system selected. Physical<br>  skill, visual skill, cognitive abilities will<br>  affect the number of items on a given<br>  display. | | Social:<br>  Receiver's acceptance<br>  Receiver's ability<br>  Receiver's knowledge/<br>  cognition<br>Physical:<br>  User's positioning<br>  User's adaptative ability<br>  Other equipment<br>  Receiver's sensory status<br>  Domains |
| Physical structure (aided)<br>  Nonelectronic or electronic | Physical status:<br>  Motor facility<br>  Positioning<br>  Movement<br>Sensory skills<br>Cognitive abilities<br>Health and disease<br>  process<br>Acceptance/motivation<br>Expectations | Selection of system made at this point in<br>relation to communication needs<br>Compatibility with symbol system<br>display<br>  Input selection<br>  Direct selection (with or without<br>  encoding)<br>  Scanning (with or without encoding)<br>  Size<br>  Flexibility/growth potential<br>  Portability<br>  Mounting<br>  Availability<br>  Reliability<br>  Output selection<br>  Voice<br>  Momentary visual indication<br>  Correctible visual display<br>  Permanent display<br>  Ascii/serial | | Social:<br>  Receiver's acceptance<br>  Receiver's ability<br>  Receiver's knowledge/<br>  cognition<br>Physical:<br>  User's positioning<br>  User's adaptative ability<br>  Receiver's sensory status<br>  Expectations |
| Symbolic interaction<br>  May be marked symbolically<br>  May continue to be marked<br>  with nonverbal signals | Motor facility (sign)<br>Cognitive abilities<br>Sensory skills<br>Experiences<br>Language knowledge<br>Interests<br>Acceptance/motivation<br>Intentions<br>Experiences<br>Situations<br>Health and disease<br>  process | System In Place<br>  User works for efficiency and effective<br>  use across all situations | | Social:<br>  Receiver's acceptance<br>  Receiver's ability<br>  Receiver's<br>  knowledge/cognition<br>Physical:<br>  User's positioning<br>  User's adaptive ability<br>  Receiver's sensory status<br>  Flexibility |

# AUGMENTATIVE COMMUNICATION SYSTEMS FOR THE ADULT

*David R. Beukelman, Ph.D.*

A. By the time nonspeaking adults are older than 21 years of age, their life styles have been sufficiently defined to allow a careful and complete assessment of their communication needs. This information is usually gathered by interviews with the client, family members, attendants, and employers (Beukelman et al, 1985; Coleman et al, 1980). The product of the assessment is an individualized list of communication needs with an indication of the urgency of each need.

B. Once the individualized need list is developed, the client's current communication approaches are assessed to determine whether the needs are met or unmet. At times the current communication approach meets all needs; however, further assessment suggests that the communication approach may become ineffective in the future, because the individual's communication needs are expected to change or the individual's capabilities are expected to change. When changes are anticipated that reduce the effectiveness of the current communication approach, the client is usually instructed about options to meet future communication needs and instructed when to reenter the evaluation process so that the "new" needs or capabilities are more clearly defined. Occasionally the communication approach is meeting an individual's needs, but a "listener" is not interacting effectively owing to impatience, uncooperativeness, or sensory disability. In these cases, the listener may require counseling, instruction, or prosthetic management such as a hearing aid or new glasses.

C. When the current communication approach does not meet the individual's communication needs, two activities are usually initiated. First, a careful assessment of the capabilities of the nonspeaking individual in terms of vision, audition, cognition, language, and motor control is completed. The product of this assessment is an individualized capability profile. When the capability profile is complete, the clinician can consider the communication options that are available to the individual based on the capability profile. From these considerations a "long list" of communication options is developed.

D. An ongoing process in the communication augmentation field is the continuous assessment of communication approaches in terms of their ability to meet communication needs. Each clinician serving nonspeaking individuals works with a formal or informal communication approach profile, which associates the communication needs that can be met with each specific communication approach. When the current approach of a client does not meet his communication needs, the clinician considers the individual's needs list in relationship to the communication approach profile and establishes a "long list" of communication options based on need (Vanderheiden, 1978).

E. Once the long list of communication options based on client capability and the long list of communication options based on client communication need have been established, a "short list" of communication options is developed that reflects both the capability and the need of the individual.

F. From this "short list" of communications options, the target option or options for the individual are selected. The narrowing of the target option(s) from the "short list" is based on a mosaic of factors, including cost, maintenance histories, availability of local repair services, cosmetics, and personal preference on the part of the client and the clinician, which at times is difficult to specify. Once the target option(s) have been selected, there is inevitably a process of individualization, which includes many factors such as mounting the equipment in a maximally effective location, selecting the appropriate symbols and messages to be included in the system, instructing the client to utilize the approach effectively, and instructing the "listeners" to interpret the output of the option appropriately and efficiently. At the conclusion of this phase of intervention, there is usually a performance assessment in which the client's ability to utilize the option is assessed and the listener's ability to interpret the communication message is assessed. Communication interaction is also assessed in this phase.

G. The last stage of communication augmentation intervention is always an extended follow-up, which includes activities related to further instruction, maintenance, and education about the changing options that are being introduced to the communication augmentation field.

## References

Beukelman D, Yorkston K, Dowden P. Communication augmentation: a case book of clinical management. San Diego: College-Hill Press 1985.

Coleman C, Cook A, Meyers L. Assessing the non-oral clients for assistive communications devices. J Speech Hear Res 1980; 45:515.

Vanderheiden G. Non-vocal communication resource book. Baltimore: University Park Press, 1978 (updates).

COMMUNICATION AUGMENTATION

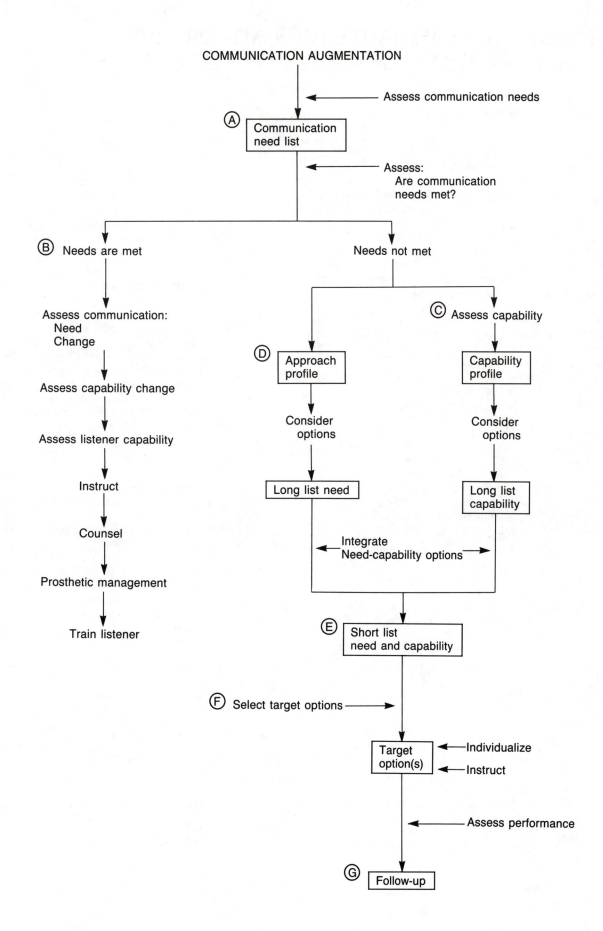

Ⓐ Communication need list

Assess communication needs

Assess:
Are communication needs met?

Ⓑ Needs are met

Needs not met

Assess communication:
Need
Change

Assess capability Ⓒ

Assess capability change

Ⓓ Approach profile

Capability profile

Assess listener capability

Consider options

Consider options

Instruct

Long list need

Long list capability

Counsel

Integrate
Need-capability options

Prosthetic management

Train listener

Ⓔ Short list need and capability

Ⓕ Select target options

Target option(s)

Individualize

Instruct

Assess performance

Ⓖ Follow-up

# UNAIDED AUGMENTATIVE AND ALTERNATIVE COMMUNICATION: GENERAL CONSIDERATIONS

*Lyle L. Lloyd, Ph.D.*
*Kathleen A. Kangas, M.S.P.A.*

Once a decision has been made that a person is a candidate for some method of augmentative and alternative communication (AAC), many aspects of aided and unaided communication must be considered. Aided communication symbols and approaches are those that require some physically external aid or device for their use, while unaided symbols and approaches do not require aids or devices (Fristoe and Lloyd, 1979; Lloyd, 1984; Lloyd and Fuller, 1986). For discussions of aided and unaided symbol sets, see Musselwhite and St. Louis (1982) and Vanderheiden and Lloyd (1987). We all make natural use of both aided and unaided communication in our daily lives, and likewise a multimodal approach is the most natural and effective approach for the AAC user (Fristoe and Lloyd, 1979; Kiernan and Jones, 1985; Kiernan et al, 1982; Vanderheiden and Lloyd, 1987). The purpose of this chapter is to discuss concerns related primarily to the use of unaided symbols and approaches to AAC.

We all use unaided AAC methods in the form of gestures, facial expressions, and nonverbal vocal sounds. Regardless of the severity of the handicapping condition, it is almost certain that the client can make some use of unaided AAC. However, decisions must be made as to the purpose of the unaided AAC (i.e., to replace speech, to augment speech, or to facilitate speech), the expected length of use, the mode to be used (i.e., receptive or expressive), and the environments in which it is to be emphasized, as well as a selection of modalities using the unaided approach itself.

A.  The clinician may use standardized testing instruments, modifications of standard tests, or informal assessments to determine the client's cognitive and receptive language support for the comprehension of speech. If these aspects are relatively intact, the emphasis for the use of AAC should be mainly expressive. If comprehension of spoken language is severely limited and if cognitive performance does not appear to be adequate for developing the comprehension of spoken language, the use of AAC should emphasize receptive skills and the facilitative effects on speech and language skills as well as the expressive use to develop early communicative behaviors.

B.  Assessment of the prognosis for developing intelligible speech would include assessment of oral motor control, the client's age, and the past use of speech therapy. If there appears to be good potential for speech that would be intelligible to an untrained listener, the use of AAC would be considered temporary and the facilitative aspects emphasized. AAC would be used to further expressive language development and to establish normalized interaction patterns with continued emphasis on improving speech. If the prognosis for intelligible speech is poor, the AAC methods should emphasize long-term effective use. Methods should be selected with the intention of using those methods indefinitely or facilitating a transition to approaches that could be used indefinitely.

C.  If vision is adequate to perceive signs and gestures, the use of unaided AAC can continue. If significant visual impairment is present, modifications of sign or gesture systems could be used. Many natural gestures consist of large movements, which may be easier to perceive. Also it should be noted that for many manual signs, the location and movement are the critical features for intelligibility as opposed to hand shape (Bornstein and Jordan, 1984). These are probably easier to perceive and discriminate visually than signs that are recognized primarily by their hand shapes. Signs can be selected or

AUGMENTATIVE AND ALTERNATIVE COMMUNICATION IS APPROPRIATE

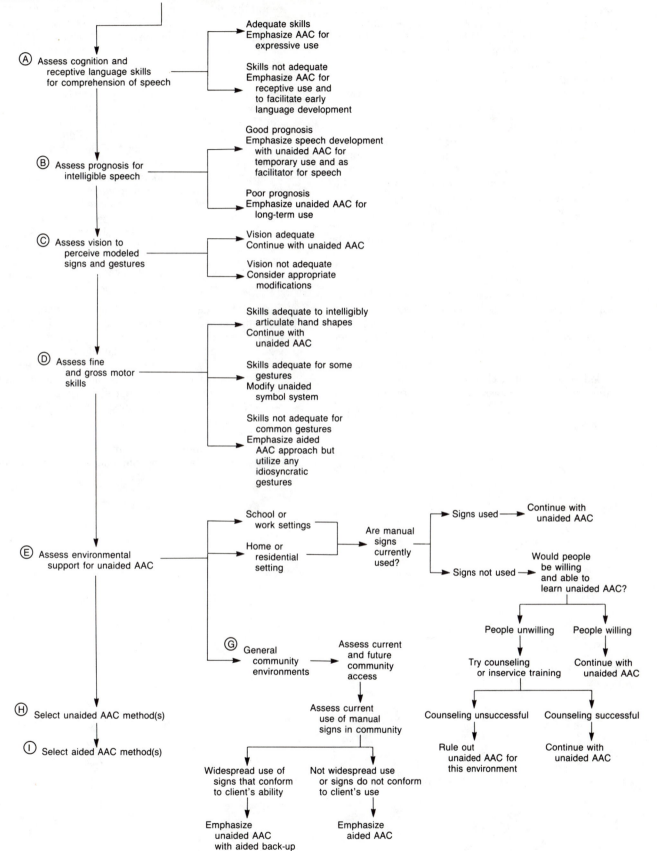

Ⓐ Assess cognition and receptive language skills for comprehension of speech

Adequate skills
Emphasize AAC for expressive use

Skills not adequate
Emphasize AAC for receptive use and to facilitate early language development

Ⓑ Assess prognosis for intelligible speech

Good prognosis
Emphasize speech development with unaided AAC for temporary use and as facilitator for speech

Poor prognosis
Emphasize unaided AAC for long-term use

Ⓒ Assess vision to perceive modeled signs and gestures

Vision adequate
Continue with unaided AAC

Vision not adequate
Consider appropriate modifications

Ⓓ Assess fine and gross motor skills

Skills adequate to intelligibly articulate hand shapes
Continue with unaided AAC

Skills adequate for some gestures
Modify unaided symbol system

Skills not adequate for common gestures
Emphasize aided AAC approach but utilize any idiosyncratic gestures

Ⓔ Assess environmental support for unaided AAC

School or work settings

Home or residential setting

Are manual signs currently used?

Signs used → Continue with unaided AAC

Signs not used → Would people be willing and able to learn unaided AAC?

People unwilling

People willing

Try counseling or inservice training

Continue with unaided AAC

Counseling unsuccessful

Counseling successful

Rule out unaided AAC for this environment

Continue with unaided AAC

Ⓖ General community environments

Assess current and future community access

Assess current use of manual signs in community

Widespread use of signs that conform to client's ability

Not widespread use or signs do not conform to client's use

Emphasize unaided AAC with aided back-up

Emphasize aided AAC

Ⓗ Select unaided AAC method(s)

Ⓘ Select aided AAC method(s)

modified to capitalize on this aspect. If the client has little or no usable vision, one might consider an approach such as a manual alphabet designed for visually impaired individuals (e.g., International Standard Manual Alphabet or Lorm Alphabet) or signs formed in the hand or vibrotactile methods (e.g., Tadoma). It is still possible for the individual to expressively sign in the usual manner to others if he understands this difference between sending and receiving modes.

D. Obviously excellent fine motor skills would be ideal for unaided AAC methods. However, these methods can be highly beneficial even when significant motor impairments are present. Signs can be selected to minimize confusion that would require good fine motor skills to differentiate, and some signs could be modified to utilize the individual's motor skills (Bornstein and Jordan, 1984). In this case, however, aided systems might receive greater emphasis by clarifying ambiguous signs or by providing a greater vocabulary. If the motor impairment is severe, conventional gestures and formalized signs might be impossible. However, facial expression and body posture and tone might still convey significant information, although these may not be interpretable to the untrained communicative partner. Even these very limited abilities should be enhanced by making others aware of their function and by teaching the client increased control and effectiveness. In this case, however, aided systems would clearly be emphasized as being more efficient for conveying message content.

E. It is critical to assess the environmental support for an AAC means of communication. If the significant people in the familiar environments are unwilling or unable to accept this approach, it will not be successful. The settings in which an AAC method is needed must also be determined. It is not uncommon for family members to report that they do not need an AAC method to communicate with the handicapped family member, because they are able to read the gestures and facial expressions and to understand the speech. The clinician must recognize that this may be true, and that insisting on an added communication method in that situation may impair more normal interactions. It should also be considered that the client may have more to say, but may not be attempting it since the means are lacking. In other words, the clinician should try to expand the client's repertoire of communication through an AAC method, but not try to complicate communication that is already effective. If persons in school, work, or home-residential environments are not initially willing to attempt to learn an unaided AAC method, a period of counseling and inservice training should be attempted. The people involved might be persuaded to participate in a short trial period during which the client could be taught a few simple messages and encouraged to use them appropriately. A successful trial period could be very effective in gaining the support of staff, co-workers, or family members.

F. The client's access to general community environments now and in the future should be considered. Even if the individual currently has no access to environments outside segregated centers for residential care or sheltered employment, wider community access should be considered. With increases in community integrated small group homes, mainstreamed education in public schools, and advances in means of training and supervising handicapped workers in nonsheltered competitive work settings, there should be increased concern for the client's ability to communicate with untrained and unfamiliar people. Thus aided symbols that are easily read by the community at large should be considered (e.g., picture communication symbols; Blissymbolics, HANDS, or Sig-symbols with printed words; or synthesized speech) along with an unaided approach. A further note regarding community access should be made. There appears to be an increasing number of people with some ability to use manual signs among the general community. However, the majority of these people have learned signs to communicate with hearing impaired individuals. In many cases, nonspeaking individuals with essentially normal hearing sign inaccurately and nonfluently, or they may sometimes use modified signs, and consequently other signers may have difficulty in understanding them. Also others may sign faster, with a greater vocabulary, or with some different signs than the handicapped individual is used to. Thus the client may be ineffective in comprehending the signing of a person accustomed to communicating with hearing impaired individuals. Thus even in a community where sign is prevalent, it is unlikely that sign alone will be an adequate method of communication.

G.  Having determined the appropriate purpose, emphasis, and settings for the use of an unaided AAC approach, one should decide which of the available systems to use.

H.  It is clear that an unaided AAC approach will be inadequate for all of a person's communication needs. Whenever an unaided AAC method is adopted as a primary approach, there should be consideration of possible aided approaches as well. Most aided approaches are frequently more effective with unfamiliar persons than many unaided AAC methods. The selection of the unaided approaches affects the choice of aided symbols. Sign-linked graphic symbols (e.g., HANDS and Sig-

symbols) may be considered for individuals using manual sign. Traditional orthography would probably be appropriate for individuals who use finger-spelling. It is not the purpose of this section to discuss the selection of aided AAC methods.

# References

Bornstein HA, Jordan IK. Functional signs. Austin: Pro-Ed, 1984.

Fristoe M, Lloyd LL. Nonspeech communication. In: Ellis NR, ed. Handbook of mental deficiency: psychological theory and research. 2nd ed. New York: Lawrence Erlbaum Associates, 1979:401.

Kiernan C, Jones M. The heuristic programme: a combined use of signs and symbols with severely mentally retarded, autistic children. Aust J of Hum Commun Disord, 1985; 13(2):153.

Kiernan C, Reid B, Jones L. Signs and symbols: a review of literature and survey of the use of non-vocal communication. London: Heinemann Educational Books, 1982.

Lloyd LL. Comments on terminology. Communicating Together, 1984; 2(1):19.

Lloyd LL, Fuller DR. Toward an augmentative and alternative communication symbol taxonomy: superordinate classification. Augmentative Alternative Commun 1986; 2:165.

Musselwhite CR, St. Louis KW. Communication programming for the severely handicapped: vocal and non-vocal strategies. San Diego: College-Hill Press, 1982.

Vanderheiden GC, Lloyd LL. Communication systems and their components. In: Blackstone SW, ed. Augmentative communication. Rockville: American Speech-Language-Hearing Association, 1987:49.

# UNAIDED AUGMENTATIVE AND ALTERNATIVE COMMUNICATION: APPROACHES

*Kathleen A. Kangas, M.S.P.A.*
*Lyle L. Lloyd, Ph.D.*

In addition to decisions relating to the appropriate emphasis of unaided augmentative and alternative communication (AAC) such as the emphasis relative to the use of aided AAC, relative emphasis of receptive and expressive use, and appropriate emphasis in various environments, it is necessary to determine the appropriate selection of unaided AAC methods. For a listing of the wide range of unaided and aided symbol sets and symbol systems available, the reader is referred to the articles by Lloyd and Fuller (1986), Vanderhieden and Lloyd (1987), and Musselwhite and St. Louis (1982).

A.  It is unlikely that one would ever choose to reverse previously learned skills and abandon an already effective approach by teaching totally different unaided symbols. More likely one would choose to use skills already present and expand both receptive and expressive skills. For example, an individual who had successfully learned to communicate basic needs through the use of gestural symbols, such as the Amer-Ind code or Generally Understood Gestures, might need a system with a more open vocabulary and greater potential for language development, such as the pedagogical signing systems of signed English or SEE-2, in order to be a more effective communicator in school or work settings. In this case, the teaching of the new symbol system would emphasize the situations and content for which the previously learned system was not adequate.

B.  If any unaided system is currently in use in the environments where the individual lives, works, or goes to school, or in the expected future environments, that system should be the basis for teaching the use of unaided AAC. It would be extremely difficult to ask other people in the environment to learn different systems, such as to learn ASL for one student and to learn SEE-2 with all 49 affix signs for another student when they are using signed English with its limited number of markers for most individuals. However, it may be necessary and relatively simple to modify a system to meet individual needs. Some examples of appropriate modifications are discussed below. One should be cautious, however, and make only those modifications that are necessary. Adherence to a standard method increases the number of potential communication partners. A more specific note with regard to ASL is in order. ASL is a complete language with its own syntax, quite different from spoken English (Vanderheiden and Lloyd, 1987; Wilbur, 1976, 1979). For the individual who is in an environment where ASL is used in a natural and communicative manner, this can be a very effective system. However, most hearing individuals and many hearing impaired individuals are in settings where most of the people they interact with are hearing and speaking. In these settings, the use of manually coded English or pedagogical systems through simultaneous communication or through signs supporting English would be more appropriate (e.g., SEE-2 or signed English).

C.  The current cognitive and receptive language skills may have an impact on selecting the unaided AAC systems. If the cognitive level and linguistic abilities are severely limited, a gestural system might be considered easier to learn. However, if a pedagogical signing system is already used in the environment, or if it is expected that the individual will be capable of using a more advanced signing system in the future, beginning with a pedagogical sign system would be preferred. If cognitive and linguistic skills are severely limited, vocabulary can be selected within any pedagogical sign system to emphasize the more iconic signs. In fact, if one is selecting a beginning vocabulary for a cognitively limited individual, there will be a great deal of similarity among all the available sign systems. Among the systems used in the United States, there is approximately 80 percent overlap of sign formation. In most cases, the simpler and more concrete vocabulary that would be appropriate for a cognitively impaired person is the same or similar across all systems, and these items will also be the most iconic and most closely related to common gestures and to some of the gesture sets and systems (e.g., Amer-Ind, Generally Understood Gestures). For example, the commonly used signs for eat, drink, and bed or sleep are very similar to natural gestures and can be easily understood even by individuals not trained in signing. Although less guessable, other common signs such as those for "more" and "come" are relatively transluscent and can be similarly effective in a beginning vocabulary when the gestural aspect of these signs is exploited (Lloyd and Karlan, 1983). If the individual has relatively good comprehension of spoken language and has relatively good cognitive skills with respect to chronologic age, a system related to spoken English would be most appropriate. In this case the vocabulary should be selected for the individual's needs and desires for expressive communication and with consideration for the comprehension by various communication partners. Cognitive skills that are at least near normal limits may also make complex coding systems possible, such as finger-spelling, gestural Morse code, or idiosyncratic codes such as an eye-blink code.

D.  Any signing or gestural system can be adapted to accomodate some motor limitations. Many signs can be adapted for one handed signing. If the fine motor skills are impaired, it may be necessary to limit the reliance on hand shapes. This can be done partly by selecting signs for which the intelligibility is based on movement or location instead of hand shape. It may be beneficial to rely more on signs selected from ASL instead of the letter cued variations that are part of the SEE-2 and signed English systems. Training people in the environment to interpret modified signs is also important. If fine and gross motor skills are severely impaired, it may be necessary to limit the use of unaided AAC to only a few commonly understood gestures, such as a head nod. In some

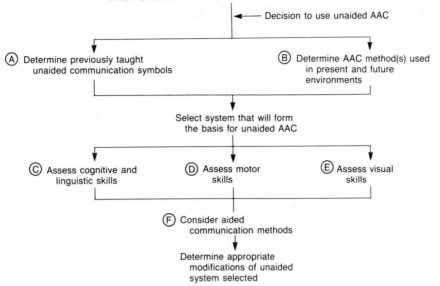

SELECTION OF UNAIDED AUGMENTATIVE
AND ALTERNATIVE COMMUNICATION APPROACHES

Decision to use unaided AAC

(A) Determine previously taught
unaided communication symbols

(B) Determine AAC method(s) used
in present and future
environments

Select system that will form
the basis for unaided AAC

(C) Assess cognitive and
linguistic skills

(D) Assess motor
skills

(E) Assess visual
skills

(F) Consider aided
communication methods

Determine appropriate
modifications of unaided
system selected

cases when the individual has such limited motor skills that common gestures are impossible, any idiosyncratic movement could be assigned a meaning. In this case aided AAC methods would be emphasized, although even the limited use of unaided gestures or signs might have a profound impact on the individual's daily functioning.

E.  It must be verified that the individual has sufficient visual skills to discriminate the unaided symbols that will be used. If vision is impaired, it may be necessary to modify signs or gestures by exaggerating movements, by emphasizing those that rely on movement and location for intelligibility, and by eliminating those that rely on slight differences in hand shapes.

F.  The most effective communication system for an individual usually is a multimodal approach incorporating several aided and unaided components, with careful consideration given to interrelating these various components (Fristoe and Lloyd, 1979; Kiernan and Jones, 1985; Kiernan et al, 1982; Vanderheiden and Lloyd, 1987). If the individual currently uses or is expected to use traditional orthography (TO), a system more closely related to written English would be appropriate. The use of TO can be very useful for the handicapped individual for writing letters, for making notes to oneself, and for computer access, and thus it should not be overlooked. Pedagogical systems such as SEE-2 and signed English are more consistent with written English than are gestural systems (e.g., Amer-Ind or Generally Understood Gestures) or ASL. Emphasis on finger-spelling and on letter cued signs within any signing system may aid the learning of TO. Also the use of signs for grammatic markers (e.g., the 14 signed morphemes of signed English or the 49 affix signs of SEE-2) may also assist in the use of TO. These markers could be incorporated gradually as the person's abilities allow. There are other ways in which aided symbols can be related to the use of unaided AAC. There are graphic symbol systems, such as HANDS and Sigsymbols, which are sign linked. The aided and unaided communication should also be linked by their training and use. If a significant amount of vocabulary is provided in both the aided and unaided approaches, each system provides a back-up method for the other. For example, a client who signs effectively finds it necessary to have another system, such as a graphic communication board, available for speaking to a person who does not know signs. Likewise, an individual who uses one or more communication devices may need an unaided system if a device is not accessible during transportation, dressing, or meal times, or if a device is in need of maintenance or repair service.

# References

Fristoe M, Lloyd LL. Nonspeech communication. In: Ellis NR, ed. Handbook of mental deficiency: psychological theory and research. 2nd ed. New York: Lawrence Erlbaum Associates, 1979:401.

Kiernan C, Jones M. The heuristic programme: a combined use of signs and symbols with severely mentally retarded, autistic children. Aust J Hum Commun Disord, 1985; 13(2):153.

Kiernan C, Reid B, Jones L. Signs and symbols: a review of literature and survey of the use of non-vocal communication. London: Heinemann Education Books, 1982.

Lloyd LL, Fuller DR. Toward an augmentative and alternative communication symbol taxonomy: superordinate classification. Augmentative Alternative Commun, 1986; 2:165.

Lloyd LL, Karlan GR. Translucency and transparency of signed English signs. Unpublished data, 1983.

Musselwhite CR, St. Louis KW. Communication programming for the severely handicapped: vocal and non-vocal strategies. San Diego: College-Hill Press, 1982.

Vanderheiden GC, Lloyd LL. Communication systems and their components. In: Blackstone SW, ed. Augmentative communication. Rockville: American Speech-Language-Hearing Association, 1987:49.

Wilbur RB. The linguistics of manual languages and manual systems. In: Lloyd LL, ed. Communication assessment and intervention strategies. Baltimore: University Park Press, 1976:423.

Wilbur RB. American sign language and sign systems. Baltimore: University Park Press, 1979.

# COMMUNICATION BEHAVIORS THAT VARY FROM STANDARD NORMS: ASSESSMENT

*Orlando L. Taylor, Ph.D.*
*Noma B. Anderson, Ph.D.*

Communication disorders diagnosticians frequently receive referrals of individuals who present communicative or linguistic behaviors that appear to deviate from norms established by the general society. The diagnostician tries to determine if the communicative or linguistic behaviors are indicative of a communication disorder, a nonstandard social dialect, a combination of the two, or neither.

A. Before assessment begins, the diagnostician is obliged to review pertinent culturally based characteristics of the cognitive, social, and linguistic behaviors of the client's speech community and to develop an appropriate assessment plan in accordance with those characteristics and requirements of federal law (Saville-Troike, 1982).

B. Within every cultural group, there is intracultural variation. Most variation is associated with such factors as gender, age, formal education, and social status. To avoid the application of overgeneralized or stereotyped cultural norms to an individual client, consideration must be given to the client's personality and its interaction with idiosyncratic representations of his or her culture.

C. Most standardized tests are biased against nondominant cultures and nonstandard English dialects. Therefore, analysis of errors and adjustments in scoring are needed in order to make these instruments culturally and linguistically fair. If norm-referenced tests are used in the assessment process, local norms should be developed for scoring purposes. In the event that local norms are not available, the raw score may be adjusted by: (1) allowing dialectal alternate responses to be scored as correct, or (2) multiplying the number of potentially biased test items by the average age equivalency of the items and adding this product to the client's score (Taylor and Payne, 1983).

D. As a final check of the validity of assessment data, the diagnostician should seek corroboration of his or her findings from the client's peers and family, or from members of the client's speech and cultural community. Corroboration should focus on both general and specific impressions of the client's communicative behavior relative to other persons of comparable age and background.

E. Prior to making a diagnostic determination, the diagnostician must ascertain what the client's cultural community considers to be pathologic communicative behavior. Cultures around the world, as well as within the United States, have different definitions and criteria for what they consider to be pathologic speech-language behavior (Taylor, 1986a).

## References

Ramirez M, Castaneda A. Cultural democracy, bicognitive development, and education. New York: Academic Press, 1974.

Saville-Troike M. The ethnography of communication: an introduction. Oxford: Basil Blackwell, 1982.

Taylor OL. Clinical practice as a social occasion: an ethnographic model. In: Cole L, Deal V, eds. Communication disorders in multicultural populations. (in press).

Taylor OL. Nature of communication disorders in culturally and linguistically diverse populations. San Diego: College-Hill Press, 1986a.

Taylor OL. Treatment of communication disorders in culturally and linguistically diverse populations. San Diego: College-Hill Press, 1986b.

Taylor OL, Payne KT. Culturally valid testing: a proactive approach. Top Lang Disord 1983; 3:8–20.

Vaughn-Cooke FB. Improving language assessment in minority children: ASHA 1983; 25(9):29–34.

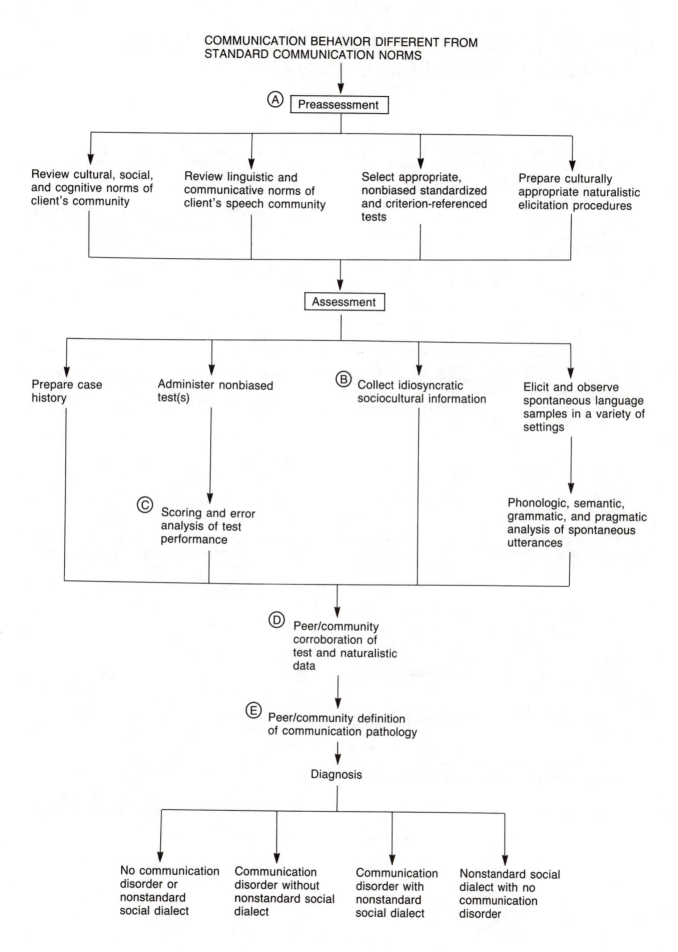

COMMUNICATION BEHAVIOR DIFFERENT FROM
STANDARD COMMUNICATION NORMS

Ⓐ Preassessment

Review cultural, social, and cognitive norms of client's community

Review linguistic and communicative norms of client's speech community

Select appropriate, nonbiased standardized and criterion-referenced tests

Prepare culturally appropriate naturalistic elicitation procedures

Assessment

Prepare case history

Administer nonbiased test(s)

Ⓑ Collect idiosyncratic sociocultural information

Elicit and observe spontaneous language samples in a variety of settings

Ⓒ Scoring and error analysis of test performance

Phonologic, semantic, grammatic, and pragmatic analysis of spontaneous utterances

Ⓓ Peer/community corroboration of test and naturalistic data

Ⓔ Peer/community definition of communication pathology

Diagnosis

No communication disorder or nonstandard social dialect

Communication disorder without nonstandard social dialect

Communication disorder with nonstandard social dialect

Nonstandard social dialect with no communication disorder

# COMMUNICATION BEHAVIORS THAT VARY FROM STANDARD NORMS: MANAGEMENT

*Orlando L. Taylor, Ph.D.*
*Noma B. Anderson, Ph.D.*

A. Prior to the initiation of treatment to address the presenting disordered speech and language behaviors, the speech-language pathologist must do considerable preparation and planning. Pretreatment activities necessitate the speech-language pathologist becoming familiar with the community's beliefs and practices regarding handicapping conditions in general, and communication disorders in particular (Taylor, 1986b).

B. The speech-language pathologist must become aware of the community's beliefs and values relative to communication disorders, the treatment of communication disorders, and appropriate practitioners from a cultural perspective. The community's culture, attitudes, and beliefs impact on its definitions and perceptions of communication disorders. It may be necessary to solicit the assistance of community practitioners and to merge conventional speech-language theories and clinical methods with the value and treatment systems of the community. It is also important to ascertain the client's and the family's perceptions and expectations about the treatment of communication disorders (Taylor and Samara, in press).

C. According to several investigators (cf. Ramirez and Casteneda, 1974), individuals differ with respect to their preferred learning style. For example, some persons appear to be more social oriented (field dependent) and prefer learning to be group oriented, humanistic, and related to life experiences in a global manner. Other persons appear to be more object oriented (field independent) and prefer to learn in independent, competitive settings that focus on details, facts, and principles.

D. Accountable and responsible clinical management includes pre- and posttreatment evaluation. The speech-language pathologist selects nonbiased criterion-referenced or standardized assessment instruments. If none are available, culturally and linguistically fair assessment items for pretreatment and posttreatment evaluations should be prepared.

E. Prior to initiating instruction in Standard English as a Second Dialect (SESD) the teacher must do considerable academic and pedagogical preparation. Among the preparation activities required of the speech pathologist is careful reading of the position of the American Speech-Language-Hearing Association concerning social dialects (ASHA, 1983).

F. Principles of second-dialect instruction are based on techniques derived from second-language instruction and on the relationship between attitudes and second-language learning. The principles are described in Taylor (1986b).

G. The acquisition of a second language or dialect occurs on a developmental continuum. In general, effective second dialect ($D_2$) instruction proceeds in the following order: (1) establishment of positive attitudes toward the learner's first dialect ($D_1$); (2) contrastive analysis between $D_1$ and $D_2$; (3) comparison of meaning differences between $D_1$ and $D_2$; (4) oral production in $D_2$ in controlled, structured and, eventually, spontaneous situations in which its use is appropriate. See Taylor (1986b) for a thorough discussion of SESD development approaches.

H. SESD instruction cannot be conducted effectively by means of random, unrelated activities. A full, integrated curriculum that is compatible with the aforementioned developmental teaching model is needed.

I. When the client presents with a communication disorder within his or her social dialect, the speech-language pathologist should treat the presenting phonologic, semantic, morphologic, syntactic, and pragmatic features that are disordered. The provision of Standard English as a Second Dialect (SESD) educational services should be offered as elective services (ASHA, 1983).

J. The learner's first dialect typically provides an important social and communicative link with his or her culture, community, or home. Therefore, SESD instruction should provide activities for the learner to maintain competence in and respect for $D_1$.

## References

American Speech-Language-Hearing Association Committee on the Status of Racial Minorities, Social dialects. ASHA 1983; 25(9):23.

Taylor OL. Nature of communication disorders in culturally and linguistically diverse populations. San Diego: College-Hill Press, 1986a.

Taylor OL. Treatment of communication disorders in culturally and linguistically diverse populations. San Diego: College-Hill Press, 1986b.

Taylor OL, Samara R. Communication disorders in underserved populations: developing nations. ASHA Reports (in press).

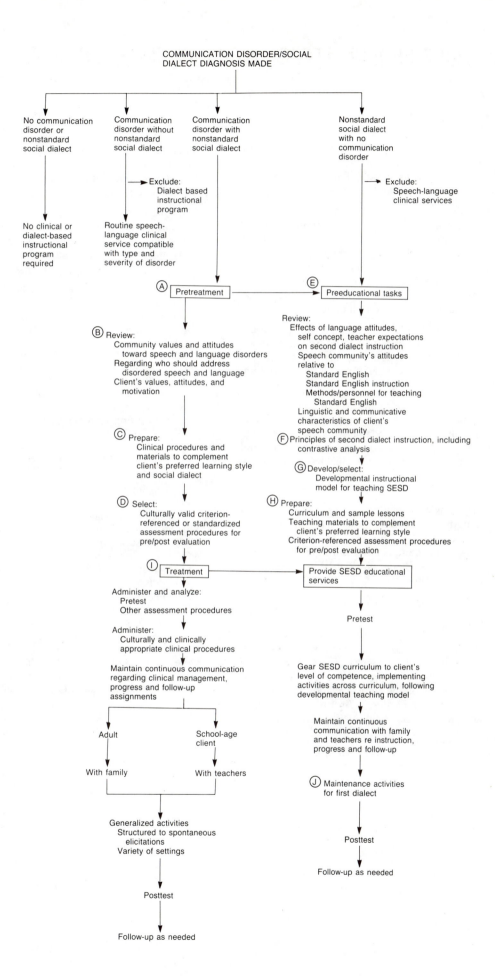

COMMUNICATION DISORDER/SOCIAL
DIALECT DIAGNOSIS MADE

No communication
disorder or
nonstandard
social dialect

Communication
disorder without
nonstandard
social dialect

Communication
disorder with
nonstandard
social dialect

Nonstandard
social dialect
with no
communication
disorder

→ Exclude:
Dialect based
instructional
program

→ Exclude:
Speech-language
clinical services

No clinical or
dialect-based
instructional
program
required

Routine speech-
language clinical
service compatible
with type and
severity of disorder

Ⓐ ◻ Pretreatment → Ⓔ ◻ Preeducational tasks

Ⓑ Review:
Community values and attitudes
toward speech and language disorders
Regarding who should address
disordered speech and language
Client's values, attitudes, and
motivation

Review:
Effects of language attitudes,
self concept, teacher expectations
on second dialect instruction
Speech community's attitudes
relative to
Standard English
Standard English instruction
Methods/personnel for teaching
Standard English
Linguistic and communicative
characteristics of client's
speech community

Ⓒ Prepare:
Clinical procedures and
materials to complement
client's preferred learning style
and social dialect

Ⓕ Principles of second dialect instruction, including
contrastive analysis

Ⓖ Develop/select:
Developmental instructional
model for teaching SESD

Ⓓ Select:
Culturally valid criterion-
referenced or standardized
assessment procedures for
pre/post evaluation

Ⓗ Prepare:
Curriculum and sample lessons
Teaching materials to complement
client's preferred learning style
Criterion-referenced assessment procedures
for pre/post evaluation

Ⓘ ◻ Treatment → ◻ Provide SESD educational
services

Administer and analyze:
Pretest
Other assessment procedures

Pretest

Administer:
Culturally and clinically
appropriate clinical procedures

Gear SESD curriculum to client's
level of competence, implementing
activities across curriculum, following
developmental teaching model

Maintain continuous communication
regarding clinical management,
progress and follow-up
assignments

Maintain continuous
communication with family
and teachers re instruction,
progress and follow-up

Adult

School-age
client

With family

With teachers

Ⓙ Maintenance activities
for first dialect

Generalized activities
Structured to spontaneous
elicitations
Variety of settings

Posttest

Posttest

Follow-up as needed

Follow-up as needed

# THE ADULT NON-NATIVE ENGLISH SPEAKER

*Karen A. Carlson, M.S.*

A.  The history of a non-native English speaker (NNES) should include information on first language ($L_1$) acquisition, hearing, general health, English training, frequency of daily use, intended goals, education, and living arrangements.

B.  Instruments are available to assess speech segments and hearing. For the NNES, observation in various speaking situations may be used to judge adequacy of prosody, language comprehension and production, pragmatics, and discourse skills. Rating scales of some of these components are available in the teaching English to speakers of other languages (TESOL) literature.

C.  Significant $L_1$ disorders (e.g., voice, motor speech, fluency, hearing, language) may have to be further assessed and/or treated before dialect management can begin. (Some clinics do not accept NNES for management unless there is an $L_1$ deficit.)

D.  Individuals who show or report no gap among English listening, reading, writing, and speaking skills probably either are still acquiring fundamental speech-language skills or desire to speak accent-free English. A referral to English as a second language (ESL) services is appropriate.

E.  It is important to estimate intelligibility of conversational speech as well as words and sentences. The Assessment of Intelligibility of Dysarthric Speakers (AIDS) (Yorkston and Beukelman, 1981) is a useful instrument to evaluate the latter two, and there is at least one clinical instrument that estimates listener effort as well as overall intelligibility of narrative speech (Carlson, 1984).

F.  Inclusion of the NNES without a first language deficit in the management caseload may depend on clinic policy or availability of services.

G.  Individuals in this category must demonstrate a significant gap between *speaking* (being easily understood) and other English skills. "Significant" decrease in intelligibility may be based on the clinician's judgment and experience with the NNES, the ESL instructor's report, or information from others in the NNES's environment.

H.  Extreme reduction in rate (Webster, 1974) and use of equal-even stress patterns allow: (1) breaking up of interfering, strongly habituated (fossilized) patterns and (2) monitoring of new articulatory gestures. Smooth blending of segments within words and among words in phrases is critical.

I.  The gradual reintroduction of more native-like rate, and stress and intonation (Allen, 1971; Taylor, 1981) must be accomplished with the focus on maintaining intelligibility, not "sounding like a native."

J.  Segmental errors and prosodic differences may be distracting (Gilbert, 1984; Acton, 1984). Usually, deletions and consonant substitutions are treated first. Be aware that word-final patterns, such as vowel off-glides or final sound devoicing, often need special attention.

K.  Training in discourse effectiveness may include such considerations as introducing a topic, conversational repair, turn taking, pause distribution, eye contact and gaze, and pause fillers. Pragmatic objectives may introduce such components as polite forms of answering, disagreeing and interrupting, and body language.

## References

Acton W. Changing fossilized pronunciation. TESOL Quart 1984; 18:71.

Allen VF. Teaching intonation, from theory to practice. TESOL Quart 1971; 4:73.

Carlson KA. Measuring speech intelligibility. Paper presented at MWTESOL Convention; Cincinnati, 1984.

Gilbert J. Clear speech. New York: Cambridge University Press, 1984 (Includes "Teacher's Manual and Answer Key" and "Students' Book").

Taylor DS. Non-native speakers and the rhythm of English. IRAL 1981; 19:219.

Webster RI. The precision fluency shaping program: speech reconstruction for stutterers. Roanoke, VA: Communication Development Corporation Ltd., 1974.

Yorkston KM, Beukelman DR. Assessment of intelligibility of dysarthric speech. Tigard, OR: CC Publications, 1981.

ADULT NON-NATIVE ENGLISH SPEAKER

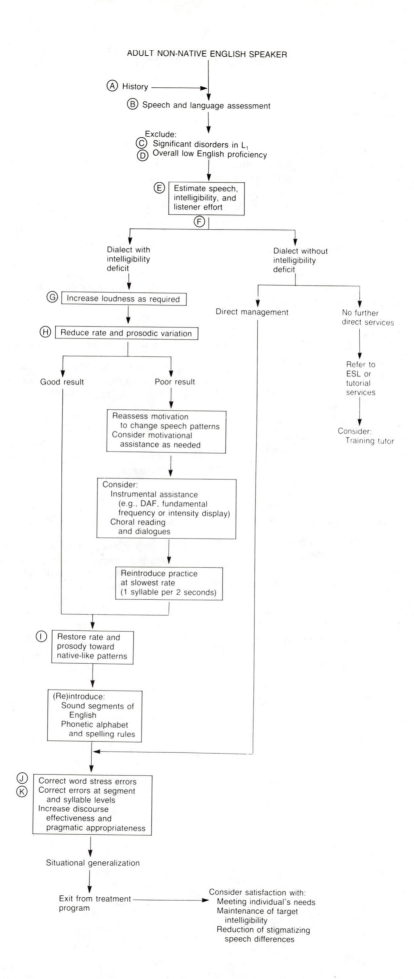

Ⓐ History

Ⓑ Speech and language assessment

Exclude:
Ⓒ Significant disorders in L₁
Ⓓ Overall low English proficiency

Ⓔ Estimate speech, intelligibility, and listener effort

Ⓕ

Dialect with intelligibility deficit

Dialect without intelligibility deficit

Ⓖ Increase loudness as required

Direct management

No further direct services

Ⓗ Reduce rate and prosodic variation

Good result

Poor result

Refer to ESL or tutorial services

Reassess motivation to change speech patterns Consider motivational assistance as needed

Consider: Training tutor

Consider:
Instrumental assistance (e.g., DAF, fundamental frequency or intensity display) Choral reading and dialogues

Reintroduce practice at slowest rate (1 syllable per 2 seconds)

Ⓘ Restore rate and prosody toward native-like patterns

(Re)introduce:
Sound segments of English Phonetic alphabet and spelling rules

Ⓙ
Ⓚ Correct word stress errors
Correct errors at segment and syllable levels Increase discourse effectiveness and pragmatic appropriateness

Situational generalization

Exit from treatment program

Consider satisfaction with:
Meeting individual's needs Maintenance of target intelligibility Reduction of stigmatizing speech differences

# THE CULTURAL-LINGUISTIC MINORITY STUDENT

Aquiles Iglesias, Ph.D.
Vera Gutierrez-Clellen, M.A.

A. School-age children with limited English proficiency often encounter communication difficulties when they enter the American educational system (Iglesias, 1985). The communication difficulties these children encounter can be due to numerous causes. Some children encounter difficulties due to communication code differences; the children speak a language that is different from that of their teacher. Other children encounter difficulties that are due to the lack of congruency between the discourse rules the children bring from home and those required for successful participation in the classroom. For still other children, the difficulties are due to cognitive and linguistic difficulties, which may be coupled with the usage of a different code, language other than English, or rules of discourse that are different from those required in the schools.

B. The teacher interview should be conducted in order to determine the type and frequency of communicative breakdowns the child is exhibiting. The interview should assess the communicative demands being placed on the child. The parental interview, to be conducted in the parents' native language, should focus on determining whether the child is exhibiting the same communicative difficulties in the home situation. Congruency between communicative demands of the home situation and those of the classroom should be evaluated.

C. An evaluation of the child's present level of functioning (static assessment) should be conducted in the setting in which the child is experiencing difficulties—the classroom, and in some cases the classroom and the home (Erickson and Iglesias, 1986). An ethnographic assessment using participant observations, informal interviews, and field notes should be used. The typology that is created is then validated. The data that emerge from this approach reflect the interaction between the child's inherent abilities and environmental experiences.

D. In order to differentiate the child's inherent abilities from environmental experiences, the child's modifiability should be assessed (Feuernstein et al, 1979). This approach evaluates the child's potential for acquiring particular skills rather than assessing skills mastered. On the basis of the results of the static assessment, the problem is identified. Changes are then made in the child's environment, and the changes in the child's performance (modifiability) are evaluated. The changes in the child's environment are those that facilitate his or her ability to learn the skills necessary to function successfully in the classroom. If the child gains those skills trained, the difficulties can be attributed to environmental experiences rather than to a true communication delay.

E. The role of the speech-language pathologist working with these normal children should be that of a classroom consultant focusing on facilitating their ability to learn.

F. If the child requires direct intervention, the clinician should be fluent in the child's native language. Monolingual speech-language pathologists could serve as classroom consultants or could work cooperatively with a bilingual professional.

## References

Erickson JG, Iglesias A. Assessment of communication disorders in non-English proficient children. In: Taylor O, ed. Nature of communication disorders in cultural and linguistically diverse populations. San Diego: College Hill Press, 1986:181.

Feuernstein R, Rand Y, Hoffman MB. The dynamic assessment of retarded performers. The learning potential assessment device. Baltimore: University Park Press, 1979.

Iglesias A. Cultural conflict in the classroom: the communicatively different child. In: Ripich DN, Spinelli FM, eds. School discourse problems. San Diego: College Hill Press, 1985:79.

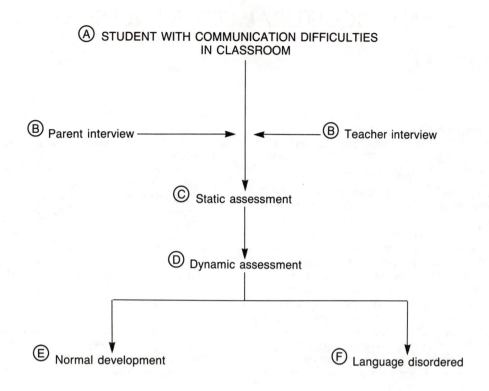

# BILINGUAL AND BICULTURAL DIFFERENCES: ASIAN

*Li-Rong Lilly Cheng, Ph.D.*

Asian language minority individuals referred to speech and language pathologists have a wide range of communicative competence in English. Some are non-English speakers (NES), some are limited-English speakers (LES), and some are fluent-English speakers(FES).

A.  These clients come from such a culturally and linguistically diverse background that clinicians need to obtain a very thorough history, including medical history, the time of arrival to this country, previous education, family history, home language(s), immigration history (refugee or landed immigrant), and psychological or adjustment history (Cheng, 1987a). The speech-language pathologist may need the help of a trained interpreter-interviewer in order to obtain a complete history of the individual. Care must be taken to examine the reason for such a referral, and a medical examination including hearing, vision, and motor skills is recommended at this time. Medical intervention may be indicated after the examinaton; the speech and language pathologist needs to follow up on the referral. On occasion, psychological evaluation and counseling may be warranted.

B.  Conduct a comprehensive speech and language evaluation to evaluate the linguistic proficiency of the individual in both English and his native language including phonology, syntax, morphology, semantics, and pragmatics (Cheng, 1987b). A speech and language screening may not be sufficient to uncover higher level difficulties in communication. The results of this investigation place the individual in one of three groups, FES, LES, or NES, based on their English proficiency.

C.  For the FES individual, a decision has to be made regarding his particular disorder, e.g., stuttering, voice, articulation, or language, and treatment needs to be provided accordingly.

D.  For the LES client who is a fluent-native-language speaker (FNS) and who does not exhibit any speech or language disorder, a decision needs to be made in conjunction with bilingual education and English-as-a-Second-Language (ESL) departments regarding proper placement and tutoring. For the LES and FNS adults with a second language acquisition problem, referrals should be made to English language centers or adult English classes. For the LES and FNS client who exhibits a communicative disorder, therapy should ideally be conducted in the client's native language. Since only a handful of speech and hearing professionals in this country are able to speak the Asian language(s), therapy may need to be conducted in English with the help of an interpretator-interviewer or a bilingual aid, and tutoring may also be indicated (Cole and Deal, 1987).

E.  For the LES student who is a limited-native-language-speaker (LNS), a decision needs to be made in conjunction with a bilingual special education department regarding proper placement. Such students require immediate attention, and priority needs to be given to the language that will most facilitate communication and learning. Special attention should be given in tutoring and cognitive assessement in the native language. For the LES and LNS adults, further cognitive and vocational evaluation may be warranted for appropriate intervention.

F.  For the NES and FNS students who do not exhibit any communicative disorder, a referral to the ESL and bilingual department is the next plan of action. For the NES and LNS students, speech and language therapy and cognitive evaluation are indicated. If the results of the cognitive evaluation indicate psychoeducational delay, a referral to a bilingual special education department is indicated. The language used for intervention needs to be selected based on the language that is conducive for interaction and communication.

## References

Cheng L. Assessing Asian language performance: guideline for evaluating limited-English proficient students. Rockville, MD: Aspen Publishers, 1987a.

Cheng L. Cross-cultural and linguistic considerations in working with Asian population. ASHA 1987b; 29(6):33.

Cole L, Deal V, eds. Communication disorders in multicultural population. Rockville, MD: America Speech–Language–Hearing Association, 1987.

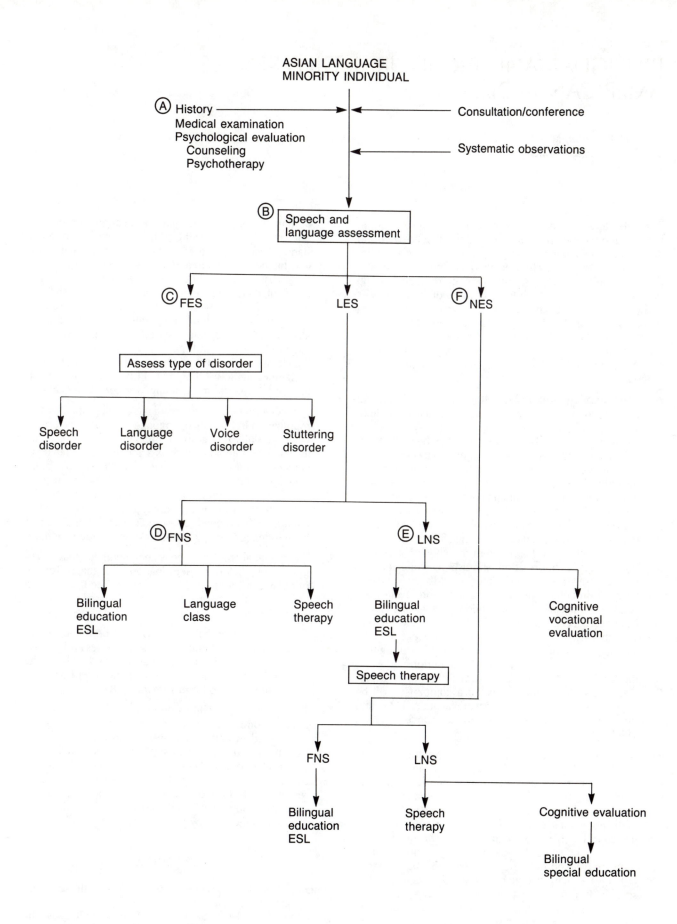

ASIAN LANGUAGE
MINORITY INDIVIDUAL

Ⓐ History ——————————→ ←—————— Consultation/conference
Medical examination
Psychological evaluation ←—————— Systematic observations
Counseling
Psychotherapy

Ⓑ Speech and
language assessment

Ⓒ FES                    LES                    Ⓕ NES

Assess type of disorder

Speech          Language          Voice          Stuttering
disorder        disorder          disorder       disorder

Ⓓ FNS                                          Ⓔ LNS

Bilingual          Language          Speech          Bilingual                    Cognitive
education          class             therapy         education                    vocational
ESL                                                  ESL                          evaluation

Speech therapy

FNS                    LNS

Bilingual                Speech                Cognitive evaluation
education                therapy
ESL
                                                Bilingual
                                                special education

93

# BILINGUAL AND BICULTURAL DIFFERENCES: AMERICAN INDIAN

Gail A. Harris, M.S.
Barbara Major, M.S.

Referral of an American Indian child for language evaluation may require competencies and procedures that are over and above those needed for the language assessment of monolingual English-speaking children who are members of the dominant culture. Language disorders are difficult to diagnose in American Indian children because of the influences of the native language and culture on language development and use of English. In addition, bilingual or monolingual tribal speakers present a challenge owing to the lack of information regarding development and structure of Indian languages and the lack of bilingual-bicultural American Indian speech-language pathologists.

A. The compilation of a case history is a critical element of appropriate assessment of minority language children. This component can provide an opportunity for the clinician to gain a comprehensive picture of the child. Medical history and other background information regarding the physical, emotional, and language development of the child, as well as knowledge about previous services must be obtained. Dominance-proficiency testing must be undertaken. Utilize the school district's bilingual evaluation team. If not available, secure information regarding child's language preference from family, classroom teacher, and directly from the child. The following linguistic information should be collected: (1) language(s) spoken in the home, (2) child's language pattern, (3) proficiency (degree of ability and level of develoment in $L_1$ and $L_2$), (4) the child's language preference (American Speech-Language-Hearing Association, 1983). With this information choices can be made regarding the language or combination of languages used during testing that allows for the child's optimal performance and the least biased assessment. Results of IQ tests or psycholinguistic measures allow for a comparison of the child's performance on tests that are language-laden and those that evaluate nonverbal performance (Mercer, 1983).

B. To appropriately assess and treat an American Indian child, the clinician must have an understanding of the cultural constraints or expectations regarding verbal communication and attitudes regarding language learning and use for this specific tribal culture. Language(s) spoken in the home must be identified including amount of time the child has been exposed to each. The phonologic, semantic, and syntactic systems of the primary language ($L_1$) may have an influence on the child's performance in English ($L_2$), even if the child is a *monolingual* English speaker. Family expectations and attitudes regarding the learning and use of English, (Anderson and Anderson, 1983) and cultural and personal orientations toward disabilities must be considered.

C. If the child is monolingual English language ($L_2$)

dominant, the speech-language evaluation must be conducted in English. Owing to the cultural bias of many standardized language tests, establishment of local norms may be required (Evard and Sabers, 1979). Linguistic features absent in the child's language may be the result of the tribal language or dialect variations of English (Wolfram, 1983; Anderson and Anderson, 1983). Features (e.g., prepositions, plural and past tense markers) that are absent in the tribal language $L_1$ may be inconsistently used in English $L_2$ and may need to be emphasized in the classroom for all students. If the child's performance is significantly lower than that of his or her age and culture peers, referral for language therapy is indicated.

D. If it is determined that the child has age-appropriate communication in his native language ($L_1$), but is lacking in language skills in English, consideration should be made for placement in an English as a Second Language (ESL) classroom. If this opportunity is not available, special instruction in the classroom to obtain these skills is recommended. If the child does *not* have age-appropriate language skills in his native language and is monolingual, there is no need to test in English; he or she must be enrolled for therapy to obtain language fundamentals.

E. The bilingual child must be tested in both languages (English and $L_1$) before a determination of language disorder or delay can be made (Mercer, 1983). The training and utilization of supportive personnel, bilingual professionals, and informed testing procedures may be required.

F. Observations in natural settings must be made to rule out test and/or examiner bias. Teacher aides and parents should be enlisted as participants in recording language samples in the classroom, playground, and home environment (Erickson and Omark, 1981).

G. The results of the child's performance on $L_2$ measures are now compared with performance on $L_1$ measures and considered in light of classroom and home data. The training and utilization of supportive personnel, bilingual professionals, (Anderson and Anderson, 1983) and informal, nonstandardized testing procedures may be required. If test performance in $L_1$ and language use in naturalistic settings (Omark, 1981) are both below normal, language therapy is indicated.

## References

American Speech-Language-Hearing Association. Bilingual language learning systems manual. Rockville, MD: ASHA 1983.

Anderson GR, Anderson SK, Omark DR, Erickson JG, eds. The bilingual exceptional child. San Diego: College Hill Press, 1983.

Evard BL, Sabers DL. Speech and language testing with distinct

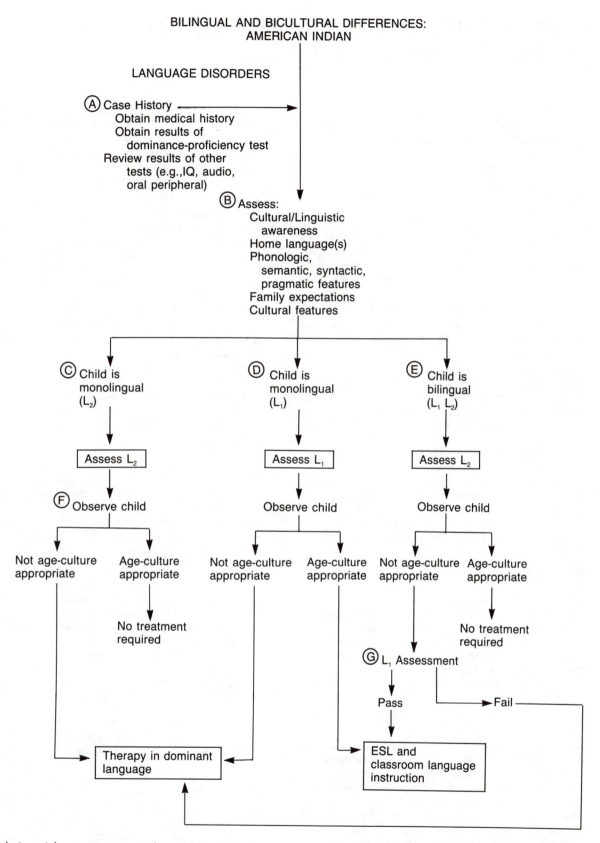

BILINGUAL AND BICULTURAL DIFFERENCES:
AMERICAN INDIAN

LANGUAGE DISORDERS

(A) Case History
   Obtain medical history
   Obtain results of
      dominance-proficiency test
Review results of other
   tests (e.g.,IQ, audio,
   oral peripheral)

(B) Assess:
   Cultural/Linguistic
      awareness
   Home language(s)
   Phonologic,
      semantic, syntactic,
      pragmatic features
   Family expectations
   Cultural features

(C) Child is
   monolingual
   (L₂)

(D) Child is
   monolingual
   (L₁)

(E) Child is
   bilingual
   (L₁ L₂)

Assess L₂

Assess L₁

Assess L₂

(F) Observe child

Observe child

Observe child

Not age-culture
appropriate

Age-culture
appropriate

Not age-culture
appropriate

Age-culture
appropriate

Not age-culture
appropriate

Age-culture
appropriate

No treatment
required

No treatment
required

(G) L₁ Assessment

Pass

Fail

Therapy in dominant
language

ESL and
classroom language
instruction

ethnic-racial groups: a survey of procedures for improving test validity. J Speech Hear Dis 1979; 44:271.

Mercer JR. Issues in the diagnosis of language disorders in students whose primary language is not English. Top Lang Disord 1983; 3 (3):46.

Omark DR. Pragmatic and ethological techniques for the ob-

servational assessment of children's communications abilities. In: Erickson JG, Omark DR, eds. Communication assessment of the bilingual bicultural child: Issues and Guidelines. Baltimore: University Park Press, 1981.

Wolfram W. Test interpretation and sociolinguistic differences. Top Lang Disord 1983; 3 (3):21.

# COMMUNICATION PROBLEMS ASSOCIATED WITH AUTISM: ASSESSMENT

*Barry M. Prizant, Ph.D.*

The types and severity of communication problems associated with the autistic syndrome vary greatly and may include processes of language comprehension, language formulation, and speech production (Fay and Schuler, 1980). The use of expressive communication abilities in social interactions is invariably affected. The full range of cognitive functioning in autism (severe cognitive impairment to normal or above normal cognitive functioning) helps to account for the wide range of ability and disability (Prizant, 1984). Principles of assessment of language comprehension and language-related cognitive function as discussed elsewhere in this book are relevant for the autistic population, as is decision making for augmentative communication. Therefore, this model focuses on expressive communicative issues due to the unique characteristics often demonstrated by individuals with autism.

A. Preassessment data gathering involves the acquisition and review of information pertinent to an individual's communicative development and current communicative functioning. With such information, the subsequent assessment process can be geared toward testing hypotheses and answering questions raised by preassessment data. It also allows the clinician to make judgments regarding the validity and reliability of assessment data as well as learning about the perceptions of the communication impairment held by significant others. Preassessment data should include results of audiologic, medical and psychological evaluations and information provided by significant others (e.g., teachers, caregivers) regarding the individual's history of communication development, effectiveness of any previous speech and language interventions, and the current communicative status.

B. When possible, an informal observation in a regularly scheduled routine activity in which the individual must engage in communication may provide further information regarding the development of hypotheses regarding the individual's communicative competence. Information may also be provided regarding environmental variables such as motivating activities and the interactive style of typical cointeractants. Informal observation should occur with no intrusion on the part of the clinician.

C. Direct assessment may involve a variety of methodologies depending upon the areas assessed and the general cognitive-communicative level of the individual. Formal assessments may include standardized tests used most typically for assessment of language comprehension and expressive abilities in individuals who are at specific language levels and function at relatively higher levels cognitively. Informal assessments are used most typically for severely cognitively impaired individuals and those at prelanguage levels and may include semistructured and unstructured situations in which communicative behaviors are elicited or enticed. Informal assessments may also be used to gather samples of spontaneous communicative and language behavior for individuals at all levels of functioning. Such samples may be gathered and recorded in a wide variety of environments with a varie-

ty of cointeractants. With the results of formal and informal assessments, the clinician should have information regarding: (1) an individual's responses to and level of comprehension of speech and language (see p 38), (2) language-related cognitive function (see p 32), (3) expressive communicative abilities, (4) communicative needs, and (5) social behavior.

D. An assessment of communicative needs derives from both preassessment data and direct formal and informal assessment. Communicative needs refers to the communicative skills (expressive or receptive) that an individual does not possess and/or are only emerging, which would enable him/her to be significantly more effective communicatively in regular communicative interactions. Variables that need to be considered include an individual's typical environments and cointeractants in those environments, the life activities that an individual cannot engage in owing to the lack of communicative skills, and the future environments that an individual will encounter, including specific communicative needs in those situations. (An example of a communicative need that is common among individuals with autism is a means to express protest or rejection in order to preclude use of aberrant means, such as self-injurious or disruptive behavior, to express these functions [Donnellan and Mirenda et al, 1984]. Another example is specific vocabulary that an individual may need to learn to request items in an employment situation). A determination of communicative needs depends upon input from a variety of persons, including primary caregivers, teachers, speech and language pathologists, and from observation of the individual involved.

E. Expressive communicative abilities are assessed most validly through recording behavioral and language samples with a variety of people in a variety of interactions. The two general questions which need to be answered are (1) what are the communicative means by which the individual expresses intent? and (2) for what functions or purposes does the individual attempt to communicate? Any behavior directed to others that influences the attitude or behavior of others may be considered communicative, including conventional and unconventional forms of nonverbal and verbal behavior. Thus, nonverbal (e.g., gestural, vocal, and gaze behavior should be described in terms of the specific means used (e.g., reaching gestures with shifting gaze) and the apparent purposes for which an individual engages in that behavior (e.g., request for food). Echolalic behaviors (immediate and delayed echolalia), a common characteristic of the speech of individuals with autism should be described as to the degree of functionality and rigidity of form (pure versus mitigated echolalia [Prizant, 1983]). For individuals beyond echolalic stages and with primarily creative language, a full assessment of language production is necessary (see p 40).

F. Assessment of social behavior provides information regarding an individual's ability to initiate, respond to, and maintain social interaction. Such assessment should

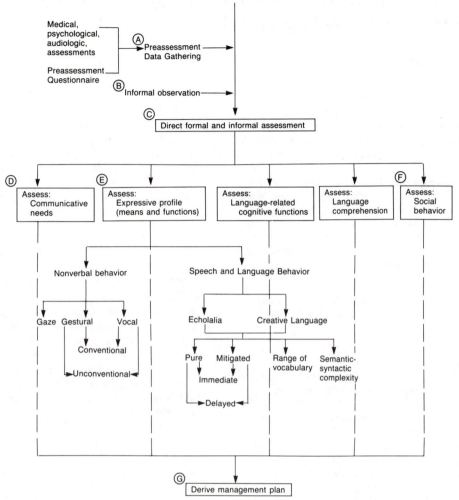

provide information derived from informal observations and informal assessments. The domains of social behavior assessed vary, depending upon development level, and may include initiation versus response strategies, sociability or desire to seek out and remain in the presence of others and for individuals with language, knowledge and use of language demonstrate nonverbal and verbal conventions of conversational interactions (Prizant, 1982).

G. Abilities of the individual in the domains of language comprehension, language related cognitive function, social behavior, and expressive communication and language production provide the primary information in determining the means of communication (e.g., speech, augmentative and alternative means) and the level of complexity of the primary means of communication to be targeted. The individual's communicative needs, as determined by preassessment information and informal assessment, provide the primary information concerning (a) environments to be considered to enhance communicative ability, (b) composition of the treatment team (e.g., parents, classroom teacher, speech and language pathologist), and (c) specific meanings and communicative functions to be targeted in the management plan.

The management plan should thus be derived by considering the developmental level of the individual, the specific problems that an individual faces due to his or her communicative impairment, and the types of skills that the individual needs to acquire, both immediately and within the long term, in order to function more independently and to participate more actively in daily communicative interactions.

## References

Donnellan AM, Mirenda P, Mesaros R, Fassbender L. Analyzing the communicative functions of aberrant behavior. Assoc Persons with Severe Handicaps; 1984: 9:201.

Fay W, Schuler AL. Emerging language in autistic children. Baltimore: University Park Press, 1980.

Prizant BM. Echolalia in autism: assessment and intervention. Sem Speech Lang 1983; 4:63.

Prizant BM. Assessment and intervention of communication problems in autism. Commun Disord 1984; 9:127.

Prizant BM. Speech-language pathologists and autistic children: what is our role? Part I. Assessment and intervention considerations. ASHA 1982; 24:463.

# COMMUNICATION PROBLEMS ASSOCIATED WITH AUTISM: MANAGEMENT

*Barry M. Prizant, Ph.D.*

The management plan is derived directly from assessment data. The plan should: (1) specify the communicative means (e.g., speech), the level of sophistication of the communicative means (e.g., single-word utterances) and the functions served and meanings expressed by the communicative means (e.g., requesting by using object nominals); (2) specify the environments and activities in which communication enhancement efforts are to be concentrated; (3) specify the service providers who are to comprise the treatment team (e.g., caregivers, special educators, speech and language pathologists), and (4) specify the mode of service delivery (e.g., one-to-one, group activities).

A.  The results of all assessments are taken into account in formulating and executing the management plan.

B.  The superordinate goal of effective management of communication problems is to help an individual acquire the skills and knowledge to communicate in a variety of environments for a variety of purposes (Prizant and Schuler, 1987a). Examples of environments or domains to be targeted include domestic, educational, vocational, leisure, and community domains (see Yoder and Villarruel, 1985 for further information). Communicative functions that address specific needs should also be identified (e.g., acceptable means to protest, to replace disruptive or aberrant means). In general, communicative functions targeted should address primary sources of frustration, behavioral problems, and specific abilities that would lead to greater independent functioning and active participation in social interactions.

C.  Functional communicative needs should be considered in reference to an individual's current communicative status as determined by assessment of expressive abilities. Discrepancies between current communicative status and functional communicative needs should be documented.

D.  Communicative means and sophistication of form to be targeted result from a consideration of current expressive level, cognitive function, language comprehension, and social behavior.

E.  Potential service providers may also influence the specific means and functions targeted. For example, the use of a communication board may not be a viable alternative if service providers will not support its use across environments, even if assessments indicate that it is the most viable means (Schuler and Prizant, 1987). Another communicative system acceptable to most service providers may have to be considered. Ideally, all service providers should be active members of the treatment team and help in decision-making processes. Furthermore, each provider must have knowledge of the communicative means and functions targeted across environments. The speech and language pathologist or other designated person should coordinate communication enhancement efforts by ensuring that all service providers are using the same communicative means or combination of means at the same level of sophistication across all environments. In addition, each service provider must address special functional needs specific to each environment.

F.  Communication enhancement occurs throughout the day across all environments (Prizant and Schuler, 1987). The mode of service delivery chosen depends upon the nature of the environment and the specific issues or needs that are addressed. For example, isolated one-to-one work with the speech and language pathologist may address issues such as motor speech problems or initial introduction of a nonspeech system. Group and incidental teaching efforts may be more conducive to enhancing communicative and social interactive ability in less structured environments (Peck and Schuler, 1983).

## References

Peck C, Schuler AL. Classroom-based language intervention for children with autism: theoretical and practical considerations for the speech and language specialist. Sem Speech Lang 1983; 4:79.

Prizant BM, Schuler AL. Facilitating communication: theoretical foundations. In: Cohen D, Donnellan A, ed. Handbook of autism and pervasive developmental disorders. New York: Wiley, 1987a.

Prizant BM, Schuler AL. Facilitating communication: Language approaches. In: Cohen D, Donnellan A, ed. Handbook of autism and pervasive developmental disorders. New York: Wiley, 1987b.

Schuler AL, Prizant BM. Facilitating communication: Prelanguage approaches. In: Cohen D, Donnellan A, ed. Handbook of autism and pervasive developmental disorders. New York: Wiley 1987.

Yoder DE, Villarreul F. Toward a system for developing communicative competence for severely handicapped children and youth. In: Children and youth with severe handicaps: effective communication. Proceedings of a Symposium. Washington, DC: U.S. Department of Education, 1985.

AUTISTIC CHILD WITH COMMUNICATION PROBLEM

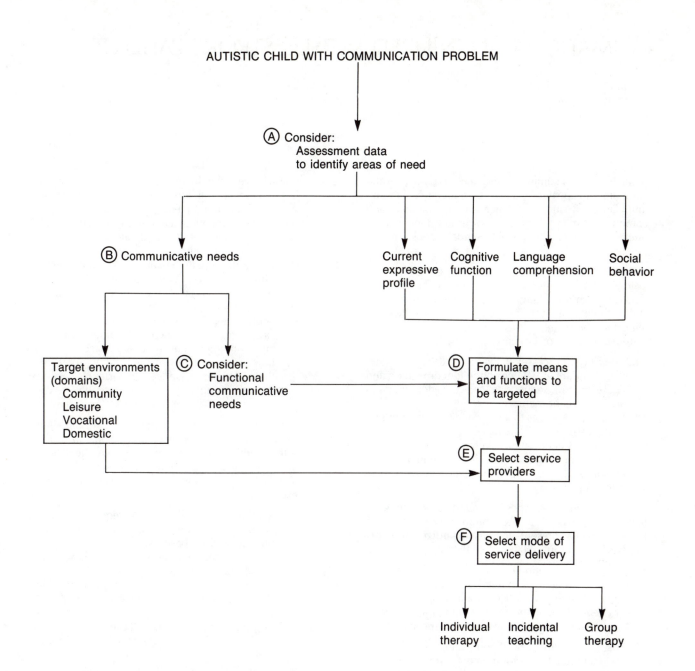

# TRAUMATIC BRAIN INJURED VERSUS STROKE PATIENTS

Frank DeRuyter, Ph.D.
Linda M. Lafontaine, M.A.
Mary R. Becker, M.A.

A. An assessment of communicative needs is basic to evaluating any nonspeaking patient. Consideration of communicative situations, manner and interaction, and communicative events or function can assist in the identification of specific augmentative goals (Beukelman et al, 1985).

B. Individuals presenting with brain injury (BI) or vascular lesions (CVA) manifest similar yet very different breakdowns in communicative abilities. Owing to the variability, three areas require specific assessment. Keep in mind that the degree of severity influences augmentative system selection and usage.

   1. Cognition. Processes to examine: alertness, selective attention, visual perception (discrimination and figure-ground), sequencing, categorization, immediate and recent memory.
   2. Language. Abilities to assess: auditory comprehension, reading, spelling, use of language.
   3. Behavior. Manifestations to characterize: initiation, disinhibition, cognitive inflexibility, stimulus bound responses, confusion, confabulation, level of cognitive functioning.

   Assessment approaches that may be used during the recovery process include observation of spontaneous behavior as well as presentation of standardized and nonstandardized stimuli (Hagen, 1984).

C. The functional evaluation is performed to determine the motor source to be used in interfacing the patient with an augmentative system. The discipline involved (OT, PT, speech) depends upon the degree of motor impairment. Areas requiring comprehensive assessment include:

   1. Positioning. Proper positioning allows effective use and control of the motor source. For nonambulatory patients, examine hip and trunk stability, feet support, and head control as they relate to positioning, wheelchair control, and lapboard use.
   2. Motor access site. When optimal positioning is obtained, potential motor sources are examined with respect to accuracy and reliability of movement, range of control, speed of movement, and endurance.

D. The following are frequently overlooked issues that are not commonly associated with these etiologies (DeRuyter and Lafontaine, 1987).

   1. Cognition. Deficits are present in both populations, but often are overlooked in CVA patients with severe language disorder. This does not preclude system selection or usage, but does influence the system decision making process and potential treatment strategies. For example:

      a. Alertness and selective attention. Deficits may be present in both populations, causing patients to have difficulty in focusing on necessary and relevant stimuli. This limits the types of systems that may be utilized.
      b. Visual perception. Deficits are noted in both populations, but BI have greater difficulty with the amount and complexity of stimuli.
      c. Categorization. Both BI and CVA exhibit deficits. This does not preclude system usage, but is important to acknowledge when developing treatment and usage strategies.
      d. Sequencing. BI exhibit difficulty in organizing, structuring, and predicting the order of presentation in augmentative system usage.
      e. Immediate and recent memory. In some BI, these deficits influence the system selection process owing to the inability to complete the multistage steps required for system access.

   2. Language. In BI the dysfunction in organization and use of language is influenced and in some instances is the result of cognitive deficits. In CVA, the deficits are language based and may involve several modalities. This influences system selection and usage. For example:

      a. Reading and spelling. CVA frequently utilize pictographic symbol systems. BI use more alphabet or word based systems.
      b. Auditory comprehension. BI often exhibit functional impairment due to immediate memory deficits. CVA exhibit classic comprehension deficits. This requires utilizing a system with less complex language.
      c. Organization of language. BI exhibit greater disorganization of language and impaired pragmatics.
      d. Expression. CVA exhibit more language impairment and grammatical problems, resulting in systems using single word communication. BI use grammatically correct language but display pragmatic problems, which affect system usage.
      e. Visual comprehension. BI exhibit visual comprehension and sequencing impairments limiting types and use of systems.

   3. Behavior. The degree and severity of behavioral manifestations influence decision making in system selection and usage, as well as treatment strategies.

      a. Initiation. BI exhibit greater reliance upon others to initiate.
      b. Inhibition: BI exhibit impulsivity of the communication act and system usage.
      c. Perseveration. This is observed in both populations, although the type of behavior varies. BI exhibit the ideational type as messages are repeated and topic shifting is difficult. CVA exhibit more motoric and verbal perseveration.

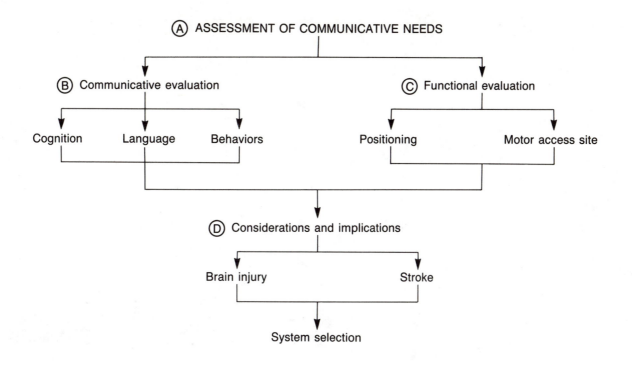

Ⓐ ASSESSMENT OF COMMUNICATIVE NEEDS

Ⓑ Communicative evaluation      Ⓒ Functional evaluation

Cognition    Language    Behaviors    Positioning    Motor access site

Ⓓ Considerations and implications

Brain injury        Stroke

System selection

d. Stimulus bound response. This behavior observed in BI results in absence of elaboration.

e. Confabulation-confusion. This behavior is not typically observed in CVA requiring augmentative system. BI responses fluctuate between appropriate and inappropriate.

f. Level of cognitive functioning. Levels should not be used with CVA. Rancho Cognitive Level III must be reached by BI before considering any system (Hagen et al, 1979).

4. Positioning. The degree of physical involvement influences system selection and motor access site. Nonambulatory BI exhibit greater physical involvement than nonambulatory CVA. This leads to more positioning problems with the BI, which may be further complicated by cognitive and behavioral deficits.

5. Motor access site. As a result of physical disability, BI require greater involvement by occupational therapy in examining potential motor sources. BI who are severely physically involved may need to utilize scanning system accessed by motor source other than finger or hand. This requires greater assessment of potentially appropriate switches. CVA typically utilize direct selection systems accessed by a finger or hand and consequently require less attention from the occupational therapist.

## References

Beukelman DR. Yorkston KM, Dowden PA. Communication augmentation: a casebook of clinical management. San Diego: College Hill Press, 1985.

DeRuyter F, Lafontaine LM. The nonspeaking brain injured: a clinical and demographic database report. Augmentative and Alternative Communication, 1987; 3:18.

Hagen C. Language disorders in head trauma. In: Holland AL, ed. Language disorders in adults. San Diego: College Hill Press, 1984.

Hagen C, Malkmus D, Durham P. Levels of cognitive functioning. In: Rehabilitation of the head injured adult: comprehensive physical management. Downey, CA: Professional Staff Association of Rancho Los Amigos Medical Center, 1979.

# III: Speech Processes and Disorders; Related Oral Function

The chapters in this section address both traditional issues in speech disorders and more recent developments and specialities. The contributions vary in length and detail, depending on the topic. Taken together, they span a large range of assessment and management problems, including general speech and oral functions, dysphagia, phonology or articulation, respiration, voice, prosody, craniofacial anomalies, motor speech disorders, dysfluent speech, and referrals. Although each chapter stands alone, the reader can derive maximum benefit from them by exploring their potential interrelationships. The subsystems of speech often interact; for example, voice may be limited by respiratory function and prosodic capability may be limited by both voice and respiration. It is appropriate, then, to view the chapters individually as specific decision-making summaries and collectively as interrelated components in a large clinical framework.

# SPEECH MECHANISM: ASSESSMENT

*Megan M. Hodge, M.S.*

A. When a speech disorder has been identified, the integrity of the speech mechanism is assessed to determine whether it is contributing to the disorder. Positive findings condition management directed at modifying the mechanism or at teaching compensatory strategies to maximize the client's use of the mechanism to produce acceptable speech. Negative findings do not implicate the mechanism in client management.

B. The most important examining tools are the clinician's eyes, ears, and fingers. Essential equipment includes a light source, tongue blades, and finger cots (to provide sterile contact with the clients's orofacial structures). A stopwatch and counter or a tape recorder are needed to measure diadochokinetic rates and maximum performance maneuver durations. Structural dimensions can be quantified with a ruler. Other useful tools include dental retractors, a dental mirror, food items, a Polaroid camera, and materials appropriate for sensory stimulation. Checklists and line drawings provide an efficient means of recording observations during the examination.

C. The format of the examination varies according to specific client characteristics. The instructions given and the interpretations made depend on the client's age, linguistic-cognitive level, and cooperation. Given knowledge of the anatomy of the speech mechanism, its associated pattern of sensorimotor innervation, and how these interact to configure the vocal tract for speech production, the enterprising clinician can design alternative procedures to use with very young or uncooperative clients to obtain the information necessary either to judge the integrity of the speech mechanism or to identify the need for further investigation. The assessment format should allow the clinician to determine how the presenting complaint, the results of previous assessments or treatments, and positive medical history (e.g., surgery, accidents, illnesses, familial syndromes, or neuromuscular, respiratory, and feeding abnormalities) relate to the present structure and function of the speech mechanism.

D. Adequate and sensitive preparation of the client prior to examination maximizes cooperation and minimizes adverse reactions to examination procedures.

The most common causes of structural and neural defects are prenatal developmental abnormalities and perinatal and postnatal trauma and disease. The effects of these conditions may be pervasive or they may be localized to specific anatomical sites, but they typically extend beyond a single structure or behavior. Therefore, prior to examination of the speech mechanism, scrutiny of the client's overall appearance for evidence of poor health, unusual physical characteristics, and positive neurological signs may reveal abnormalities that will condition subsequent observations, interpretations, and recommendations regarding the speech mechanism. Siegel-Sadewitz and Shprintzen (1982) describe genetic syndromes associated with communicative disorders.

Bateman and Mason (1984) review the postnatal development of the head and neck and provide normative information for the dimensions of the craniofacial skeleton.

E. The challenge facing the clinician is to combine knowledge of embryology, anatomy, and neurology and knowledge of speech production with discerning observational skills and client rapport to direct a comprehensive and efficient examination of the mechanism. Crelin (1976) reviews the embryologic development of the upper respiratory system. Perkins and Kent (1986) review the anatomy and neurology of the speech mechanism and discuss these in relation to speech production.

The logic of the examination typically flows from global to localized observations of physical structures and their function (Tables 1 and 2), and then to observations of how these structures interact to meet the postural and movement demands of speech production (Table 3). As observations accumulate, the clinician scans these for patterns that suggest the presence and the extent of structural or neuromuscular abnormality. When such patterns emerge, initial observations are refined by detailed examination of structures related by embryological origin or by common innervation. On the basis of these hypotheses the clinician devises additional nonspeech and speech tasks to probe suspected aspects of function and continues this cycle of observation, analysis, synthesis, and hypothesis testing until all necessary and sufficient information is available to judge the integrity of the mechanism for speech production.

F. The structures of the speech mechanism are of two basic types: those that do not move or move by passive forces alone (e.g., teeth, hard plate, lymphatic tissue) and those that actively move via muscular composition (e.g., lips, tongue, velum) or by muscular attachments (mandible, hyoid bone, laryngeal cartilages). Similar principles guide the examination of each, although for the latter type, observation during movement may be required to rule out possible structural restrictions imposed by attachments or scar tissue. Bateman and Mason (1984) provide views of the speech mechanism, including dental occlusal relationships, and describe in detail the relevant landmarks of craniofacial and oronasopharyngeal structures. Table 1 specifies characteristics of tissue that indicate potential abnormalities. Bain, Carter, and Morton (1985) provide numerous photographs of normal and abnormal oral cavity structures. Visual inspection and palpation are used to examine accessible structures. The integrity of inaccessible structures can be judged by inference based on the results of nonspeech or speech function tests. Referral for visual imaging procedures can provide information about suspect inaccessible structures. Observations of structures may reveal abnormalities that have obvious effects on speech, such as a cleft of the hard or soft palate. Other identified abnormalities, such as dental malocclusions, may or may not have functional significance for the dynamic processes of

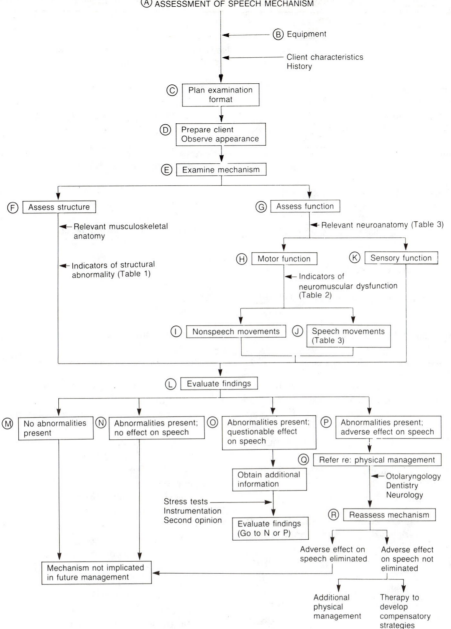

speech. Conversely, structural abnormalities may not be apparent, but the requisite actions of these structures for speech may be impaired by abnormalities in neuromuscular function.

G. The anatomic structures composing the speech mechanism are also components of the digestive and respiratory systems. Although the specific function of each structure varies with the system under consideration, the sensorimotor innervation extending from the cranial or spinal nerve nuclei to each structure (listed in Table 3) is constant.

H. Nonspeech and speech movements can be used to exa-

mine the neuromuscular integrity of the peripheral mechanism and can be alternated to check the reliability of an observation. It is assumed that damage to a cranial or spinal nerve will affect function of its associated musculature similarly for nonspeech and speech movements, that have equal force and temporal specifications. For example, significant weakness of the expiratory musculature affects the ability to generate and maintain specified subglottal pressures for blowing and speech production. However, it cannot be assumed that nonspeech and speech movements involving similar structures have the same neuromuscular specifications. For example, while swallowing and production of non-

## TABLE 1   Characteristics of Tissue Indicating Potential Structural Abnormalities

| Characteristic | Example |
| --- | --- |
| Unusual color | Red (inflammation); bluish tint (absence of underlying tissue, as with a submucous cleft; cyanosis) |
| Rough, fissured, or furrowed texture | Ulceration; atrophy of muscular structure |
| Unexpected discontinuities in surface or underlying structure (especially at sites of midline union of structures) | Pits or notches in lips; clefts; fistulas; bifid uvula |
| Absence of structure | Velar musculature inserts anteriorly into hard plate, i.e., no palatal aponeurosis; missing teeth |
| Disproportionate size in relation to surrounding structures | Short velum in relation to depth of oropharynx; enlarged palatine tonsils occlude oropharynx |
| Asymmetry in shape or size of bilateral structures | Unilaterally reduced muscle bulk or wasting of tongue; depressed nasal ala |
| Misalignment of adjacent or functionally related structures | Mandibular retrusion; dental malocclusion |
| Unusual contour (elevations or depressions in tissue where not expected | Peaked hard palate; torus on hard palate |
| Constrained range of muscular structures | Lingual or labial frenum attached over extended area of structure |

nasal sounds both require closure of the velopharynx, the site of closure and the muscular actions involved differ, so one cannot infer function for one of these actions from the other. Table 2 lists movement characteristics that indicate potential neuromuscular dysfunction. The reader is referred to current neurology textbooks for more detailed information about identifying the site of a neurological lesion from patterns of motor dysfunction of the head and neck.

I.  Observation of nonspeech movements permits the clinician to detect signs of neuromuscular abnormalities divorced from an auditory signal and may be the only source of information if the client cannot or will not speak. Because the number of potential movements of vocal tract structures greatly surpasses those used in any one spoken language, observation of nonspeech movements increases the sample of behaviors available to judge the integrity of the mechanism. Limits of function such as maximal strength, maximal rate, maximal duration for sustaining postures, and maximal range of motion can also be determined using nonspeech tasks. The application of maximal performance measures to speech production is most appropriate for measures of diadochokinetic rate. Speech movements are rapid but typically use small amounts of force and a limited range of motion and are of short duration.

J.  Table 3 summarizes speech movements associated with various structures of the speech mechanism, examples of speech sounds produced in isolation or in CV's using these movements, and the innervation associated with these movements. Most speech sounds require the participation of more than one structure and so reflect the interaction and coordination of several structures. The enterprising clinician can use a phonetic chart that classifies sounds by their place and manner of articulation (see Figure 7.7 in Perkins and Kent, 1986) to guide the selection of individual and concatenated speech sounds

to probe the actions of the various combinations of articulators.

For example, production of /s/ requires coordination of a laryngeal devoicing gesture with tight closure of the velopharyngeal valve and fine force control of the tongue tip to direct the airstream over the cutting edge of the teeth. The phonetic features of the sound actually produced by the client (i.e., the presence of voicing, nasal emission, or sibilant distortion) direct the clinician to probe the function of the structure or structures associated with these respective features. Production of alternating voiced–voiceless phones (e.g., tititititi) taps the devoicing gesture; production of alternating nonnasal-nasal phones (e.g., dinidinidini) taps the velopharynx, and production of alternating stop-sibilant phones (e.g., tisitisitisi) may tap the fine force control of the tongue tip required for /s/ but not /t/. This is only one illustration of how a knowledge of speech production can be used to probe systematically the integrity of the mechanism. Poorer performance for nonspeech than for speech movements may indicate lack of cooperation or misunderstanding of directions by the client. Poorer performance for speech than for nonspeech movements, especially when this poorer performance is characterized by sequencing or initiation errors, may indicate neurological damage at the cortical level. (The reader is referred to page 154 for detailed information regarding the differential diagnosis of motor speech disorders.)

K.  The relationship between the cutaneous and proprioceptive sensibility of the structures of the vocal tract and their sensory function during speech production has not been definitively established, although investigations of reflex activity and cortical processing of oral sensory information (oral stereognosis) have been reported. Thus, the clinician does not typically conduct tests of sensory function of vocal tract structures. However, when the integrity of a specific cranial nerve is questionable on the basis of observations of motor function, observation of its

**TABLE 2   Characteristics Indicating Potential Neuromuscular Dysfunction**

| Characteristic | Example |
|---|---|
| Reduced or absence of movement | Paralysis of levator palatini results in little or no elevation of soft palate |
| Weakness, i.e., unable to resist pressures applied to muscular tissues; unable to sustain a position | Muscle wasting or paralysis of the tongue—cannot resist tongue blade pushed against it; can attain initial closure of velopharyngeal port, but cannot maintain this for continuous nonnasal speech |
| Low muscle tone or flaccidity | Lips parted, drooping at rest (drooling may accompany this) |
| Spontaneous involuntary movements observed at rest or during voluntary movements | Fasciculations of tongue; involuntary "chewing" movements |
| Absence of reflexes | No gag or cough reflexes; no jaw jerk when muscles are stretched |
| Asymmetrical movement due to deviation of bilateral structures | Asymmetrical retraction of lips due to unilateral facial nerve paralysis |
| Compensatory use of a structure | Use of jaw movements to assist tongue; unable to dissociate movement of tongue from that of jaw |
| Slow labored movements on rapid alternating movement tasks | Fastest rate at which patient can open and close jaw is once per second |
| Inaccuracy of movement; under- or overshooting of intended motion; inconsistency in velocity, amplitude, or rhythm of repetitive movements | Side to side movements of tongue directed at touching tongue blade positioned at each corner of mouth demonstrate lack of coordination |
| Breakdown in performing a sequence of several different movements | On attempting to repeat sound sequence "puh tuh kuh" rapidly, cannot maintain sequence or cannot shift from one movement to next |

associated sensory function can substantiate such suspicions. For example, deviation of the jaw to one side on closing and paresthesia of the facial skin and oral and nasal mucosa on the side of deviation corroborate damage to cranial nerve V.

L.  The clinician evaluates the examination findings to reach one of four conclusions about the contribution of the mechanism to the speech disorder and then makes appropriate recommendations.

M.  Conclusion 1. No abnormalities are observed and therefore no management specific to the mechanism is indicated.

N.  Conclusion 2. Abnormalities are observed that do not adversely affect speech production. No management of the mechanism is indicated for speech, but if these abnormalities are risks to the client's health (e.g., inflamed or ulcerated oral mucosa, dental caries, undiagnosed neurological signs that are not affecting speech), recommendations for appropriate follow-up are made.

O.  Conclusion 3. Abnormalities are observed, but the clinician lacks adequate information or expertise to make a judgment about their impact on speech. The clinician may obtain additional information by probing the limits of questionable aspects of the mechanism using stress tests. Because the majority of observations made regarding the mechanism are qualitative in nature, and because each mechanism is unique, clinical experience is directly related to the reliability of the judgements made. In some instances, the clinician needs to augment his observations by using instrumentation, which can extend the variety and sensitivity of the observations or by consulting with more experienced clinicians to determine the effect of observed abnormalities on the speech disorder. Using the information obtained from these sources, the clinician reaches a definitive conclusion (N or P).

P.  Conclusion 4. Abnormalities in structure and function adversely affect speech production. Management recommendations specific to the mechanism are indicated.

**TABLE 3   Musculoskeletal Anatomy and Innervation of Speech Mechanism**

| Structure | Speech Function | Associated English Speech Sounds or Suprasegmentals[†] | Innervation[‡] |
|---|---|---|---|
| Nasal cavity (R) | Provides chamber for nasal resonance | /m/ /n/ /ŋ/ | M: Cranial VII to nares<br>S: Cranial V |
| Lips (A) (R) | Round<br>Spread<br>Compress<br>Elevate lower lip | /u/ /o/ /w/<br>/i/ /ɛ/ /æ/<br>/b/ /p/ /m/<br>/f/ /v/ | M: Cranial VII<br>S: Cranial V |
| Mandible (A) (R) | Lower<br>Raise<br>Retract | /a/ /r/ /j/<br>/s/ /z/<br>/f/ /v/ | M: Cranial V<br>S: Cranial V |
| Maxilla (A) (R) | Separates oral from nasal cavity, anteriorly | All sounds | S: Cranial V |
| Alveolar ridge | Provides contact surface for tongue | /n/ /t/ /d/ /l/ | |
| Hard palate | Provides contact surface for tongue | /j/ / ʃ / / ʒ / | |
| Teeth (A) | Provide sharp cutting edge for air stream<br>Contact for tongue | /s/ /z/<br><br>/ θ / /ð/ | S: Cranial V |
| Tongue (A) (R) | Shapes oral and pharyngeal cavities | | M: Cranial XII<br>S: Cranial V;<br>Taste: Cranial VII to anterior two thirds<br>Cranial IX to posterior two thirds |
| Tip | Lowers<br>Raises<br>Extends<br>Retroflexes | /i/ /ɛ/ /æ/<br>/t/ /d/ /n/<br>/ θ / /ð/<br>/r/ / ɝ / | |
| Dorsum | Lowers<br>Raises<br>Flattens<br>Elevates borders<br>Groves midline | / ɔ / /o/<br>/i/ / ʃ / /k/ /æ/ /j/<br>/ θ / /ð/ / ʃ / / ʒ /<br>/ ɝ /<br>/s/ /z/ | |
| Root | Shapes pharyngeal cavity | /i/ vs /u/<br>/a/ vs /æ/ | |
| Faucial pillars | Anterior (Palato glossus)<br>Posterior (palatopharyngeus) | (See elevation of tongue dorsum)<br>Nonnasal sounds (aids in velopharyngeal closure) | M: Cranial IX, X, XI |
| Velopharynx (A) (R) | Couples nasal cavity to rest or vocal tract | | M&S: Cranial IX, X, IX |
| Velum | Raises<br>Lowers | All nonnasal sounds<br>/m/ /n/ / ŋ / | |

**TABLE 3  Musculoskeletal Anatomy and Innervation of Speech Mechanism (Continued)**

| Structure | Speech Function | Associated English Speech Sounds or Suprasegmentals† | Innervation‡ |
|---|---|---|---|
| Pharynx | Inward and forward movement when velum raises | Nonnasal sounds | |
| | Outward and backward movement when velum lowers | Nasal sounds | |
| | Tenses | Vowels | |
| Hyoid bone (A) (R) | Attachment for extrinsic lingual and laryngeal musculature involved in vertical movements of tongue and larynx | All but labial sounds | |
| Glottis (P) | Adducts vocal folds | Voiced sounds | M: Cranial X |
| | Abducts vocal folds | Voiceless sounds | S: Cranial X |
| | Changes mass and tension of vocal folds | Voice quality, pitch, and loudness | |
| | Constricts vocal tract | /h/ | |
| Chest wall | Displaces lung volume | All sounds | |
| | With larynx, generates subglottal pressure requirements for speech | | |
| Abdomen | Expiration | | M: Thoracic VII to lumbar II |
| Rib cage | Expiration and inspiration | | M: Thoracic I to XI |
| Diaphragm | Inspiration | | M: Cervical III to V; thoracic X to XII |

\* Capital letters after structure name indicate the processes the structure participates in for speech production, i.e., A = articulation, P = phonation, R = resonance.
† Examples; not intended to be an exhaustive listing.
‡ M = motor, S = sensory.

Q.  Referrals for consideration of physical management of structures in the head and neck are typically made to otolaryngology and dentistry. (See page 128 for management of disorders of respiratory structures in the torso.) Referrals for assessment and management of neuromuscular dysfunction are made to the neurology department.

R.  When the recommended management has been carried out (e.g., surgical, prosthetic, chemical), the client is reassessed to determine the success of these management procedures for speech production. If the adverse effect of the mechanism on speech has been eliminated, no further management of the mechanism is indicated. If the adverse effect has not been eliminated, futher physical management may be considered, or a period of therapy may be recommended to teach the client strategies to compensate for the abnormal mechanism or to augment speech with other modes of communication.

# References

Bain J, Carter P, Morton R. Color atlas of mouth, throat and ear disorders in children. San Diego: College-Hill Press, 1985.

Bateman HE, Mason RM. Applied anatomy and physiology of the speech and hearing mechanism. Springfield IL: Charles C Thomas, 1984.

Crelin ES. Development of the upper respiratory system. Clinical symposia, 28, No. 3. Summit NJ: CIBA Pharmaceutical, 1976.

Perkins WH, Kent RD. Functional anatomy of speech, language and hearing: a primer. San Diego: College-Hill Press, 1986.

Siegel-Sadewitz V, Shprintzen RJ. The relationship of communicative disorders to syndrome indentification. J Speech Hear Disord, 1982; 47:338.

# FEEDING DISORDERS IN THE INFANT AND YOUNG CHILD

*Marilyn Seif Workinger, Ph.D.*

This decision tree deals with infants and young children referred to the speech/language pathologist for evaluation and treatment of feeding disorders. Causes for these disorders generally fall into one of four categories: structural, neuromuscular, developmental, and behavioral. No matter what the cause, feeding disorders can be devastating problems. The caregiver's primary responsibility is to feed and nurture the child. When a feeding disorder interferes with this process, the caregiver-child interaction and relationship can be seriously disrupted (Morris, 1977b). Even if a behavioral component is not a primary factor, it may develop secondarily.

At birth, the feeding process consists of five basic reflexes: root, suck, swallow, gag, and bite (Radtka, 1977). At birth, the term infant uses a sucking pattern of tongue movement to express liquid from the bottle. Sucking has been defined by Morris (1977c) as "the rhythmical raising and lowering of the body of the tongue as a method of obtaining liquid." For sucking, lip approximation on the nipple is firm. A suckle pattern develops at approximately 1 to 2 weeks. During suckling, more anterior-posterior movement of the tongue is observed, and lip approximation on the nipple is loose. Sucking or suckling triggers a swallow. Sucking, swallowing, and breathing are well coordinated in the term infant, and little or no coughing or choking occurs during feeding. The infant progresses from a single suckle per swallow sequence to a sequence of several suckles before a swallow is triggered.

Between 1 and 6 months, the suckling pattern of tongue movement predominates in taking liquid from the bottle or solids from a spoon. Solids placed on the gums elicit a munching pattern. The lips become more active, particularly in removing food from a spoon. Choking and gagging are not uncommon during this period. The rooting, sucking, and biting reflexes generally are integrated and disappear during this time.

From 7 to 12 months, the youngster becomes progressively more sophisticated at using the lips, tongue, and jaw during feeding. True sucking becomes the prominent pattern in taking liquid from the bottle. Suckling is still seen in removing food from a spoon and in the new experience of cup drinking. The upper and lower lips are active in food removal from a spoon. Tongue lateralization accompanies maturation of chewing. The first pattern seen at approximately 7 months of age is a gross rolling lateralization which refines to a more mature side-to-side movement. A sustained bite through a soft solid is first seen at approximately 10 months of age.

Several abnormal movement patterns can be seen in children with feeding disorders. The most common pathologic behaviors that are not a part of the normal developmental sequence are: jaw thrust, tongue thrust, lip retraction, tonic bite reflex, tongue retraction, and nasal regurgitation.

Jaw thrust is a forceful downward extension of the mandible, which can be seen both during or outside the feeding situation. It is often elicited upon presentation of food. At times, the jaw seems to be locked in this position momentarily. The jaw thrust interferes with efficient removal of food or liquid from the spoon, bottle, or cup.

A tongue thrust is the forceful protrusion of the tongue from the mouth. The tongue may appear thick and the extension phase of movement is longer than the retraction phase. Tongue thrusting not only interferes with acquisition of food or liquid, but also prevents efficient oral transit of material to the pharynx.

In a lip retraction pattern, the upper lip appears pulled upward and the lips are retracted almost as if in a smile. This interferes with use of the lips in removal of food or liquid from the cup, bottle, or spoon and use of the lips in retaining food and saliva in the mouth.

A tonic bite reflex is triggered by stimulation to the teeth or gums. It is a strong clenching of the jaws, with the child frequently unable to release for several seconds.

In tongue retraction, the tongue is pulled back into the pharynx and range of movement limited. This also interferes with removal of food from utensils and efficient oral transit.

Nasal regurgitation, loss of food or liquid through the nose, can occur in children with structural or motor deficits. In children with a cleft or short palate, the structure is inadequate to provide closure. In children with a submucous cleft palate or those with coordination problems, the structure is present, but the timing of movement or the range of movement is inadequate.

A. The first step in assessment is to obtain a history, both from the caregiver and from medical personnel and/or records. It is necessary to establish that this is not a problem requiring medical attention, such as lack of appetite caused by illness or fatigue due to heart failure. Information obtained from the caregiver should include: foods attempted and the child's response, time involved in feeding, the amount of food the child can eat in one feeding, interventions attempted to date, and the child's behavior during feeding. The caregiver should also be asked to indicate the primary concern regarding the feeding problem.

B. Assessment should include observations made while the child is being fed by both the caregiver and the examining clinician. Feeding by the caregiver should be made as normal as possible using equipment, utensils, and positioning that are the same as in the home environment. The clinician assesses the following parameters: movement patterns affecting the feeding process, positioning and handling, types and amounts of foods, manner of presentation of foods, primitive or pathological feeding patterns, behaviors interfering with the feeding process, and the caregiver's response to these behaviors. The clinician will wish to feed the child in order to assess further the nature of the problem and also to use treatment techniques in a diagnostic manner and, thus, determine interventions that may be useful. In some instances, particularly if aspiration is suspected, a modified barium swallow videofluoroscopy study should be obtained.

C. Goals of the treatment program for a feeding disorder are: (1) to make feeding more efficient and pleasurable for the child and for the caregiver; (2) to minimize danger

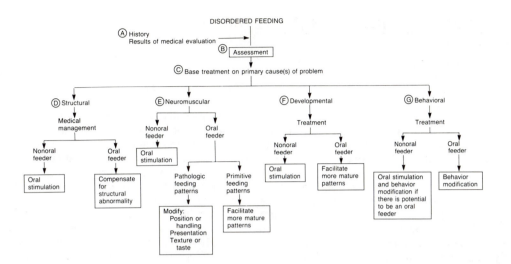

of aspiration; (3) to reduce or modify pathologic behaviors; and (4) to facilitate more mature feeding behaviors. Some authors suggest that work on oral-motor function in feeding disorders will also improve oral-motor function for speech (Morris, 1977a; Alexander, 1987; and Mueller, 1972). Although this may well be true, it has not as yet been documented in the literature. Therefore, clinicians should use caution in setting goals and expectations for both the child and the caregiver.

The treatment approach is directly dependent upon the outcome of the assessment. As a general rule, the clinician deals with behavioral aspects of the problem first. Work to reduce or modify pathologic behaviors can follow this, and then more mature feeding patterns can be facilitated. If the youngster requires a supplementary form of nutrition or is determined to be a non-oral feeder, a program of oral stimulation should be instituted unless medically contraindicated. The goal of oral stimulation in this situation is to reduce the likelihood of development of oral hypersensitivity. Procedures for oral stimulation are described by Morris (1977d) and Alexander (1987).

D. Those feeding problems determined to be structural, such as those seen in cleft lip and palate, should be managed medically, if possible. If the youngster is determined to be an oral feeder, methods to compensate for the structural abnormality should be explored. This may involve fabrication of a prosthesis, trial of various types of nipples or bottles, or changing texture of food (Brookshire et al, 1980).

E. When a child is determined to have feeding problems with a neuromuscular cause, the clinician must determine whether the feeding behaviors are primitive or pathologic in nature. Primitive behaviors are those which are part of the normal developmental sequence. Pathological behaviors, such as jaw thrust and tongue thrust, are not seen as part of the normal developmental sequence.

Four aspects of the feeding process can be modified in treatment: (1) behavior, (2) positioning and handling, (3) method of presentation of foods, and (4) textures and tastes of foods. Treatment is usually most successful when that aspect of the problem causing most concern to the caregiver is addressed first. Specific suggestions for treatment are available in numerous sources (Alexander, 1987; Finnie, 1975; and Morris, 1977d).

F. Feeding problems that are determined to be developmental in nature frequently can be treated by facilitation of more mature feeding patterns. Techniques used are the same as those for feeding disorders with neuromuscular bases. It is important to remember that if a child is showing uniform delays in all areas of development, it may not be appropriate to expect age-appropriate feeding skills.

G. Some feeding behaviors, including rejection of some types or textures of foods may be determined to be behavioral problems. Behavior modification is appropriate in these instances. Approaches to treatment of a variety of behavioral feeding problems are discussed by Morris (1977d).

The reader is cautioned to seek training in assessment and treatment of feeding disorders before implementing such a program.

# References

Alexander R. Prespeech and feeding development. In: McDonald E, ed. Treating cerebral palsy: for clinicians by clinicians. Austin, TX: Pro-Ed, 1987:133.

Brookshire B, Lynch J, Fox D. A parent-child cleft palate curriculum: developing speech and language. Tigard, OR: CC Publications, 1980.

Finnie N. Handling the young cerebral palsied child at home. New York: EP DuHon, 1975.

Morris S. Abnormalities of oral-motor function and the development of speech. In: Wilson J, ed. Oral-motor function and dysfunction in children. Chapel Hill: University of North Carolina, 1977a:194.

Morris S. Interpersonal aspects of feeding problems. In: Wilson J, ed. Oral-motor function and dysfunction in children. Chapel Hill: University of North Carolina, 1977b:106.

Morris S. Oral-motor development: normal and abnormal. In: Wilson J, ed. Oral-motor function and dysfunction in children. Chapel Hill: University of North Carolina, 1977c:23.

Morris S. Program guidelines for children with feeding problems. Edison, NJ: Childcraft, 1977d.

Mueller H. Facilitating feeding and prespeech. In: Pearson P, Williams C, eds. Physical therapy services in the development of disabilities. Springfield: Charles C Thomas, 1972:283.

Radtka S. Feeding reflexes and neural control. In: Wilson J, ed. Oral-motor function and dysfunction in children. Chapel Hill: University of North Carolina, 1977:96.

# DYSPHAGIA IN THE ADULT

*Jeri A. Logemann, Ph.D.*

*Swallowing* requires fine neuromuscular coordination of structures in the oral cavity, pharynx, larynx, and esophagus. The oral preparatory and oral stage of the swallow are under voluntary neurologic control. Tongue control of the bolus is the most important aspect of both oral preparation of the food (mastication) and the oral stage of the swallow. The pharyngeal or "reflexive" stage of the swallow is considered to be involuntary, although it can be modified volitionally in a number of ways. The "swallowing reflex" is now thought to be a patterned neuromuscular response to a specific stimulus or pattern of stimuli in the oropharynx. In all probability, the stimulus consists of the voluntary tongue movement of the oral stage in combination with the food or liquid bolus (Larson, 1985; Miller, 1982). The swallow center in the brainstem programs the various neuromotor components of the pharyngeal swallow, including velopharyngeal closure, pharyngeal peristalsis, airway protection (both laryngeal elevation and closure), and opening of the upper esophageal sphincter by the cricopharyngeus muscle. Swallowing disorders may result from neurologic or structural damage to the upper aerodigestive tract, from systemic disease, or rarely from psychogenic origins (Logemann, 1983).

A.  Review the patient's medical history and nutritional and respiratory status. Assess the oral structures and function of the lips, facial musculature, tongue (tip and back), pharynx, larynx, oral sensation (light touch), and the gag and palatal reflexes (Linden and Siebens, 1983). These reflexes permit assessment of symmetry and strength of the pharyngeal motor response. They do not predict the presence or adequacy of the swallow. Note the patient's level of alertness and ability to follow directions. With currently available techniques, the bedside assessment is highly inaccurate in evaluating the neuromuscular components of the reflexive-pharyngeal swallow, aspiration, or the etiology of aspiration.

B.  Assess the oral preparatory, oral, and pharyngeal stages of deglutition with a radiographic procedure, the modified barium swallow, recorded on videotape (videofluoroscopy) or on movie film (cinefluoroscopy) (Logemann, 1983;1985). Initially, view the oral cavity, pharynx, larynx, and cervical esophagus in the lateral plane while the patient swallows a small amount (one-third teaspoon) of each of at least three consistencies (liquid, paste, and masticated material [cookie]). The small amount of material facilitates viewing the movement patterns of the desired structures while minimizing the chance of aspiration. The fluorographic tube should not follow the bolus but should continuously view the oral cavity, pharynx, and larynx to assess the patient's reaction to residual food remaining in the pharynx (i.e., does aspiration occur after the swallow? If so, why? Does the patient dry swallow to clear residue, indicating normal pharyngeal sensation?). Follow the examination in the lateral plane with several swallows in the anterior plane. The symmetry of the swallow can be examined in the anterior view.

C.  Aspiration is a generic term that indicates the entry of material into the airway below the true vocal folds. Entry of material into the laryngeal vestibule but not below the true vocal folds is not considered aspiration. In order to eliminate aspiration, its neuromuscular or structural etiology must be defined. Aspiration may occur for any of the following reasons: reduced tongue control of the bolus during chewing or the initiation of the swallow, delayed or absent triggering of the pharyngeal swallow, reduced pharyngeal peristalsis, unilateral pharyngeal dysfunction, reduced laryngeal elevation, or cricopharyngeal dysfunction. Aspiration may also occur well after the swallow if food is refluxed up and out of the esophagus into the pharynx.

D.  In normal individuals oral transit time is approximately 1 second and pharyngeal transit time is 1 second or less (Mandelstam and Lieber, 1970). A patient who takes more than 10 seconds to swallow a single bolus of all consistencies, is unable to get sufficient nutrition by mouth to maintain his weight (Logemann, 1983).

E.  Postural changes affect the way food falls into and through the oral cavity and pharynx, in combination with gravity. With the head down, the tongue falls forward because of gravity, the epiglottis falls backward in a more overhanging position over the airway and the valleculae is widened. This posture is helpful for patients with a delayed swallowing reflex or reduced laryngeal closure. Tilting the head back facilitates oral transit by using gravity to help drain food from the oral cavity. Turning the head to one side closes the pyriform sinus on that side and directs food down the opposite side, facilitating the swallow in patients with a unilateral pharyngeal dysfunction. Turning the head to the damaged side also improves vocal fold adduction in patients with unilateral damage to laryngeal closure. Tilting the head to one side uses gravity to keep food on one side of the oral cavity and pharynx. Lying down can eliminate aspiration after the swallow that is caused by reduced pharyngeal peristalsis.

F.  Food consistencies vary in the way they drain or fall through the oral cavity and pharynx. Liquid is easiest for patients with reduced peristalsis or cricopharyngeal disorders and most difficult for patients with oral control problems or a delayed swallowing reflex. Thin paste is easiest for patients with oral control problems. Pureed (thick pastes) and solid foods are easiest for patients with delayed triggering of the pharyngeal swallow and laryngeal closure problems.

G.  Therapy techniques that are quick and require little teaching can be attempted during the fluorographic study to assess their effectiveness. Currently two such techniques exist: thermal stimulation (sensitization) of the swallowing reflex and voluntary airway protection (the supraglottic swallow). Thermal stimulation involves stroking the anterior faucial arch with an iced size 00 laryngeal mirror. This stimulation is designed to increase the patient's oral sensation so that when the patient swallows after the thermal stimulation, the pharyngeal stage of the swallow will be triggered faster. The supraglottic swallow,

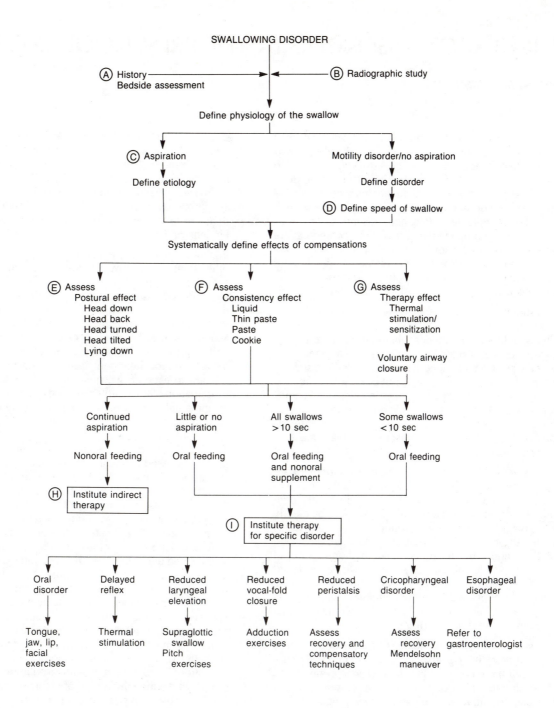

SWALLOWING DISORDER

(A) History — Bedside assessment

(B) Radiographic study

Define physiology of the swallow

(C) Aspiration → Define etiology

Motility disorder/no aspiration → Define disorder → (D) Define speed of swallow

Systematically define effects of compensations

(E) Assess
Postural effect
Head down
Head back
Head turned
Head tilted
Lying down

(F) Assess
Consistency effect
Liquid
Thin paste
Paste
Cookie

(G) Assess
Therapy effect
Thermal stimulation/sensitization → Voluntary airway closure

Continued aspiration → Nonoral feeding → (H) Institute indirect therapy

Little or no aspiration → Oral feeding

All swallows >10 sec → Oral feeding and nonoral supplement

Some swallows <10 sec → Oral feeding

(I) Institute therapy for specific disorder

| Oral disorder | Delayed reflex | Reduced laryngeal elevation | Reduced vocal-fold closure | Reduced peristalsis | Cricopharyngeal disorder | Esophageal disorder |
| Tongue, jaw, lip, facial exercises | Thermal stimulation | Supraglottic swallow Pitch exercises | Adduction exercises | Assess recovery and compensatory techniques | Assess recovery Mendelsohn maneuver | Refer to gastroenterologist |

also known as voluntary airway protection, requires the patient to hold his or her breath while swallowing.

H. Indirect swallowing therapy involves neuromuscular exercises without giving food (e.g., oromotor exercises for chewing and tongue movement to initiate the swallow, thermal sensitization or stimulation of the pharyngeal swallow, and laryngeal adduction exercises).

I. Select and initiate therapy techniques that are appropriate for the patient's particular swallowing disorder(s), usually in three short sessions per day. Some disorders, such as reduced pharyngeal peristalsis and cricopharyngeal dysfunction, recover spontaneously over a 2- to 4-month period. Patients with these disorders should be reassessed monthly with the modified barium swallow to determine progress in recovery and expand diet when possible.

## References

Larson C. Neurophysiology of speech and swallowing. In: Logemann J, ed. Seminars in speech and swallowing 1985; 6(4):275.

Linden P, Siebens A. Dysphagia: predicting laryngeal penetration. Arch Phys Med Rehabil 1983; 64:281.

Logemann J. Evaluation and treatment of swallowing disorders. San Diego: College Hill Press, 1983.

Logemann J. A manual for videofluorographic examination of dysphagia. San Diego: College Hill Press, 1985.

Mandelstam P, Lieber A. Cineradiographic evaluation of the esophagus in normal adults. Gastroenterology 1970; 58:32.

Miller A. Deglutition. Physio Rev 1982; 62:129.

# ARTICULATION DISORDERS IN THE PRESCHOOL CHILD

*Rachel E. Stark, Ph.D.*

A. Overall assessment of both speech and language must first be carried out by means of standardized tests and clinical observation. If a language disorder is found to be present as well as an articulation disorder, the decision must be made: Is language intervention to be provided in conjunction with treatment for the speech disorder or separately? Pragmatic disorders are not as likely to be accompanied by articulation problems as are semantic-syntactic disorders. If present, however, a pragmatic disorder needs to be identified in the initial evaluation and priority given to planning for its treatment. The same is true for voice and fluency disorders.

B. Questionnaires have been prepared by Morris (1982) and others that aid the speech-language pathologist in identifying delays or difficulties relating to feeding. If such difficulties are reported or are still present, they may suggest the presence of a speech motor disorder. The severity of an articulation disorder may not be closely correlated with the extent of a coexisting feeding problem. If a history of neuromotor deficits, oral structural anomalies, or middle ear disease is documented, referral to the appropriate specialist or multidisciplinary team must be considered.

C. Assessments of level of speech motor development are carried out differently depending upon whether the child is in a prelinguistic or early language developmental period. The onset of the latter period is marked by clearly recognizable attempts to produce referential words. Prelinguistic levels of speech motor skill are described by Stark and Oller in the book by Yenikomshian et al (1980). Characteristics of early phonologic development are described by Ingram (1981) and others. Normative data for level of speech production skill in the early language period are provided by the Templin-Darley Picture Test of Articulation (1969).

D. The speech-language pathologist (SLP) must be alert to signs of delay in cognitive and social maturity. Psychometric (IQ) data may be required to enable the SLP to determine to what extent a child's developmental misarticulations are related to overall developmental delay; hence, the need for psychological evaluation. If speech production skill is at the child's cognitive level, speech intervention may not be indicated. The need for audiologic evaluation is determined on the basis of hearing screening and acoustic immittance screening. Medical referral is indicated by a history of seizures, otitis media, movement disorder, emotional disturbance, attentional deficit disorder, hyperactivity, and other conditions that have not yet received medical attention. Educational referral may be appropriate if a child is clearly unable to attend to, or participate in, activities in preschool or kindergarten.

E.
F. In depth examination of oral structure and of feeding and other nonspeech movements helps the SLP identify a speech motor disorder. Regardless of whether a speech motor disorder is thought to be present, questions about the level of functioning in speech sound production should be addressed as indicated under the Speech-Oral Motor Disorder heading. A careful description of the child's phonatory repertoire is essential to this part of the assessment. Treatment approaches are suggested in relation to each of five possible levels of functioning. Examination of the child's response to speech and to environmental sounds is included in a number of infant communication scales, e.g., Sequenced Inventory of Communication Development (Hedrick, Prather and Tobin, 1984). Comprehension of spoken language should also be assessed by means of such tests as the Peabody Picture Vocabulary Test (PPVT: Dunn and Dunn, 1981) and the Preschool Language Scale (Zimmerman et al, 1979). Their use may indicate the presence of a delay or disorder of speech reception. Regardless of whether such a disorder is indicated, the questions about level of function in speech sound reception should be asked as indicated under the Speech Reception Disorder heading. This step is necessary because the child may have adopted some useful compensatory strategies in responding to conversational speech even when he has a marked speech discrimination problem. Treatment approaches are suggested in relation to each of five possible levels of functioning. If a mixed disorder is found to be present, both the speech-oral motor disorder and the speech reception disorder must be addressed in treatment. The SLP must decide which type of disorder to emphasize, but in most cases a combined approach may be designed. Treatment for each type of disorder must be carefully matched at the child's level of functioning. Within each level the SLP sets specific treatment goals. The child may be moved up to a next higher level of treat-

# ASSESSMENT AND MANAGEMENT OF ARTICULATION DISORDER IN THE PRESCHOOL CHILD

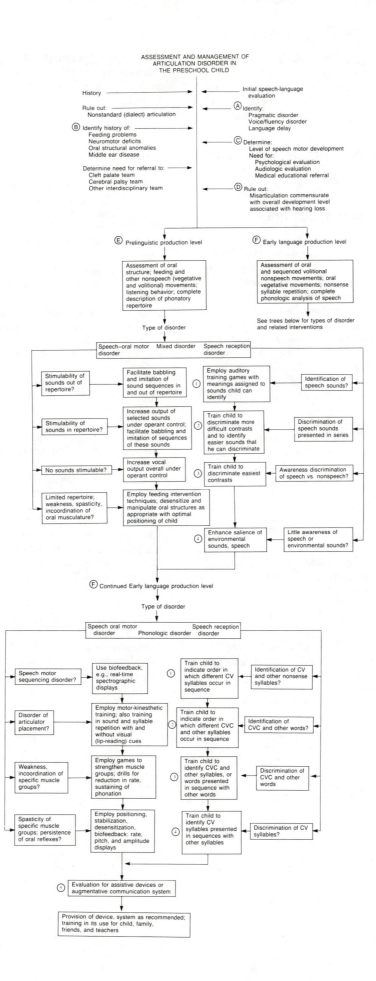

ment as he meets criteria set for these goals, or down to a next lower level if he is not successful in meeting criteria at the selected entry level. Reevaluation must be carried out at intervals to ensure that progress is being made.

## Notes on Suggested Levels of Intervention for Prelinguistic Child

### Speech-Oral Motor Disorder

1. Babbling and imitation are best facilitated through games in which the SLP first imitates the child and then rewards the child for taking further turns in the imitation game. Puppets may be made to bounce or to bang, shake or wave toys in accompaniment to the sounds produced as motivation. Consonant-Vowel (CV), CVCV, and other sequences should be assigned meanings as soon as the child is able to exercise some degree of control over their production. Meanings should at first be general (nonreferential), e.g., "ha" for "hot" or "m+ vowel" for "me" or "mine"; only later are more specific meanings (referential) assigned, e.g., "ba" for "ball" or "da" for "dog."
2. When the child produces a specific sound-sequence selected for training, he or she may be reinforced for its production by means of a social reward (smiling, tickling, praise), a tangible reward (food or a toy from a dispenser), or a play activity or activation of a mechanical toy.
3. When the child produces any speech sound from his repertoire (i.e., not crying, laughing, coughing, or sneezing), he may be reinforced for its production by means of a social, tangible, or activity reward as in (2) above.
4. Treatment at this level is described in texts on the neurodevelopmental approach, e.g., Morris (1982).
5. Manual signing is usually considered first unless the child has a severe motor deficit affecting the upper limbs. Assistive devices may include communication boards or simple E-tran devices as well as sophisticated electronic devices (e.g., those with synthetic speech output). Messages may be conveyed in the form of pictures, nonconventional symbols, or printed words, phrases, and sentences. Alternatively, they may be encoded so that letters and numerals in different combinations are made to convey sentence-length messages (Blackstone and Bruskin, 1986).

### Speech Reception Disorder

1. Identification may be assessed by having a child (1) press a button whenever he hears a target speech sound or word, e.g., /ba/ or "ball," and (2) ignore other contrasting sounds or words, e.g., /ma/ or /da/ or "dog" and "bat" presented in series (one at a time) with the target sound. The meanings assigned in auditory training games may be general (nonreferential); e.g., the child may be trained to respond to the word "open" by opening a bag of toys, a door, or a picture book. Referential meanings may be introduced in play routines as soon as the child responds reliably and consistently to a number of words (at least 10) used nonreferentially.
2. Discrimination training should not be attempted within a same versus different paradigm if the child's speech reception abilities are at a prelinguistic level. Instead the child may be trained to respond to a change in background stimulation (from one CV or other syllable to another) by a head turn or a button press. The child may then be trained to identify a speech sound in the presence of the contrasting sound included in the discrimination task. The responses required may be a button press for the target sound and no response or the word "No" or a head shake for the nontarget sound.
3. Discrimination training should be within the paradigm described in (2) above. Easier contrasts to be presented first may be vowels or CV syllables vs. an environmental sound; or a CV syllable babbled by a baby vs. the same CV syllable spoken in isolation by an adult. Harder contrasts include initial stops vs. initials nasals, e.g., /pa/ vs. /na/ and initial /f/ vs. initial /th/, e.g., (/fa/ vs. /tha/) in CV syllables.
4. The child may be trained to respond to environmental or speech and speechlike sounds with a related activity, e.g., dancing to music, taking the telephone off the receiver and pretending to have a conversation when the telephone rings, or kissing the clinician's hand when he or she pretends to be hurt and says "ouch" with ap-

propriate emphasis and accompanying actions. These sounds are presented one at a time only, not within a discrimination paradigm, at this level.

5. Manual signing should be considered if a severe speech reception disorder is documented, even if peripheral hearing is normal (as in the case of verbal agnosia, Rapin et al, 1977). Assistive devices that may be considered include an auditory trainer at a very mild gain setting and a tactile aid.

## Notes on Suggested Levels of Intervention for Early Language Production*

### Speech-Oral Motor Disorder

1. Real time spectrographic displays are effective in teaching hearing impaired children to sequence speech sounds motorically. Our experience suggests that this approach may also be useful with normal hearing children who have a speech motor sequencing disorder.

2. In case of an articulatory placement disorder, indicating target positions of the articulators through touch and visual demonstration may be useful. Manipulation of the child's tongue, lips, and jaw may also be tried.

3. Exercises and drills are described in the cerebral palsy literature from the 1950s and 1960s. Delayed auditory feedback may be useful in helping the child to reduce rate of production.

4. The procedures recommended reflect a neurodevelopmental approach (Morris, 1982). They may be carried out most usefully in cooperation with other disciplines (e.g., physical therapy, occupational therapy).

5. See prelinguistic production level.

### Speech Reception Disorder

The steps outlined are designed to train the child to listen to speech and nonspeech sounds. Notice that the child is not asked to identify, discriminate, or sequence phonemes, skills that are probably acquired by most children after they enter school.

1. The child is trained to respond to two nonsense syllables. These may be presented one at a time (A or B) or two at a time (in the sequences AA, AB, BA, or BB). The child selects an A target (picture, symbol, or button press) for the A syllable and a B target for the B syllable. Training at this level is not appropriate unless the child's language abilities are at least at a 5-year-old level.

2. Identification at this level is by selecting or finding a picture or object in response to a word. The child may also be trained (a) to indicate the number of syllables in words of no more than three syllables that are in his vocabulary and (b) to indicate the order in which the syllables occur by repeating the words or, in special cases, by pointing to pictures or objects corresponding to the syllables, e.g., to "dog" and "house" for the word "doghouse."

3. The child is trained to respond to one nonsense syllable in the presence of another nonsense syllable when they are presented one at a time. He must select an A target (picture, symbol, or button press) in response to the A syllable and ignore the B syllable, or vice versa (respond to the B syllable and ignore the A syllable).

4. The child is trained to select a target (picture, symbol or object) in response to a previously trained word (e.g., "dog") and to ignore all other words (real or nonsense) presented in sequence with the target word, "dog." Contrasting items should at first be very different from the target word (e.g., "man"), and should later be more similar to the target word (e.g., "bog" or "dig").

5. See prelinguistic production level.

---

* For management of phonologic disorder see Shriberg, p118.

## References

Blackstone SB, Bruskin D. Augmentative communication: an introduction. Rockville: American Speech-Language-Hearing Association, 1986.

Dunn LM, Dunn LM. Peabody picture vocabulary test. Circle Pines, MN: American Guidance Service, 1981.

Hedrick DL, Prather EM, Tobin AR. Sequenced inventory of communications development. Seattle: University of Washington Press, 1984.

Ingram D. Procedures for the phonological analysis of children's language. Baltimore: University Park Press, 1981.

Morris S. The normal acquisition of oral feeding skills: implications for assessment and treatment. Boston: Therapeutic Media, 1982.

Rapin I, Mattis S, Rowan AJ, Golden GS. Verbal auditory agnosia in children. Dev Med Child Neurol, 1977; 19:197.

Yenikomshian GH, Ferguson CA, Kavanagh JF. Child phonology. Vol 1. Production. New York: Academic Press, 1980.

Zimmerman IL, Steiner VG, Pond RE. Preschool language scale. Columbus, OH: Charles E Merrill, 1979.

# PHONOLOGIC ASSESSMENT IN THE YOUNG CHILD

*Lawrence D. Shriberg, Ph.D.*

A phonologic disorder is suspected when a parent, physician, or teacher refers a preschool child because (a) the child's speech is delayed in onset, (b) the child's speech is difficult to understand, or (c) the child's speech contains one or more noticeable speech sound errors. Assessment tasks are divided into two interdependent areas: procedures to obtain causal-correlates data and procedures to obtain speech data.

## IDENTIFICATION AND SEVERITY

A. The causal-correlates diagnostic battery includes tasks to assess hearing and speech mechanism functioning, cognitive-linguistic functioning, and psychosocial functioning. Hearing and speech mechanism tasks include procedures to assess capacity for normal speech perception (audiologic, acoustic immittance) and speech production (diadochokinesis, oral-peripheral examination, nonverbal oral gestures). Cognitive-linguistic tasks include formal and informal tests for comprehension and production of semantic, syntactic, and pragmatic forms and functions. Psychosocial tasks include behavioral information from the developmental history, parent interview, and relevant medical, educational, and social records. Speech assessment includes an articulation test, a continuous speech sample, stimulability testing, and probe lists to obtain multiple tokens of selected words and phrases.

B. A developmental phonologic disorder is identified and rated in severity from the speech data. Information from both the speech tasks and causal-correlates task is used to classify the nature of the disorder (Shriberg et al, 1986). If the child performs below the cut-off score on a standardized articulation test or below three severity-level criteria based on errors tallied during a continuous speech sample, the child has a developmental phonologic disorder. These criteria, which involve three analyses from the PEPPER software package (percentage of consonants correct, suprasegmental ratings, and an intelligibility index) yield a severity of involvement category ranging from mild to severe (Shriberg, 1986, Shriberg and Kwiatkowski, 1982a; 1982b).

## DIAGNOSTIC CLASSIFICATION

C. Diagnostic classification of a child identified as having a developmental phonologic disorder begins with an inspection of the results of natural process analysis of the continuous speech sample. The subtype of phonologic disorders is determined by the child's age in relation to his or her phonologic stage of development. School-aged children whose errors are restricted to speech sound distortions consistent with Phonological Stage IV (Ingram, 1976) are classified as having *residual errors*. Children older than 4 years whose errors include, but are not limited to, phoneme deletions and substitutions consistent with Phonological Stage III, are classified as having *delayed speech*.

D. Probe list procedures to assess children's underlying forms and nonnatural process errors provide information on past or current constraints on speech acquisition. If the results of these analyses suggest that the child has some underlying forms that are not adult-like (Elbert and Dinnsen et al, 1984) or that some sound changes cannot be categorized as natural phonologic processes (Shriberg and Kwiatkowski, 1983), each datum in the causal-correlates assessment battery should be considered for its possible role as an original, contributing, or maintaining cause of the speech problem. Computer-based procedures for rating the intake data and all other assessment information allow classification of children into seven diagnostic categories. The most frequent classification category observed when using this system is speech delay in association with language production delay. Other provisional classifications include speech delay in association with early fluctuant hearing deficits, craniofacial deficits, motor speech deficits, intellectual deficits, and deficits affecting intrapersonal or interpersonal functioning.

E. Management considerations weigh the information in A and B in relation to options in the community. Children with residual errors or mild speech delays who indicate the potential to normalize without management should be monitored. Children who do not indicate this potential should be provided with speech services, with the goal of normalizing speech before school age. Especially for children with reduced intelligibility, whatever the suspected origin, intensive speech services should be provided during preschool years.

## References

Elbert M, Dinnsen D, Weismer G. Phonological theory and the misarticulating child. ASHA Monographs, No. 22, 1984.

Ingram D. Phonological disability in children. London: Edward Arnold, 1976.

Shriberg L. PEPPER: programs to examine phonetic and phonologic evaluation records. Madison, WI: University of Wisconsin Software Development and Distribution Center, 1986.

Shriberg L, Kwiatkowski J. Phonological disorders I: a diagnostic classification system. J Speech Hear Disord 1982a; 47: 226.

Shriberg L, Kwiatkowski J. Phonological disorders III. A severity metric. J Speech Hear Disord 1982b; 47: 256.

Shriberg L, Kwiatkowski J. Computer assisted natural process analysis (NPA): recent issues and data. In: Locke J, ed. Assessing phonological disorders: current issues. Sem Speech Lang Hear, 1983.

Shriberg L, Kwiatkowski J, Best S, Hengst J, Terselic-Weber B. Characteristics of children with phonologic disorders of unknown origin. J Speech Hear Dis 1986; 51:140.

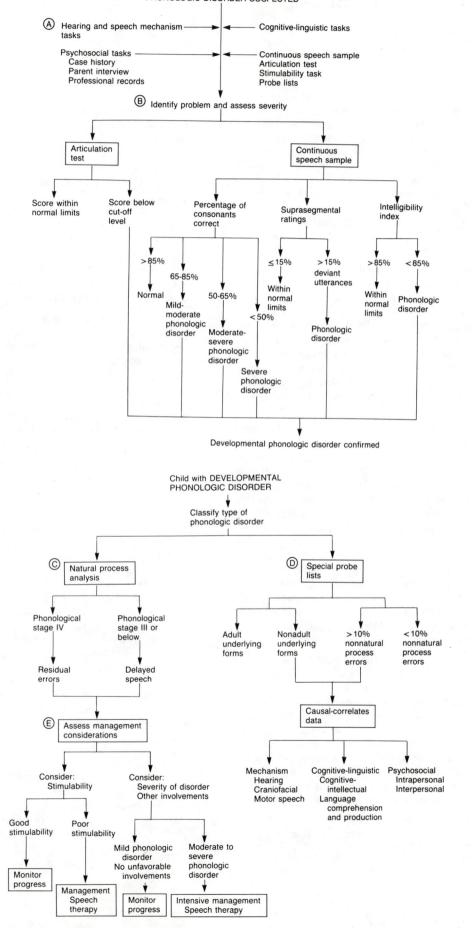

PHONOLOGIC DISORDER SUSPECTED

Ⓐ Hearing and speech mechanism tasks ⟶ ⟵ Cognitive-linguistic tasks

Psychosocial tasks ⟶ ⟵ Continuous speech sample
  Case history          Articulation test
  Parent interview      Stimulability task
  Professional records  Probe lists

Ⓑ Identify problem and assess severity

Articulation test

Continuous speech sample

Score within normal limits

Score below cut-off level

Percentage of consonants correct

Suprasegmental ratings

Intelligibility index

>85%
Normal

65-85%
Mild-moderate phonologic disorder

50-65%
Moderate-severe phonologic disorder

<50%
Severe phonologic disorder

≤15%
Within normal limits

>15% deviant utterances
Phonologic disorder

>85%
Within normal limits

<85%
Phonologic disorder

Developmental phonologic disorder confirmed

Child with DEVELOPMENTAL PHONOLOGIC DISORDER

Classify type of phonologic disorder

Ⓒ Natural process analysis

Phonological stage IV

Phonological stage III or below

Residual errors

Delayed speech

Ⓔ Assess management considerations

Consider: Stimulability

Consider: Severity of disorder Other involvements

Good stimulability

Poor stimulability

Mild phonologic disorder No unfavorable involvements

Moderate to severe phonologic disorder

Monitor progress

Management Speech therapy

Monitor progress

Intensive management Speech therapy

Ⓓ Special probe lists

Adult underlying forms

Nonadult underlying forms

>10% nonnatural process errors

<10% nonnatural process errors

Causal-correlates data

Mechanism
Hearing
Craniofacial
Motor speech

Cognitive-linguistic
Cognitive-intellectual
Language comprehension and production

Psychosocial
Intrapersonal
Interpersonal

# SPEECH INTELLIGIBILITY

*Raymond D. Kent, Ph.D.*

Speech may be defined as the vocalization of information. From this definition, it follows that intelligibility can be defined as the information that a listener can recover from the speech signal. Because intelligibility is the essential feature of speech communication, the assessment of intelligibility is an issue of fundamental clinical importance. Improvement of intelligibility is an overarching goal of much of speech-language management, and the measurement of such improvement is therefore an integral part of various therapies. This chapter reviews the major clinical approaches to the assessment of intelligibility (see also, Yorkston and Beukelman, 1978).

A. Scaling and identification are the two major methods of intelligibility assessment. Generally, scaling offers the advantage of economy. Most scaling methods applied clinically are easily used and require relatively little time from client or clinician. Identification methods are more time consuming, but provide more information about the client's intelligibility deficit. The two general approaches can be combined to provide a comprehensive evaluation in which the overall level of intelligibility is determined by scaling and a more detailed analysis is accomplished by an identification test.

B. The chief scaling methods of interest clinically are direct magnitude estimation (DME) and interval scaling (IS) (Schiavetti et al, 1983). With DME, listeners scale stimuli by assigning numbers that are proportional to the ratios of stimulus magnitudes along the continuum to be scaled. With IS, listeners assign to stimuli numbers that correspond to a linear partition of the continuum to be scaled. Some evidence indicates that DME is preferable to IS for intelligibility scaling insofar as intelligibility is a prothetic continuum, or one that can be described as degrees of a magnitude or quantity (Schiavetti et al, 1981). Whatever scaling procedure is used, further decisions have to be made about details of the procedure, e.g., selection of a standard or modulus (required for DME), range of numbers available for scaling, and reliability of the listener(s).

C. The selection of speech materials should recognize client capabilities, representativeness of the stimuli to communication situations, and time-personnel constraints on the scaling method. Questions to consider include: Can the client read? If so, at what level? Is reading likely to be affected by factors that contaminate the assessment of intelligibility? If conversation is to be used as the sample, who will converse with the client and about what topics? If picture description or a similar task is to be used, what materials will be used as stimuli and what instructions will be given to the client?

D. For many clinical situations, the clinician is the sole source of scaling data. Unfortunately, clinician's judgments can be biased by increasing familiarity with the client's speech patterns and by a conscious or unconscious desire to record improvement (or the lack of it). Ideally, a panel of impartial judges would be recruited as listeners. If this ideal is not practicable, steps should be taken to minimize biases in the scaling procedure, or at least to recognize that biases may exist.

E. Identification methods require that a listener respond to stimuli by transcribing what was heard, by selecting an item from an open- or closed-response set, or by identifying in some other way the item presented. Most identification tasks use nonsense syllables, words, or sentences as stimuli. Particularly when syllabic or word stimuli are used, thought should be given to the syllabic structure of the items (Porter and Dickerson, 1986).

F. The clinician can choose from published materials or construct stimuli as desired. An advantage of some nonsense syllable or word lists is that errors can be analyzed in terms of phonetic patterns. An advantage to sentential items is that they may approach typical communicative situations more closely than nonsense syllables or words. Another alternative is the use of sentences in which one word (usually the final word in the sentence) is the target word to be identified (Kalikow et al, 1977).

G. Typically, the results of identification tests represent the percent of correct responses. Depending on the nature of the test, this score can be complemented by additional information, such as phonetic analyses of the errors made.

H. For various purposes, it may be appropriate to consider further tests or additional analyses. For example, if intelligibility data were collected for a speech sample that was not representative of the client's communicative needs, the clinician may choose to repeat the task with other materials; or, if a scaling method was used initially and the clinician wants to confirm or quantify the intelligibility deficit, an identification method may be used. Phonetic analyses may be conducted, if not already completed, to ascertain the particular errors that contribute to an intelligibility deficit. Finally, it may be appropriate to conduct another kind of test, such as a test of communicative competence (Politzer and McGroarty, 1983) to gain a broader perspective on a client's speech communication ability.

## References

Kalikow DN, Stevens KN, Elliott LL. Development of a test of speech intelligibility in noise using sentence materials with controlled word predictability. Acoust Soc Am 1977; 61:1337.

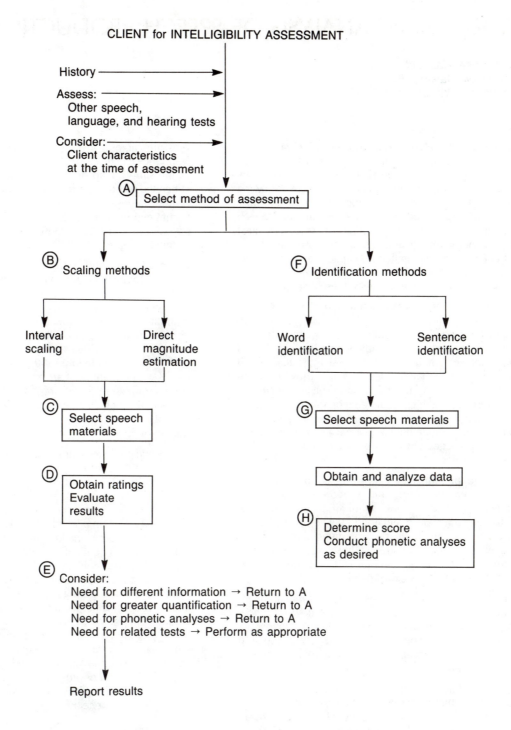

CLIENT for INTELLIGIBILITY ASSESSMENT

History

Assess:
Other speech,
language, and hearing tests

Consider:
Client characteristics
at the time of assessment

Ⓐ Select method of assessment

Ⓑ Scaling methods

Interval scaling

Direct magnitude estimation

Ⓒ Select speech materials

Ⓓ Obtain ratings Evaluate results

Ⓔ Consider:
Need for different information → Return to A
Need for greater quantification → Return to A
Need for phonetic analyses → Return to A
Need for related tests → Perform as appropriate

Report results

Ⓕ Identification methods

Word identification

Sentence identification

Ⓖ Select speech materials

Obtain and analyze data

Ⓗ Determine score Conduct phonetic analyses as desired

Politzer RL, McGroarty M. A discrete point test of communicative competence. Int Rev Appl Ling Lang Teach 1983; 21:179.

Porter KA, Dickerson MV. Syllabic complexity and its relation to speech intelligibility in a deaf population. Am Ann Deaf 1986; March:36.

Schiavetti N, Metz DE, Sitler RW. Construct validity of direct magnitude estimation and interval scaling of speech intelligibility: evidence from a study of the hearing impaired. J Speech Hear Res 1981; 24:441.

Schiavetti N, Sacco PR, Metz DE, Sitler RW. Direct magnitude estimation and interval scaling of stuttering severity. J Speech Hear Res 1983; 26:568.

Yorkston K, Beukelman D. A comparison of techniques for measuring intelligibility of dysarthric speech. J Commun Disord 1978; 11:499.

# AERODYNAMIC ANALYSIS OF SPEECH PRODUCTION

W. Michael Hairfield, D.D.S.
Rodger M. Dalston, Ph.D.
Donald W. Warren, D.D.S., Ph.D.

A. Aerodynamic analysis has been used principally to assess velopharyngeal closure. Other uses have included studying pharyngeal pressure-flow patterns, oral port size, nasal airway impairment, speech alterations following surgery of the dentofacial complex, respiratory volume exchanges during speech, nasal valve function, speech appliance function, and timing of velopharyngeal closure. Aerodynamic analysis can be performed in any patient who has the intellectual capacity and neuromuscular integrity needed to perform the tasks required. A normal 5 year old would satisfy these criteria.

B. Impaired nasorespiratory function and mouth breathing under certain circumstances may alter facial growth, leading to a retrognathic mandible, protruding maxillary anterior teeth, high palatal vault, constricted V shaped maxillary arch, and flaccid perioral musculature. All these variables may influence the aerodynamics of speech. Oral or nasal breathing may result from increased nasal resistance, which would concomitantly affect nasal emission and resonance. If a patient manifests an abnormal breathing mode but has normal airway patency, behavioral management may be necessary to reestablish nasal breathing.

C. Subglottic pressures can be assessed using a body plethysmograph, airway interruption techniques, or tracheal puncture. At conversational speech levels, subglottal pressures are maintained between 6 and 10 cm of water and generally do not differ very much in magnitude among consonants. These pressures must be maintained for a minimum of 5 to 10 seconds in order to sustain normal speech prosody.

D. Glottal aerodynamic variables available for analysis include transglottal pressure, resistance, flow rate, flow volume, voicing duration, and onset time. Vocal fold activity during voicing produces a significant pressure drop across the vocal tract and has an important influence on intraoral pressure.

E. Supraglottal aerodynamic variables available for analysis include the pressure, resistance, flow rate, flow volume, and minimal cross sectional area of the oral, nasal, and pharyngeal portions of the vocal tract. Cross sectional area measurements are made most commonly for the velopharyngeal orifice, the oral port, and nasal valve. Heated pneumotachographs are used to measure flow rate. Volume is determined by integration of flow over time. Inductive plethysmography is a noninvasive technique that can be used to measure ventilatory movements. Data collected utilizing these transducers are subsequently analyzed by both analog and digital instrumentation. The hydrokinetic equation, area = rate of airflow / k × SQRT [2(differential pressure)/density of air], can be applied to estimate effective minimal cross sectional area whenever the rate of air flow and the differential pressure across a constriction can be measured. Resistance can be calculated from Ohm's law, $R = \triangle P/\dot{V}$, as the simple ratio of pressure difference to flow rate. When the resistance calculation is not linear over a range of flow values, it indicates the presence of turbulence in that region, and the functional relationship between pressure and flow can be described by a quadratic polynomial.

F. Normal plosive and fricative consonants are typically produced with high intraoral pressures (3 to 8 cm of water) and essentially no nasal air flow. Nasal consonants have low intraoral pressures (0.5 to 1.5 cm of water) and high rates of nasal air flow (100 to 300 cc per second). Vowel sounds have negligible intraoral pressures and nasal air flow. Individuals with palatal incompetence frequently demonstrate lower intraoral pressure (3 to 4 cm of water) and high nasal air flow (150 to 800 cc per second) for pressure consonants. Oral and nasal cavity abnormalities such as open bite malocclusion or nasal obstruction can influence these values and affect the quality of speech.

G. Diagnostic guidelines for velopharyngeal cross sectional area measured during nonnasal consonant production are as follows:
  0.00—0.049 sq cm adequate closure
  0.05—0.099 sq cm adequate-borderline closure
  0.10—0.20 sq cm borderline-inadequate competency
  >0.20 sq cm inadequate closure
"Static" assessment of velopharyngeal function is achieved, for example, during the production of the utterance *papa*, and dynamic or timing assessments are most easily made during the utterance *hamper*. If only phoneme specific nasal emission is present, both studies would show velopharyngeal adequacy. Speech therapy is the preferred method of treatment in such cases. If either study is borderline, trial speech therapy and subsequent reassessment are indicated. If either study is inadequate, surgical or prosthetic management is in order. Such treatment would also be appropriate if trial speech therapy proves ineffectual for borderline patients.

Supported in part by grants DE06957, DE06061, DE07105, DE0129, and, DE02668, NIDR.

## References

Dalston RM, Warren DW. The diagnosis of velopharyngeal inadequacy. Clin Plast Surg, 1985; 12(4):685.

Warren DW. Aerodynamics of speech. In: Lass NJ, McReynolds LV, Northern JL, Yoder DE, eds. Speech, language and hearing. Philadelphia: WB Saunders, 1982.

AERODYNAMIC ANALYSIS OF SPEECH PRODUCTION

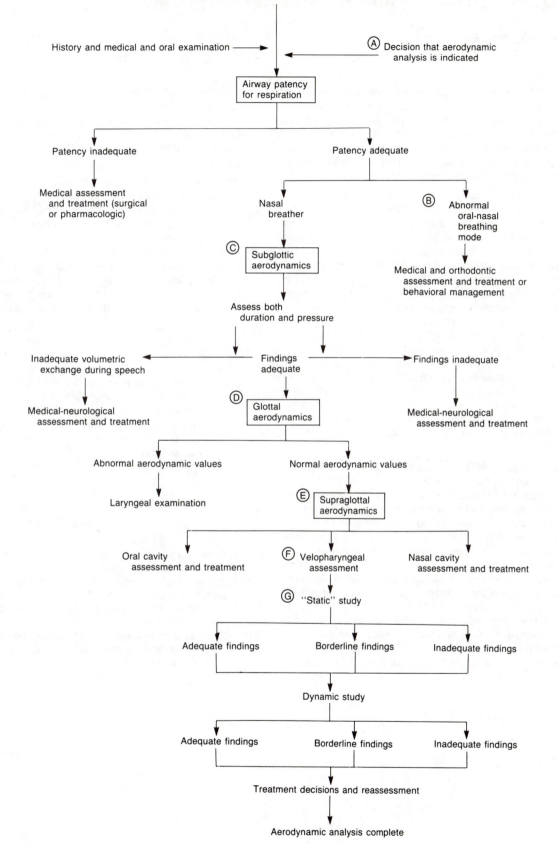

# ACOUSTIC ANALYSIS OF SPEECH

*Gary Weismer, Ph.D.*

Intelligibility scores have often been used as an index of severity in assessing speech disorders. Unfortunately, the typical intelligibility score does not provide information on the basis of a patient's intelligibility deficit. Attempts to determine the acoustic basis of intelligibility deficits (and by inference, the physiologic basis) can help to focus remediation efforts within a rational physiologic framework.

A. In many cases multiple hypotheses regarding the basis of a patient's intelligibility deficit can be advanced, so the speech sample will have to include several items from those listed here (e.g., diphthongs, stops, corner vowels). Efforts should be made to construct the speech sample in a compact way (i.e., a small number of unique utterances), because each utterance in the sample should be repeated by a patient no fewer than five times. The repetition is necessary because persons with speech disorders often produce vocal tract output that is more variable than that in persons with normal speech. Multiple repetitions of each utterance (and, thus, multiple data points for each measurement) provide a relatively stable statistical estimate of the patient's speech production behavior. The process depicted here is probably not very useful for patients with severe intelligibility deficits (i.e., < 30 percent on single word intelligibility tests), because acoustic analysis of such disorders is typically tedious and unreliable.

B. Texts (Pickett, 1980) and chapters (Weismer, 1980) discuss types of acoustic measurement and instruments that can be used to make the measurements. Several computer programs that run on microcomputers are available to make the same kind of measurements that have traditionally been obtained using the sound spectrograph or storage oscilloscope. Most programs include a waveform editor, which allows the user to mark a speech waveform in time and thus make accurate temporal measurements. Many of the programs also include a special digital approach to determining formant frequencies, which would be useful for plotting the "vowel space" or measuring formant transition characteristics. This approach, called linear predictive code (LPC) analysis, poses some problems in the determination of correct formant frequencies when the speaker's voice quality is characterized by excessive noise (vocal roughness) or hypernasality. Because many persons with speech disorders have "noisy" vocal fold vibration or are hypernasal, LPC analysis in these patients should be approached with caution.

C. When displaying data and comparing findings to normal, it is important to recognize that a given acoustic measurement may be affected by many variables. Thus, it is inappropriate to speak of a single value for an acoustic measurement that should be considered as "normal." Some of the factors that contribute to variability of acoustic measures in the normal population are as follows: age, sex, and size of speaker; speaking rate; stress level of syllable; "style" of speech (formal vs. casual); and phonetic context of target segment.

D. A distinct advantage of the acoustic approach in focusing physiologically based remediation efforts is that the measurement strategies used originally to guide remediation can serve as an ongoing index of progress resulting from therapy. For example, the clinician could plot, throughout therapy, the expansion of a previously "collapsed" vowel space. In some situations, acoustic indexing of remediation efforts may reveal progress (change in the desired direction) that is difficult to detect using perceptual techniques.

## References

Kent RD. Isovowel lines for the evaluation of vowel formant structure in speech disorders. J Speech Hear Disord 1979; 44:513.

Kent R, Rosenbek JC. Acoustic patterns of apraxia of speech. J Speech Hear Res 1983; 26:231.

Pickett JM. The sounds of speech communication. Baltimore: University Park Press, 1980.

Weismer G. Acoustic descriptions of dysarthric speech; perceptual correlates and physiological inferences. Sem Speech Lang 1984; 5:293.

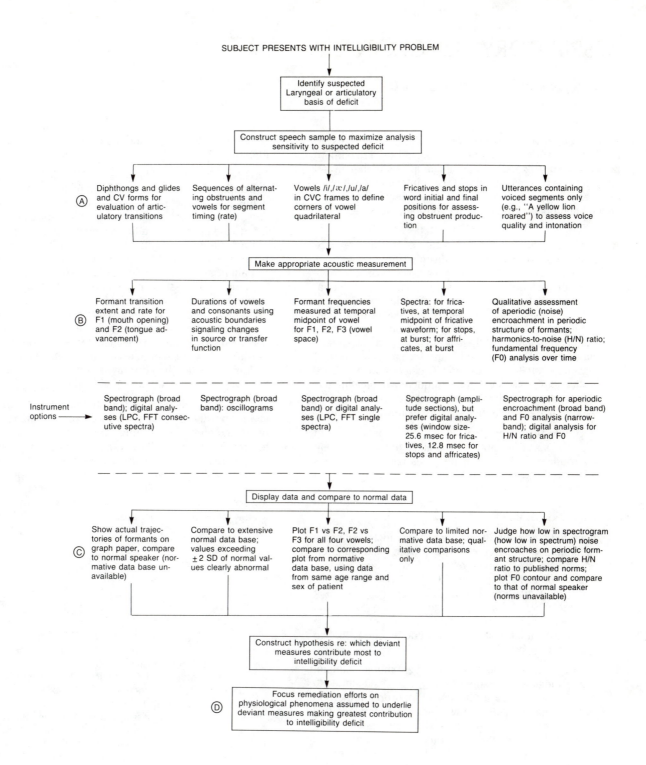

SUBJECT PRESENTS WITH INTELLIGIBILITY PROBLEM

Identify suspected
Laryngeal or articulatory
basis of deficit

Construct speech sample to maximize analysis
sensitivity to suspected deficit

(A) Diphthongs and glides and CV forms for evaluation of articulatory transitions

Sequences of alternating obstruents and vowels for segment timing (rate)

Vowels /i/,/æ/,/u/,/a/ in CVC frames to define corners of vowel quadrilateral

Fricatives and stops in word initial and final positions for assessing obstruent production

Utterances containing voiced segments only (e.g., "A yellow lion roared") to assess voice quality and intonation

Make appropriate acoustic measurement

(B) Formant transition extent and rate for F1 (mouth opening) and F2 (tongue advancement)

Durations of vowels and consonants using acoustic boundaries signaling changes in source or transfer function

Formant frequencies measured at temporal midpoint of vowel for F1, F2, F3 (vowel space)

Spectra: for fricatives, at temporal midpoint of fricative waveform; for stops, at burst; for affricates, at burst

Qualitative assessment of aperiodic (noise) encroachment in periodic structure of formants; harmonics-to-noise (H/N) ratio; fundamental frequency (F0) analysis over time

Instrument options →

Spectrograph (broad band); digital analyses (LPC, FFT consecutive spectra)

Spectrograph (broad band): oscillograms

Spectrograph (broad band) or digital analyses (LPC, FFT single spectra)

Spectrograph (amplitude sections), but prefer digital analyses (window size- 25.6 msec for fricatives, 12.8 msec for stops and affricates)

Spectrograph for aperiodic encroachment (broad band) and F0 analysis (narrowband); digital analysis for H/N ratio and F0

Display data and compare to normal data

(C) Show actual trajectories of formants on graph paper, compare to normal speaker (normative data base unavailable)

Compare to extensive normal data base; values exceeding ± 2 SD of normal values clearly abnormal

Plot F1 vs F2, F2 vs F3 for all four vowels; compare to corresponding plot from normative data base, using data from same age range and sex of patient

Compare to limited normative data base; qualitative comparisons only

Judge how low in spectrogram (how low in spectrum) noise encroaches on periodic formant structure; compare H/N ratio to published norms; plot F0 contour and compare to that of normal speaker (norms unavailable)

Construct hypothesis re: which deviant measures contribute most to intelligibility deficit

(D) Focus remediation efforts on physiological phenomena assumed to underlie deviant measures making greatest contribution to intelligibility deficit

# RESPIRATORY FUNCTION

*Stephen A. Cavallo, M.S., B.S., Ph.D.*

A comprehensive assessment of ventilatory function is indicated when prior evaluation has revealed short maximum phonation time, reduction in breath-group length, diminished vocal intensity, poorly regulated vocal intensity, dysphonia, dyspnea during speech production, basal ganglia disorder, or general neuropathologies (e.g., amyotrophic lateral sclerosis, multiple sclerosis).

A. Ventilatory abnormalities indicate either the presence of a more global neurologic disorder (timing functions and chest wall movements) or incompetence of respiration for metabolic needs (dead space, forced expiratory volume (FEV), vital capacity (VC), inspiratory capacity (IC); expiratory reserve volume (ERV); airway resistance; maximum expiratory and inspiratory flow; gas partial pressures). Both may adversely affect speech production. Expected values are: I-fraction $\cong$ 0.4; tidal volume (TV) $\cong$ 450–600ml (10 percent of VC) above resting expiratory level (REL); frequency of breathing 11 to 14 breaths per minute under basal conditions; all will vary with age, sex, and body size (Comroe et al, 1962).

B. Repeat tests specified in C, D, E and F across the breath group for speech sample and sustained phonation, where appropriate. For evaluation purposes, passage reading is recommended rather than spontaneous conversational speech samples, in order to control for linguistic context and elicit more systematic (i.e., less variable) ventilatory behavior.

C. Expected prespeech ventilatory behavior includes: inspiratory time $\cong$ 10 percent of breath group duration (average duration of inspiration = 0.6 sec); lung volume change of 10 to 20 percent of VC above REL; oppositional chest wall adjustment; minimal change of lung volume after inspiration— a significant expiratory lung volume change accompanying chest wall posturing may indicate ventilatory-laryngeal discoordination (Baken and Cavallo, 1981).

D. During *sustained phonation* the patient should maintain stable subglottal pressure ($P_S$) of $\geq 5$ cm $H_2O$ almost to the end of phonation (the airway interruption method [Sawashima et al, 1983; Sawashima and Honda, 1987] is recommended for estimating alveolar pressure during phonation); vocal intensity should be maintained (with no sudden instability) almost to the termination of phonation. During *speech production* (at normal conversational loudness in an upright posture) utterance should proceed throughout the midvolume range (approximately 40 to 60 percent VC); expect lung volume excursions between 10 and 20 percent of VC with utterance termination at or slightly below REL; $P_S$ at utterance onset should be $\geq 5$ cm $H_2O$ and maintained throughout the utterance.

E. Rib cage and abdominal movements should be cooperative during speech expiration. From relative motion diagrams evaluate: the relative contributions of the rib cage and abdomen (normal patients typically displace volume using both the rib cage and abdomen with rib cage displacement predominating; relative contributions of the rib cage and abdomen will vary, however, from patient to patient and as a function of lung volume level and utterance loudness); slope of utterance tracings (slope should be relatively constant at least for expiratory limbs not involving extreme lung volume excursions); and mechanical efficiency of the chest wall. Utterance tracings should be located to the left of the relaxation characteristic, i.e., rib cage size should be larger and the abdomen smaller than during relaxation at a particular lung volume level (Hixon et al, 1976).

F. Evaluate the patient's ability to generate and maintain various positive alveolar pressures. Expect utterances to begin and end at higher lung volume levels as target intensity ($P_S$) level increases. Expect more positive chest wall efforts as vocal intensity increases. Evaluate the patient's ability to produce rapid and brief expiratory muscle efforts associated with linguistic prominence during speech production. In 1985, Weismer provided a review of normal and disordered speech breathing behavior.

## References

Baken RJ, Cavallo SA. Prephonatory chest wall posturing. Folia Phoniatrica 1981; 33:193.

Comroe JH, Forster RE, Dubois AB, Briscoe WA, Carlsen E. The lung: clinical physiology and pulmonary function tests. Chicago: Year Book Medical Publishers, 1962.

Hixon T, Mead J, Goldman M. Dynamics of the chest wall during speech production: function of the thorax, rib cage, diaphragm, and abdomen. J Speech Hear Res 1976; 19:297.

Sawashima M, Honda K. An airway interruption method for estimating expiratory air pressure during phonatin. In: Baer T, Sasaki C, Harris K, eds. Laryngeal function in phonation and respiration. San Diego: College-Hill Press, 1987:439.

Sawashima M, Kiritani S, Sekimoto S, et al. The airway interruption technique for measuring expiratory air pressure during phonation. Ann Bull RILP 1983; 17:23.

Weismer G. Speech breathing: contemporary views and findings. In: Daniloff RG, ed. Speech science. San Diego: College-Hill Press, 1985:47.

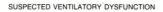

SUSPECTED VENTILATORY DYSFUNCTION

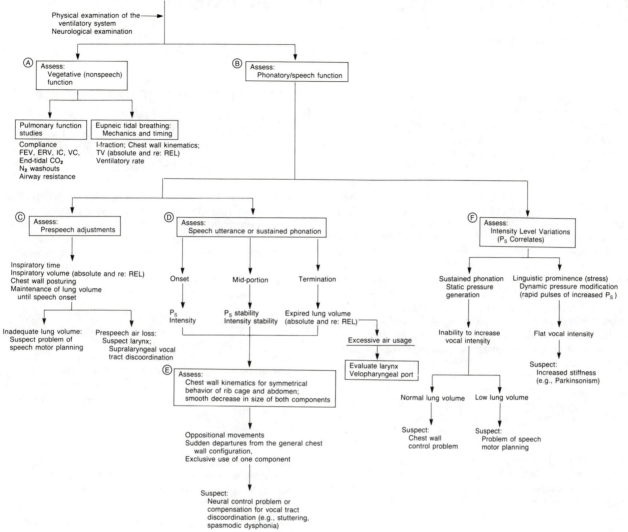

Physical examination of the
ventilatory system
Neurological examination

Ⓐ Assess:
Vegetative (nonspeech)
function

Ⓑ Assess:
Phonatory/speech function

Pulmonary function
studies

Compliance
FEV, ERV, IC, VC,
End-tidal CO$_2$
N$_2$ washouts
Airway resistance

Eupneic tidal breathing:
Mechanics and timing

I-fraction; Chest wall kinematics;
TV (absolute and re: REL)
Ventilatory rate

Ⓒ Assess:
Prespeech adjustments

Inspiratory time
Inspiratory volume (absolute and re: REL)
Chest wall posturing
Maintenance of lung volume
until speech onset

Inadequate lung volume:
Suspect problem of
speech motor planning

Prespeech air loss:
Suspect larynx;
Supralaryngeal vocal
tract discoordination

Ⓓ Assess:
Speech utterance or sustained phonation

Onset

P$_S$
Intensity

Mid-portion

P$_S$ stability
Intensity stability

Termination

Expired lung volume
(absolute and re: REL)

Excessive air usage

Evaluate larynx
Velopharyngeal port

Ⓔ Assess:
Chest wall kinematics for symmetrical
behavior of rib cage and abdomen;
smooth decrease in size of both components

Oppositional movements
Sudden departures from the general chest
wall configuration,
Exclusive use of one component

Suspect:
Neural control problem or
compensation for vocal tract
discoordination (e.g., stuttering,
spasmodic dysphonia)

Ⓕ Assess:
Intensity Level Variations
(P$_S$ Correlates)

Sustained phonation
Static pressure
generation

Linguistic prominence (stress)
Dynamic pressure modification
(rapid pulses of increased P$_S$ )

Inability to increase
vocal intensity

Flat vocal intensity

Suspect:
Increased stiffness
(e.g., Parkinsonism)

Normal lung volume

Suspect:
Chest wall
control problem

Low lung volume

Suspect:
Problem of speech
motor planning

# RESPIRATORY DYSFUNCTION: MANAGEMENT

*Anne H. B. Putnam, Ph.D.*

Management options are presented for vegetative and speech breathing when functional integrity of the chest wall is impaired by acute dysfunction (e.g., crises of poliomyelitis, myasthenia gravis, or Guillain-Barré syndrome), chronic deficit (e.g., paralytic sequelae to spinal cord trauma or disease), or progressive deterioration (e.g., motor neuron disease, multiple sclerosis, tabes dorsalis). Normally, the respiratory system is a slave to the linguistic constraints of connected speech. When the chest wall or one of its component parts is paretic or paralyzed, linguistic utterance is constrained by the limitations of prespeech inspiration (INSP) and available expiratory pressures. Specifically, when inspiratory (INSP) muscles are paretic or paralyzed, INSP gestures may be abnormally prolonged, less efficient, or both. Further, these muscles may be less competent to counteract relaxation pressures in the expiratory direction. When voluntary expiratory (EXP) muscle power is reduced or lost, overall speech loudness, relative loudness contrasts associated with linguistic stress, and breath group durations are limited by available muscular pressure (if any), available relaxation pressure, and/or the duration of the EXP cycle of an external mechanical ventilator on which the speaker may be dependent. In the face of these limitations, speakers tend to be, or may be trained to be, frugal with the air obtained on every INSP gesture. They must rely on laryngeal control of segmental duration and pitch to mark linguistic stress. "Heroic" efforts to minimize air loss at the laryngeal valve may produce a strained-strangled voice quality. Obstruent consonants wasteful of air (voiceless fricatives, affricates, stops) may be shortened, elided, or replaced with glottal stops. Intrautterance pauses may be defined by glottal stops, and pauses for INSP refills between breath groups are more frequent and may occur at linguistically inappropriate places in continuous utterance. Speakers may even adopt a telegraphic utterance form (Hixon et al, 1983; Hixon and Putnam, 1983). Augmentative or alternative communication devices may be necessary speech complements.

References to counseling about the liabilities of chest wall muscle dysfunction in the management charts imply that clinicians must decide if speech breathing behaviors under these conditions are maladaptive and detrimental to socially useful communication, or if they should be instituted as compensatory strategies to maximize communication efficiency. References to (re)training imply management strategies that may include, where available and appropriate, (re)habilitation of INSP and/or EXP muscle power via exercise against resistive airway loads, repeated trials of isocapnic hyperpnea, and/or pursuit tracking of a visible analog of respiratory behavior (e.g., electromyogram, respiratory pressure, or chest wall kinematic pattern)(Gross et al, 1980; Netsell and Daniel, 1979; Rosenbeck and LaPointe, 1985).

## MANAGEMENT OF EXTREME OR PROGRESSIVE CHEST WALL PARESIS OR TOTAL PARALYSIS: OPTIONS FOR VEGETATIVE AND SPEECH BREATHING ASSISTANCE

A. External mechanical INSP devices include pumps that deliver an inflatory positive pressure pulse at an airway opening (mouth; nose; tracheostoma), and tank- or cuirass-style devices that create negative pressure externally around the torso, thereby encouraging it to assume a larger size and inflating the pulmonary apparatus. INSP also may occur via passive recoil from external mechanical compression in the EXP direction (see B, below).

B. External mechanical EXP devices include various chest wall compressors in the form of pneumatic vests, cuffs, or belts that "squeeze" the chest wall (usually the abdominal component) in the EXP direction below the upper level of the functional residual capacity (FRC). Expiration (EXP) also may occur via passive recoil from external mechanical ventilation in the INSP direction above FRC.

C. Both INSP and EXP gestures can be elicited by a rocking bed on which a patient lies supine. Upswing of the bed from horizontal to about 45 degrees encourages footward displacement of the diaphragm and INSP. Downswing to horizontal encourages headward displacement of the diaphragm and EXP.

D. Speech may be produced on the EXP side of any of these mechanically-induced breathing cycles. If the speaker has a patent tracheostomy tube, it must be plugged to route EXP flow through the laryngeal and upper airways. Respiratory pressure for speech production derives from the relaxation pressure associated with passive recoil in the EXP direction following ventilator-assisted INSP or during the downward swing of a rocking bed. When pneumatic chest wall compressors effect EXP, speech may be produced on the pressure generated during the compressive cycle.

E. For individuals who are chronically dependent on an external mechanical ventilator, INSP nevertheless may be accomplished temporarily in a free-breathing mode via elevation of the rib cage using the muscles of the neck and shoulders, glossopharyngeal pumping, or a combination of both (Hixon et al, 1983). EXP in the free-breathing mode occurs via passive recoil and may include speech as long as relaxation pressure is sufficient

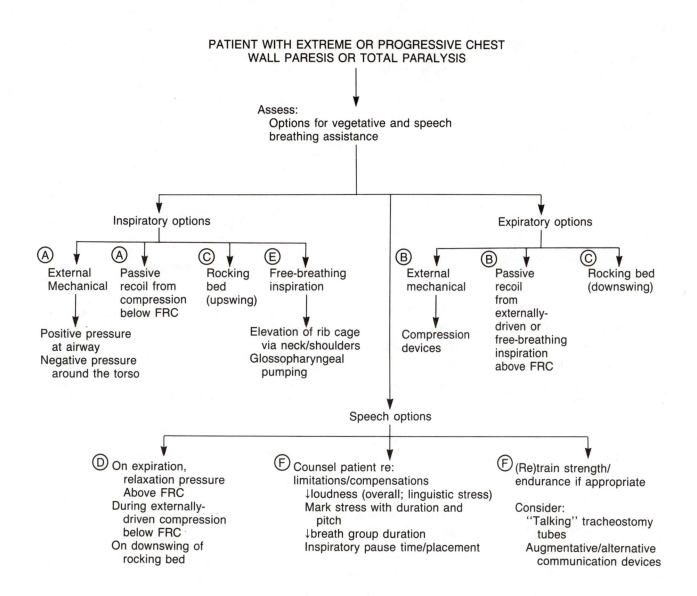

PATIENT WITH EXTREME OR PROGRESSIVE CHEST
WALL PARESIS OR TOTAL PARALYSIS

Assess:
Options for vegetative and speech
breathing assistance

Inspiratory options

Ⓐ External
Mechanical

Positive pressure
at airway
Negative pressure
around the torso

Ⓐ Passive
recoil from
compression
below FRC

Ⓒ Rocking
bed
(upswing)

Ⓔ Free-breathing
inspiration

Elevation of rib cage
via neck/shoulders
Glossopharyngeal
pumping

Expiratory options

Ⓑ External
mechanical

Compression
devices

Ⓑ Passive
recoil
from
externally-
driven or
free-breathing
inspiration
above FRC

Ⓒ Rocking bed
(downswing)

Speech options

Ⓓ On expiration,
relaxation pressure
Above FRC
During externally-
driven compression
below FRC
On downswing of
rocking bed

Ⓕ Counsel patient re:
limitations/compensations
↓loudness (overall; linguistic stress)
Mark stress with duration and
pitch
↓breath group duration
Inspiratory pause time/placement

Ⓕ (Re)train strength/
endurance if appropriate

Consider:
"Talking" tracheostomy
tubes
Augmentative/alternative
communication devices

to support sound production in the larynx and upper airways. Note that a patent tracheostoma precludes successful glossopharyngeal INSP. Also, both methods of temporary free-breathing under conditions of extreme chest wall paresis or total paralysis require functional integrity of laryngeal, lingual, labial, velopharyngeal, and some cervical muscles.

F. Counseling about the limitations imposed by any of these breathing conditions on speech and appropriate compensations is essential. (Re)training respiratory muscle strength-endurance may not be an option unless some component of the chest wall remains functional (e.g., the diaphragm in some quadriplegias [Gross et al, 1980]). For chronic ventilator dependents, consider "talking" tracheostomy tubes and/or the use of augmentative-alternative communication devices to complement speech.

## MANAGEMENT OF CHEST WALL COMPONENT PARESIS OR PARALYSIS: OPTIONS FOR VEGETATIVE AND SPEECH BREATHING ASSISTANCE

G. Abdominal (AB) wall paresis and/or paralysis may result in reduced EXP power, particularly below FRC, and reduced INSP efficiency due to loss of a stable partner against which the diaphragm may work (Hixon and Putnam, 1983; Hixon et al, 1983; Rosenbek and LaPointe, 1985). AB paresis and/or paralysis during INSP may be managed by externally-applied binding or girdling. However, these devices pose medical risks to the user and should be applied only with a physician's approval and scrupulous attention to the details of their use (Rosenbek and LaPointe, 1985). Self support of the AB wall during INSP may be accomplished by the individual who can use the arms to stabilize the anterior wall or hold a pillow against it. One also may lean forward against a fixed support on a wheelchair, desk, or lap board to stabilize the AB during inspiration. During EXP, AB paresis may be complemented by external mechanical compression devices (pneumobelts, vests, or cuffs), arm compression, gradual postural inclination against a fixed support during the expiratory cycle, or the downswing of a rocking bed on which a person lies supine. Counsel the patient and significant others that any activities below FRC (i.e., vital capacity maneuvers, productive coughs, laughter, maximum phonation or speaking tasks, or extended breath group durations in conversation) may be limited, more or less, by AB paresis and/or paralysis. Further, apprise that a weak or flaccid AB wall also may compromise the efficiency of the diaphragm; INSP time may increase, or need to be increased, to maintain adequate ventilation or achieve a pre-speech INSP level adequate to support desired breath group duration. (Re)train strength and endurance as appropriate.

H. Diaphragm (DI) paresis and/or paralysis results in reduced INSP power and efficiency (Hixon and Putnam,

1983; Hixon et al, 1983). When the DI is paretic, its mechanical advantage may be optimized by the supine body position or AB wall stabilization, both of which tend to displace it headward. Its INSP gesture also may be complemented by positive pressure at an airway opening, negative pressure around the torso, the upswing of a rocking bed on which a person lies supine, or elevation of the rib cage via accessory muscles of the neck and shoulders. Counsel the patient about the effects of reduced INSP efficiency on ventilation as well as speech breathing: specifically, reduced potential for EXP recoil force, desired loudness, and normal breath group durations. INSP pause time may be increased or may need to be increased to counteract these effects, and speakers so impaired may need training in the placement of more frequent or longer INSP refill pauses during continuous utterance at linguistically-appropriate places. (Re)train strength and endurance as appropriate (Gross et al, 1980).

I. Rib cage (RC) paresis and/or paralysis may compromise both INSP and EXP gestures, thereby limiting muscular efficiency and power in both directions (Hixon and Putnam, 1983). RC muscle paresis may be complemented during INSP by positive pressure at an airway opening, negative pressure around the torso, the upswing of a rocking bed on which a person lies supine, or elevation of the RC via accessory muscles of the neck and shoulders. During EXP, efforts of paretic RC muscles may be complemented by external mechanical compression via pneumatic devices or the arms (usually applied across the abdominal wall), as well as the downswing of a rocking bed cycle. The liabilities of decreased RC muscle abilities to INSP efficiency and EXP power for breath group durations and loudness in speech are comparable to those already enumerated for DI and AB weaknesses and must be explained to the impaired speaker and relevant listeners (Rosenbek and LaPointe, 1985). Institute or train compensatory strategies, and (re)train strength and/or endurance of muscles where appropriate (Netsell and Daniel, 1979).

## References

Gross D, Ladd HW, Riley EJ, Macklem PT, Grassino A. The effect of training on strength and endurance of the diaphragm in quadriplegia. Am J Med 1980; 68:27.

Hixon TJ, Putnam AHB. Voice disorders in relation to respiratory kinematics. Sem Speech Lang 1983; 4:217.

Hixon TJ, Putnam AHB, Sharp JT. Speech production with flaccid paralysis of the rib cage, diaphragm, and abdomen. J Speech Hear Dis 1983; 48:315.

Netsell R, Daniel B. Dysarthria in adults: physiologic approach to rehabilitation. Arch Phys Med Rehabil 1979; 60:502.

Rosenbek JC, LaPointe LL. The dysarthrias: description, diagnosis and treatment. In: Johns DF, ed. Clinical management of neurogenic communicative disorders. 2nd Ed. Boston: Little, Brown, 1985:97.

PATIENT WITH CHEST WALL COMPONENT PARESIS OR PARALYSIS

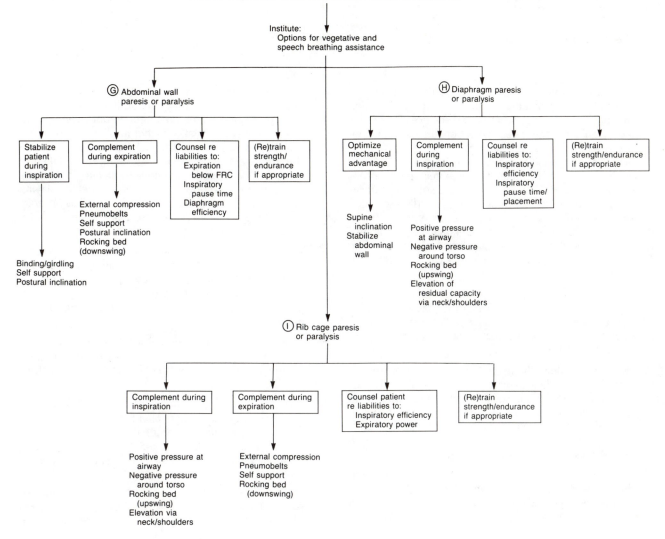

# VOICE: ASSESSMENT

*Celia R. Hooper, Ph.D.*

The assessment of voice is particularly challenging because voice disorders, like other communication disorders, intersect the biophysiologic and behavioral sciences. The voice diagnostician needs the assistance of both the medical community and the client's insightfulness. Often a measurable, physical abnormality exists as a direct or indirect result of psychogenic factors in a chain of cause-effect relationships (Nation and Aram, 1977). Sometimes the voice disorder is a behavioral manifestation of an underlying disease better managed by some other professional, either with or without the ongoing assistance of the speech-language pathologist. Key steps in the decision-making process take place when the speech-language pathologist identifies and describes the client's voice.

A. When the client presents with the complaint of a voice problem, an initial screening history, either oral or written, enables the speech-language pathologist to construct a preliminary hypothesis regarding the causal factors of the presumed disorder.

B. The history allows the referral for laryngoscopic examination to be made with more information. The individual performing the laryngoscopic examination, usually an otolaryngologist, documents the condition of the vocal folds through indirect laryngoscopy. In indirect laryngoscopy the larynx is viewed through a mirror, a right-angle telescope, or flexible fiberoptic nasendoscope.

C. Many clients actually enter the decision tree at this point, having seen the physician first. The speech-language pathologist takes a voice history, such as those described in the voice disorder literature (Boone, 1977; Aronson, 1985) and similar to that described by Johnson in this text (see p 134). One cautionary note regarding the assessment of adult voice disorders: many of these clients may not have had a communication disorder per se and may be more concerned with physical discomfort than with the sound of the voice.

D. Several types of measurement can be used to describe the voice for identification of a disorder or for documentation during treatment. A high-quality calibrated tape recording during all interview and measurement tasks allows the clinician to analyze voice data at a later time. Perceptual observation includes voice profiles or scales and frequency counts of pitch, loudness, and quality behavior. Acoustic measurement of a compact voice sample (see pp 126, 136) can be made from the tape recording. Vocal intensity and vocal fundamental frequency are the two most widely used clinical descriptors and are greatly influenced by the procedures and instrumentation used to collect the data. As for intelligibility measures, computer programs that run on microcomputers, which utilize an analog-to-digital converter for digital records, are available. Average fundamental frequency, jitter, and shimmer measurements are beginning to be taken in clinical voice research. Additionally, electroglottography produces a record of vocal fold contact area displaying time-varying waveforms for analysis as well as observations of the actual vibratory mode of the larynx. Aerodynamic measurement is described on page 122.

E. All of the previous data enable the voice clinician to construct a hypothesis regarding the chain of cause-effect relationships in voice disorders. Several avenues may be taken depending upon the prognosis for change in either the voice behavior or the underlying histological condition.

F. One avenue is further referral if the primary causal or contributing factor is better treated by some other professional, such as a psychologist, otolaryngologist, or neurologist.

G. A decision not to treat the client with traditional voice therapy may be made either after E (hypothesis construction) or after F (further referral). If this option is chosen, the client is either counseled and dismissed or monitored for spontaneous improvement or maintenance before dismissal.

H. A decision to treat a client is always accompanied by repeated reevaluation(s) or voice probes to document the effectiveness of treatment. If a normal voice or acceptable voice is the result, a repeated laryngoscopic examination is recommended before dismissal. If the voice disorder remains, the client may be either reenrolled in voice therapy for a different treatment plan or referred to another professional for alternative or additional management.

## References

Aronson AE. Clinical voice disorders. 2nd ed. New York: Thieme, 1985.

Boone DR. The voice and voice therapy. 2nd ed. Englewood Cliffs, NJ: Prentice Hall, 1977.

Keith RL, Darley FL. Laryngectomee rehabilitation. 2nd ed. Houston: College-Hill Press, 1986.

Nation JE, Aram DM. Diagnosis of speech and language disorders. St Louis: CV Mosby, 1977.

CLIENT PRESENTS WITH VOICE PROBLEM

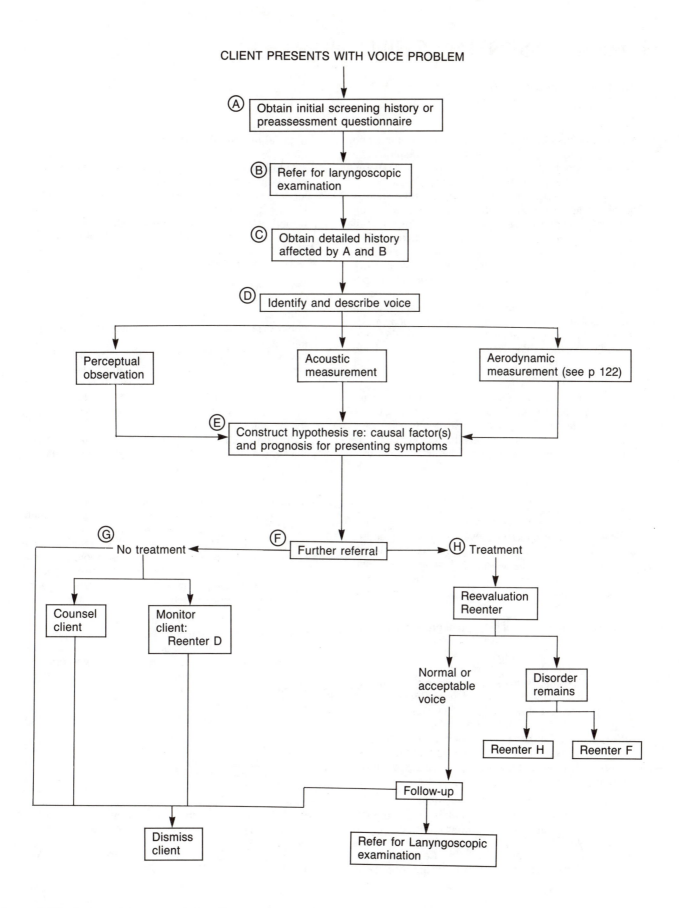

* Client can enter system at A or C.

# HOARSENESS IN THE CHILD

*Thomas S. Johnson, Ph.D.*

A. Vocal roughness in children is a symptom that must be seriously considered. Such symptoms can be indicative of serious medical-physiologic disturbances; however, more often the symptoms are related to simple hyperfunctional vocal behaviors. Pathologic disorders such as vocal nodules, vocal polyps, thickened cords, contact ulcers, polypoid degeneration, and hyperkeratosis may all be due to vocal use, abuse, or misuse behaviors. Childhood hoarseness is a frequently occurring symptom and most of the time is related to transient upper respiratory infection or inflammation. Hence, the initial clinical consideration must be to determine whether the symptoms are chronic and persistent or transient. A useful rule of thumb is that if a child is continually hoarse for 3 weeks, the problem is considered to be persistent and the child should have a medical laryngoscopic examination. If the condition is a benign hyperfunctional problem, a full voice evaluation should be completed.

B. A complete voice evaluation consists of complete case history data, perceptual description and profiling of the voice, respiratory and acoustic measurements of vocal phenomena, determination of possible susceptibility factors, and determination of specific levels of vocal use, abuse, and misuse. The susceptibility factors include potential histologic differences, presence of invading pathogens, vocal conditioning factors, environmental or situational toxicity factors, and the presence of an overlay of some physiologic component (e.g., SICCA). Two critical activities in specifying levels of vocal use, abuse, and misuse include the pinpointing of specific contributing hyperfunctional behaviors and determining high probability time periods in which those behaviors occur. The voice evaluations pulls together all these contributing factors.

C. Continuous monitoring of perceptual profiles and more objective measurements of vocal phenomena are important in tracking clinical progress as clinical intervention proceeds. These data include profile scales (Frank Wilson voice profile, Buffalo voice profiles), respiratory measures (vital capacity, 50-word index, maximum duration of sustained blowing), phonatory measures (maximum phonation time, phonation volume, /s/-/z/ ratio, jitter, shimmer, fundamental frequency), and other appropriate measurement parameters. Currently there is considerable research under way to determine clinically sensitive measures.

D. The susceptibility factors should be treated to the extent possible. One cannot do much about basic tissue histologic differences at this time; however, it is apparent to know that such differences are there because of the wide variation in tissue response to vocal abuse or misuse. Invading pathogens should be treated as appropriate by medical referral. Bacterial pathogens may require antibiotic therapy, and new pharmacologic viral agents are also holding promise. Allergy is also a factor that must be considered. Voice intervention is difficult if active allergies are present. The extent to which vocal conditioning is a factor in the problem should also be considered if there is any indication of extensive change in vocal usage. Other possible environmental-situational and physiologic factors also should be considered with respect to childhood problems.

E. Once the contributing vocal use, abuse, or misuse behaviors have been pinpointed and specific high probability time periods determined as to when those behaviors frequently occur, the clinical intervention program is aimed at gaining behavioral control of those behaviors in each high probability time period in a systematic fashion. A program including self-monitoring of use, abuse, and misuse behaviors has been found to be especially successful with children (VARP program; Johnson, 1985). Once behavioral control is established, the vocal roughness usually diminishes as a result of the reduction or elimination of the vocal nodules, polyps, thickening, contact ulcers, or other hyperfunctional disorders originally caused by vocal use, abuse, or misuse behaviors.

F. Some clients continue to remain hoarse even after the vocal disorder has been reduced or eliminated. A variety of "facilitative approaches" are available that optimize the production of "good" vocal quality. Once the vocal physiology is in optimal condition, these approaches may be used to evoke units of good vocal quality behavior and a progression program employed to generalize the "good" vocal quality behavior.

G. All the components of the voice evaluation should be considered again at the end of the intervention program. The perceptual description-profiles, the respiratory-acoustic measurements, and the laryngoscopic re-evaluation should all show improvement before a client is released from the intervention process.

## References

Boone DR. The voice and voice therapy. Englewood Cliffs: Prentice Hall, 1983.

Johnson TS. VARP: vocal abuse reduction program. San Diego: College Hill Press, 1985.

Johnson TS. Voice disorders: the measurement of clinical progress. In: Costello JM, Holland AL. Handbook of speech and language disorders. San Diego: College-Hill Press, 1986.

Wilson DK. Voice problems of children. 3rd ed. Baltimore: Williams & Wilkins, 1987.

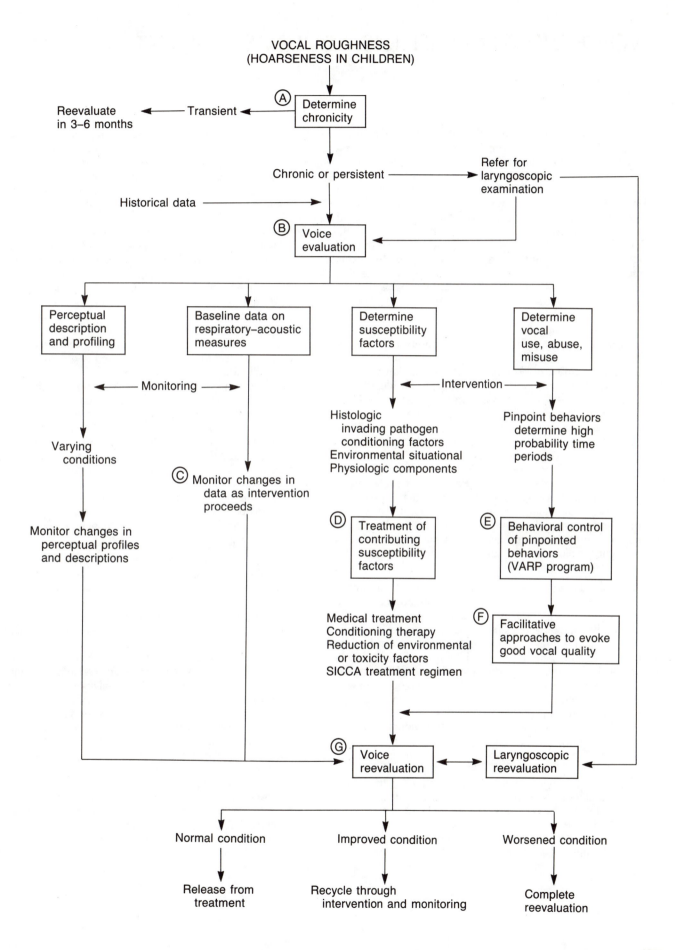

VOCAL ROUGHNESS
(HOARSENESS IN CHILDREN)

Ⓐ Determine chronicity

Reevaluate in 3–6 months ← Transient ←

Chronic or persistent → Refer for laryngoscopic examination

Historical data →

Ⓑ Voice evaluation

Perceptual description and profiling

Baseline data on respiratory–acoustic measures

Determine susceptibility factors

Determine vocal use, abuse, misuse

← Monitoring →

← Intervention →

Varying conditions

Histologic
invading pathogen
conditioning factors
Environmental situational
Physiologic components

Pinpoint behaviors determine high probability time periods

Ⓒ Monitor changes in data as intervention proceeds

Monitor changes in perceptual profiles and descriptions

Ⓓ Treatment of contributing susceptibility factors

Ⓔ Behavioral control of pinpointed behaviors (VARP program)

Medical treatment
Conditioning therapy
Reduction of environmental or toxicity factors
SICCA treatment regimen

Ⓕ Facilitative approaches to evoke good vocal quality

Ⓖ Voice reevaluation ↔ Laryngoscopic reevaluation

Normal condition

Improved condition

Worsened condition

Release from treatment

Recycle through intervention and monitoring

Complete reevaluation

# VOICE DISORDERS IN THE ADULT: ASSESSMENT

*Diane M. Bless, Ph.D.*

A voice disorder may be defined as (1) an alteration in vibratory characteristics of the vocal folds resulting in a psychoacoustic percept that differs from those of other adults of similar age, sex, size, cultural background, and geographic locations, or (2) vocal characteristics that fail to meet an individual's needs (even though in some cases the characteristics may fall within the norms for the individual). Altered vocal characteristics may arise from a large variety of medical, social, psychological, and behavioral problems. The various connections and interrelations among these factors require an interdisciplinary approach and extensive testing by clinicians knowledgeable about both normal and disordered voice production (Aronson, 1985; Boone, 1982; Hirano, 1981; Moore, 1982).

Voice evaluation requires five basic steps: interviewing; observing; describing voice; comparing observations to standards and normal values; and integrating information to determine treatment disposition. All five evaluation steps are done before therapy is initiated, and are not considered completed until a medical diagnosis from an otolaryngologist has been made. The medical diagnosis determines the type and extent of therapy.

Because dysphonia is a broad term covering many voice disorders, their causes, and their symptoms, no single test, value, or measure can provide an accurate diagnosis of the etiologic bases of the dysphonia. Rather, the battery of tests in this chapter is a diagnostic aid, to be used along with the case history, laryngologist's report, physical examination findings, and perceptual judgments of voice production, to design the best treatment program. To consider a technique as a diagnostic aid does not mean that technique must always yield a specific diagnosis.

A. Current status of the individual and presenting complaint are obtained from a case history. Information about the nature of the problem includes: description of the problem, the patient's perception of its onset, duration, and cause; previous treatment if any; medical history; habits; occupation; social and living conditions. The clinician should note the course of the problem (acute, chronic, progressive), whether its onset co-occurred with any identifiable event, associated symptoms (e.g., dysphagia, hearing problems, weakness, breathing difficulties), factors that might place the individual at risk for developing and maintaining a voice disorder (e.g., talking in noisy environments, laryngeal irritants [see Sataloff, 1987, for further discussion]). The clinician should use questionnaires designed for populations with unique characteristics or problems related to voice, such as professional voice users. These various sources of information are used to form hypotheses about the cause or maintenance of the voice problem, the prognosis, and the appropriate treatment.

B. Successful treatment of persons suffering from dysphonia depends upon the ability to assess the type and degree of vocal impairment and to monitor the subsequent progress throughout treatment. This requires use of a standardized battery of subjective and objective voice measures by an experienced speech pathologist, laryngologist, and other team members. A major objective is to describe habitual vocal behavior and the vocal capabilities. Tape recordings are made under three conditions: natural conversational speech, phonatory tasks that test maximum performance and flexibility of phonation, and experimental treatment programs. The experimental treatment tasks differ according to the pathology and phonatory pattern presented. The recordings may be used to make perceptual judgments and acoustic analysis and saved for therapy baseline data. Two baselines of all tasks and measures are obtained to determine individual variability, and to save for comparisons with posttreatment samples. The first baseline is made during the first evaluation, and the second baseline is made at a later time before administration of treatment. The clinician should note the frequency of the problem, the effect of situation variables (person, place) and of specific phonetic contexts, pitches, changes in loudness, duration of problem, severity of problem, and variability over time of day and year. The clinician should model requested tasks to insure that the patient understands them and to help decrease patient anxiety. Three trials should be used to assess reliability of performance.

C. A simple but standardized classification is used to describe vocal quality (Hirano, 1981). With this scale, which is easily learned and used, the clinician rates on a four-point system (0 = normal, 3 = extreme problem) the five voice parameters: grade, rough, asthenic, strained, and breathy. Each parameter is rated individually. Judgments of pitch and loudness are made in relation to the speaking environment and the speaker's age, sex, and size. Observations of speech breathing and maximum sustained phonation times are used to make judgments concerning respiratory-laryngeal coordination, and observations of phonation breaks, prosody, and abnormal resonance are used to make judgments about vocal control. Observe whether voice used for coughing, laughing, crying, or singing differs significantly from speaking voice. Perceptual judgments are used to decide whether a voice problem exists and to provide an indication of inadequate or excessive glottal closure; however, when used alone these judgments are insufficient to provide a differential diagnosis because similar perceptual profiles may have different etiologic bases.

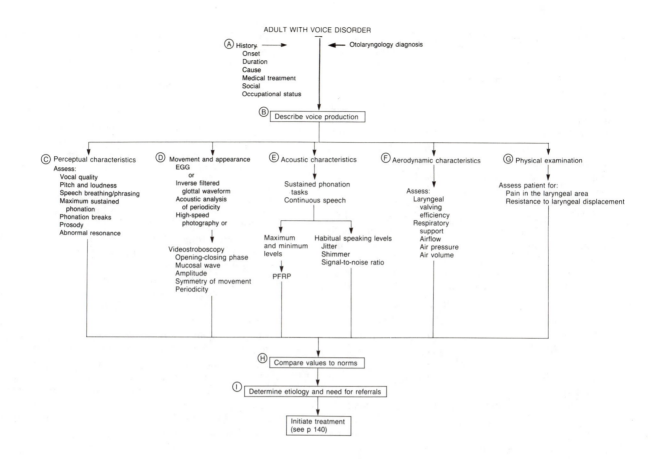

ADULT WITH VOICE DISORDER

(A) History. →                    ← Otolaryngology diagnosis
Onset
Duration
Cause
Medical treatment
Social
Occupational status

(B) Describe voice production

(C) Perceptual characteristics
Assess:
Vocal quality
Pitch and loudness
Speech breathing/phrasing
Maximum sustained
  phonation
Phonation breaks
Prosody
Abnormal resonance

(D) Movement and appearance
EGG
  or
Inverse filtered
  glottal waveform
Acoustic analysis
  of periodicity
High-speed
  photography or

Videostroboscopy
Opening-closing phase
Mucosal wave
Amplitude
Symmetry of movement
Periodicity

(E) Acoustic characteristics

Sustained phonation
  tasks
Continuous speech

Maximum
and minimum
levels

PFRP

Habitual speaking levels
Jitter
Shimmer
Signal-to-noise ratio

(F) Aerodynamic characteristics

Assess:
Laryngeal
  valving
  efficiency
Respiratory
  support
Airflow
Air pressure
Air volume

(G) Physical examination

Assess patient for:
Pain in the laryngeal area
Resistance to laryngeal displacement

(H) Compare values to norms

(I) Determine etiology and need for referrals

Initiate treatment
(see p 140)

D.  Movement may be assessed indirectly by several techniques including electroglottography (EGG), inverse filtered glottal waveform, acoustic analysis of periodicity of waveform, and movement and appearance by high-speed photography and videostroboscopy. These techniques provide information about regularity and closure patterns. The most practical clinical measure of these is videostroboscopy. With videostroboscopy one is able to directly observe the apparent motion of the larynx. Parameters observed include opening-closing phase, mucosal wave, amplitude, symmetry of movement, and periodicity (see Fig. 1).
    Movement is recorded at normal pitch and loudness, at high-pitch and low-pitch productions, and at loud and soft productions, during quiet breathing, and during laryngeal diadochokinesis tasks. In healthy larynges, movement varies in predictable manners with changes in pitch and loudness. As pitch is raised, the vocal folds elongate and become thinner, amplitude, mucosal wave, and closed phase become reduced. As loudness is increased, the vocal folds become shorter and thicker in appearance, amplitude and mucosal wave become larger, and the closed phase is increased. A few representative examples of typical deviations are as follows. With vocal fold edema, amplitude and mucosal wave are reduced. In cases of paralysis, movements depend in part

on the type and degree of paralysis present. On the paralyzed side, vocal fold movement may be irregular and the vertical displacement of the mucosal wave increased because of the flaccid muscle, which renders the body and cover homogenous (for explanation of body-cover and its relation to vibratory characteristics see Hirano and Bless, 1987). A return of a regular mucosal wave is indicative of reinnervation. Bilateral superior laryngeal nerve paralysis is characterized by short closed phase, reduced but clearly present mucosal wave, and reduced amplitude and is frequently accompanied by the clinical complaint of aspiration and an asthenic quality. Bilateral recurrent laryngeal nerve paralysis is rarely seen by speech pathologists, since airway maintenance (not voice) is the primary problem. During hyperfunction of the larynx, the closed phase is increased, and the mucosal wave is reduced; during hypofunction the amplitude is small, the closed phase short, and the mucosal wave small.

E.  Acoustic analysis of voice production permits quantitative analysis of the multidimensional physical characteristics of the voice signal and inference about the underlying physiological mechanism. Acoustic characteristics of the normal voice are age- and sex-dependent. Analysis is completed during sustained phonation tasks and during continuous speech (see Baken, 1986; Fritzell and Fant, 1987; and Hirano, 1981). Physiological frequency range of phonation (PFRP) is determined by having the speaker produce his or her frequency range at maximum and minimum intensity levels. The range is expressed in semitones. The resultant frequencies are plotted against intensities to yield a PFRP or phonetogram (Schutte, 1983). Measures of jitter, shimmer, and signal-to-noise ratio are determined for habitual speaking levels. Information concerning tongue position and resonance characteristics are determined from spectral analysis of sustained vowels. Normal individuals should exhibit an intensity range of 30 dB and a frequency range of at least 24 semitones. Voice treatment is indicated for individuals with reduced vocal ranges, low signal-to-noise ratios, fundamental frequency incompatible with age and sex, inappropriate habitual intensity level, high perturbation scores, inappropriate vocal tract configurations, and inconsistency in performance in what person habitually does versus what he or she is able to do.

F. Airflow, air pressure, and air volume measures are obtained to provide an indication of the laryngeal valving efficiency and respiratory support (see Baken, 1986; and Hirano, 1981). During sustained vowel productions, high airflows are indicative of poor laryngeal valving. Low airflows suggest hyperfunction, obstruction, low effort, or poor respiratory support. Low airflows coupled with a loud voice and normal or high intraoral pressures help rule out poor respiratory support and reduced effort. Similarly high glottal resistance is indicative of excessive closure from the presence of an obstruction; or musculoskeletal tension, stiff structure, and associated compensatory movements; low glottal resistance is indicative of incomplete approximation of the vocal folds.

G. Physical examination includes observation of the larynx and oral facial structures, palpation of the superhyoids, strap muscles, thyroid cartilage and submental musculature, and digital manipulation of the larynx (see Aronson, 1985 and Morrison et al, 1986). In the absence of laryngeal disease, resistance to laryngeal displacement and pain in response to pressure may indicate chronic laryngeal muscle tension.

H. Values obtained from the quantitative and qualitative measures are compared to age- and sex-based norms (Hirano, 1981; Baken, 1987). Normal physiologic alterations with age include: reductions in mean airflow, air pressure, phonation times, signal to noise ratio, maximum performance tasks, vital capacity; changes in the morphological appearance of the larynx; changes in the vocal quality; and increase in dryness of the mucosa resulting in poorer vibratory source. It is impossible to mention here all of the potential dysphonic combinations of normal and abnormal values that are clinically useful, but in general, the clinician should look for results that point to incomplete glottal closure, excessive glottal closure, problems of motor control, or inconsistency

in physiologic use of the mechanism. If results are inconsistent reevaluate the history to exclude psychologic, neurologic, or other medical problems.

I. Diagnoses of voice disorders are used to determine the cause of a voice disorder, the degree and extent of the causative disease, the degree of disturbance in phonatory function, the prognosis, and indications for a therapeutic program (Hirano, 1981). This requires direct input from a laryngologist who provides the medical diagnosis and status of the laryngeal structure; in some cases it may also require input from a neurologist, internist, mental health professional, audiologist, or significant others in the patient's environment in addition to extensive testing of vocal function under a variety of conditions. Determining the prognosis, type and length of therapy program, requires integrating information concerning the degree and severity of the problem, speaker's age, stress, etiology, site and extent of lesion, duration of problem, concomitant medical problems, and motivation. Indications for behavioral management of voice therapy may be as either a primary approach to alleviate the laryngeal pathology, to assist in the adaptation to anomalies that cannot be changed, and to help realize good voice with nonorganic problems, or as a supplementary approach to precede or follow an operation or prothesis in combination with other treatments (e.g., psychological or neurologic). Therapy may include direct management of the vocal symptom, supportive counseling, and vocal hygiene.

# References

Aronson A. Clinical voice disorders. New York: Thieme, 1985.

Baken R. Clinical measurement of speech and voice. San Diego: College Hill Press, 1986.

Boone D. The voice and voice therapy. Englewood Cliffs, NJ: Prentice-Hall, 1982.

Fritzell B, Fant G, eds. Voice acoustics and dysphonia. J Phonet 1986; 14.

Gottfried EL, Wagar EA. Laboratory testing: a practical guide. DM 1983; 29:9.

Hirano M. Clinical examination of voice. New York, Vienna: Springer-Verlag, 1981.

Hirano M, Bless DM. Videostroboscopy of the larynx. San Diego: College Hill Press 1987.

Moore P. Voice disorders. In: Shames GH, Wiig EH, eds. Human communication disorders: an introduction. Columbus: Charles E. Merrill, 1982:141.

Morrison MD, Nichol H, Rammage LA. Diagnostic criteria in functional dysphonia. Laryngoscope 1986; 94:1.

Schutte HK, Seichner W. Recommendations by the Union of the European Phoniatricians (UEP): standardized voice area measurement/phonetography. Folia Phoniatr 1983; 35:286.

Sataloff R. Care of the professional voice. Ear Nose Throat J, Special Issue 1987:66.

Tucker HM. The larynx. New York: Thieme, 1987.

# University of Wisconsin
# STROBOSCOPIC ASSESSMENT OF VOICE

| GLOTTIC CLOSURE | Complete | Posterior | Irregular | Spindle | Anterior | Hourglass | Incomplete |
|---|---|---|---|---|---|---|---|

| | | | | | | | |
|---|---|---|---|---|---|---|---|
| **SUPRAGLOTTIC ACTIVITY** | (0) None | (1) slight compres. of ventricular folds | (2) | (3) | (4) | | (5) Dysphonia plica Ventricularis- VFolds not visible |
| **VERTICAL LEVEL OF VF APPROX IMATION** | (0) Glottic Plane | (1) | (2) | (3) | (4) | | (5) OFF Plane |
| **VOCAL FOLD EDGE** LEFT | (0) Smooth Straight | (1) | (2) | (3) | (4) | | (5) Rough Irregular |
| RIGHT | (0) | (1) | (2) | (3) | (4) | | (5) |
| **AMPLITUDE** LEFT | (0) Normal | (1) Slightly Decreased | (2) Moderately Decreased | (3) Severely Decreased | (4) Barely Perceptable | | (5) No Visible Movement |
| RIGHT | (0) | (1) | (2) | (3) | (4) | | (5) |
| **MUCOSAL WAVE** LEFT | (0) Normal | (1) Slightly Decreased | (2) Moderately Decreased | (3) Severely Decreased | (4) Barely Perceptable | | (5) ABSENT |
| RIGHT | (0) | (1) | (2) | (3) | (4) | | (5) |
| **NON-VIBRATING PORTION** LEFT | (0) None | (1) 20% | (2) 40% | (3) 60% | (4) 80% | | (5) 100% |
| RIGHT | (0) | (1) | (2) | (3) | (4) | | (5) |

| **PHASE CLOSURE** | (−5) (−4) Open Phase Predominates (Whisper dysphonia) | (−3) (−2) | (−1) (0) (1) **Normal** | (2) (3) | (4) (5) Closed Phase Predominates (Glottal fry- extreme hyper adduction) |
|---|---|---|---|---|---|

| | | | | | | |
|---|---|---|---|---|---|---|
| **PHASE SYMMETRY** | (0) regular | (1) irregular during end or begin tasks | (2) irregular during extremes pitch or loud | (3) irregular during 50% + | (4) generally irregular 75% + | (5) always irregular |
| **REGULARITY** | (0) | (1) | (2) | (3) | (4) | (5) |

NAME_____
HOSPITAL ID #_____
DATE _____
COMPLAINT_____
_____
_____
_____
_____
Abuse_____
_____
Allergies_____
Arthritis _____
Aspiration _____
Esophageal reflux_____
Neurological _____
_____
Psychological _____
_____
Thyroid _____
Other health problems_____
_____
_____

**STROBE COMMENTS AND**
**INTERPRETATIONS** _____
_____
_____
_____
_____
_____
_____
_____
_____

**AERODYNAMICS** _____
Flow _____ Volume _____
Pressure_____
**ACOUSTICS**_____
Frequency_____ Intensity _____
**PERCEPTUAL QUALITY**_____
Pitch_____ Loudness_____
Stridor_____ GRBAS_____
Breaks Pitch/Phonation_____
**RECOMMENDATIONS** _____
_____
_____
_____
_____
_____

**Figure 1** Questionnaire for stroboscopic assessment.

# VOICE DISORDERS IN THE ADULT: TREATMENT

*Diane M. Bless, Ph.D.*

A.  Successful treatment depends upon the ability to assess the type and degree of vocal impairment, determine the appropriate treatments, and monitor progress once treatment has been initiated. The first step in treatment is diagnosis. Specific treatment to meet the individual needs of the patient may be initiated once there is medical clearance and the etiology of the disorder has been ascertained. Occasionally, it is necessary to initiate treatment working on the most probable etiology because nothing definitive can be determined. Although there may be recovery in more than one parameter of vocal function, direct symptom management is usually initiated to modify one parameter at a time. A shotgun approach that provides several therapeutic strategies simultaneously may be both confusing and counterproductive. The parameter selected for beginning treatment is usually the problem that appears easiest to treat. Goals of therapy should be agreed upon by patient and clinician. A brief overview of some of the major categories of voice disorders and associated treatment, as they pertain to decision making strategies based on diagnostic laboratory results is given in the following (for a more detailed description of vocal pathologies and treatment see Aronson, 1985; Boone, 1982; Moore, 1982; and Tucker, 1987).

B.  A person with normal voice seeking help generally needs counseling and reassurance that the voice is appropriate for age and sex. Vocal education about factors that affect good vocal function and a referral for voice training to further develop the voice to meet individual social and occupational needs may be helpful.

C.  Laboratory tests at or near normal (Baker, 1986; Fritzell and Fanta, 1987, and Hirano, 1981), loss of upper portions of register, normal appearing larynx or reduced mucosal wave in midmembranous area of vocal folds, musculoskeletal tension, history of vocal abuse, high normal habitual intensity, and low normal habitual frequency are symptoms of dysphonia caused by vocal abuse. Vocal abuse is managed with vocal hygiene and direct symptom management. Vocal hygiene is aimed at reducing or eliminating factors that may affect laryngeal physiology (e.g., abusive use of voice, laryngeal irritants, dehydrating drugs or chemicals, and high-risk enviromental situations such as noise and smoky bars). Referrals for medical management of contributing factors such as allergies and for singing lessons for problems with singing techniques may be indicated. If patient is responsive to treatment, change may be noted within 2 weeks. If there are no other concomitant problems, treatment is rarely needed beyond 8 weeks.

D.  Reduction in vocal fold approximation includes vocal fold paralysis and hypofunctionally based disorders. Diagnostic indicators of reduced vocal fold closure include high airflow, short or absent closed phase, low signal-to-noise ratio, reduced intensity range, short maximum phonation duration, and breathy quality. Adduc-tion and respiratory coordination exercises may be initiated. If no change can be measured or benefits are minimal, suggest supplementing adduction exercises with amplification and referral back to laryngologist to determine if patient is a good candidate for a medialization procedure. Patients with central nervous system diseases are resistant to treatment.

E.  Musculoskeletal tension dysphonia is typically seen in a younger to middle-aged person who uses the voice extensively. External features indicative of muscle tension dysphonia include visible and palpable muscular tension around the larynx, which is most easily assessed by palpating the suprahyoid muscles. At rest, the fingers sink into the mandibular arch from below, but on phonation the muscles (digastric, mylohyoid, geniohyoid) tighten increasingly with elevation in pitch. The tightness is accompanied by an observable elevation of the larynx, with jutting forward of the chin, and a large posterior glottic chink accompanied by a breathy and rough vocal quality. Laboratory tests of vocal function may be at or near normal. (see Morrison et al, 1986 for complete description) Initiate tension reduction exercises and vocal hygiene program.

F.  If onset is acute and associated with a traumatic event, if patient appears to be getting secondary gain from voice problem, if voice production is inconsistent with non-speech phonatory tasks such as coughing and humming, or if vocal folds vibrate normally during some of test tasks, consider loss secondary to psychological stress or trauma or faulty learning. Work directly on the symptom, provide support, and refer to a psychiatrist or counselor as indicated.

G.  When the presenting dysphonia is secondary to medical problems such as esophageal reflux or sinus infection, a medical referral is indicated. Initiation of voice treatment should be deferred until the medical problem has been remedied or is no longer a major precipitating factor. If the voice problem persists, direct management of the vocal symptoms is indicated.

H.  Dysphonia secondary to hearing impairment may be exhibited as a hypo- or hyperfunctional disorder. The type and severity of hearing loss and how it has been managed will to a large part determine the presenting voice symptoms. Direct management of the vocal symptoms using visual feedback is indicated. If other hearing-impaired persons are in the speaker's environment and vocal fold edema or other tissue changes in the larynx are present, vocal hygiene programs and amplification may be needed to help reduce vocal abuse and irritation to the larynx.

I.  Dysphonias secondary to neurologic disease are complex, rarely are limited to laryngeal involvement in isolation, and are resistant to treatment (for description of symptoms and suggested treatments see Aronson, 1985).

ADULT WITH VOICE DISORDER

Assessment (p 136)

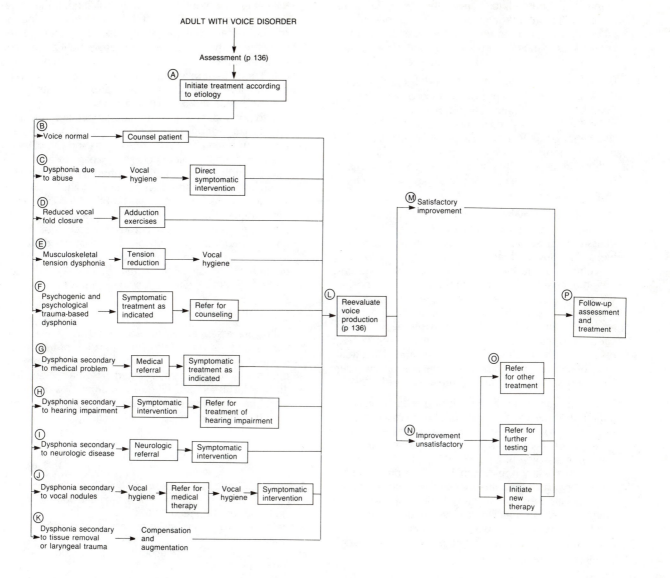

Ⓐ Initiate treatment according to etiology

Ⓑ Voice normal — Counsel patient

Ⓒ Dysphonia due to abuse → Vocal hygiene → Direct symptomatic intervention

Ⓓ Reduced vocal fold closure → Adduction exercises

Ⓔ Musculoskeletal tension dysphonia → Tension reduction → Vocal hygiene

Ⓕ Psychogenic and psychological trauma-based dysphonia → Symptomatic treatment as indicated → Refer for counseling

Ⓖ Dysphonia secondary to medical problem → Medical referral → Symptomatic treatment as indicated

Ⓗ Dysphonia secondary to hearing impairment → Symptomatic intervention → Refer for treatment of hearing impairment

Ⓘ Dysphonia secondary to neurologic disease → Neurologic referral → Symptomatic intervention

Ⓙ Dysphonia secondary to vocal nodules → Vocal hygiene → Refer for medical therapy → Vocal hygiene → Symptomatic intervention

Ⓚ Dysphonia secondary to tissue removal or laryngeal trauma → Compensation and augmentation

Ⓛ Reevaluate voice production (p 136)

Ⓜ Satisfactory improvement

Ⓝ Improvement unsatisfactory

Ⓞ Refer for other treatment

Refer for further testing

Initiate new therapy

Ⓟ Follow-up assessment and treatment

The goal of therapy may be to maintain voice rather than to return it to normal, to decrease the speed of deterioration, or to provide augmentative vocal-speech aids when phonation is impossible. Successful treatment generally demands intensive and vigilant therapy. Therapy should be coordinated with other treatment.

J. It is presumed in cases of vocal nodules and selected cases of vocal fold polyps that programs of vocal hygiene combined with symptomatic intervention of excessive musculoskeletal tension and loudness or other vocal abusive behaviors will correct the problem, that voice will return to normal, and the nodules will be eliminated. If the nodules and dysphonia persist after 6 weeks of voice therapy from a cooperative patient, medical treatment may be indicated.

K. Voice therapy may be used as a primary rehabilitation technique for dysphonias resulting from surgical removal of tissue because of carcinoma, papillomas, or laryngeal webs. Therapy is directed at teaching compensatory movements to produce the most audible voice of best possible quality. Structural limitations make normal voice unfeasible in most cases. Alternate sources of vibration including the ventricular folds, arytenoids, epiglottis, and artificial larynges may be indicated. Laboratory tests are important for measuring change resulting from treatment. Symptoms exhibited and treatment objectives depend on the shape, tension, size, surface, and speaker's control of the vocal folds.

L. Voice is reevaluated at the conclusion of each treatment paradigm to determine if there has been satisfactory improvement. Minimal tests should include baseline comparisons of aerodynamic, acoustic, and perceptual measures. If voice problems persist, additional testing may be necessary (see A-H, p 136). If improvement is satisfactory, patient may be dismissed from treatment and seen for follow-up examinations. When improvement is unsatisfactory, the clinician attempts to determine the reason for failure to improve and either initiates new therapy or refers to other health care professionals for additional testing or treatment.

M. Measurement of success of treatment is determined from changes in vocal function, knowledge of voice, reduction in pathology or dysphonia, or patient satisfaction (Fig. 1). Criteria for measurement of success and termination of treatment are determined during the initial therapy session. Success criteria are based upon knowledge of anatomy and potential for change through treatment.

N. When no measurable change is observed or patient is dissatisfied with results, progress is considered unsatisfactory. If improvement is unsatisfactory, suspect that inappropriate treatment or instructions have been provided, patient is unmotivated or unable to follow the treatment regimen, patient and clinician goals are mismatched, or there may be a concomitant medical problem needing to be resolved.

O. If the voice problem is resistant to treatment because of a concomitant medical or psychological problem, refer the patient for other treatment as indicated. If the voice problem has been successfully treated but medical or psychological problems persist, refer the patient to appropriate counseling or medical management as needed.

If treatment is successful and patient is to be terminated from therapy, refer the patient back to the otolaryngologist for laryngoscopic examination. If treatment is not successful and the reason for lack of success is not due to poor patient motivation or cooperation, or to inappropriate administration of behavioral management techniques, refer for further testing as indicated.

If the voice problem persists and prognosis is favorable for further change, initiate a new therapy program to treat another disordered parameter. The parameter selected for treatment is again based on the clinician's best judgment as to what will be the easiest to modify. If treatment is unsuccessful because the technique selected was inappropriate, initiate new treatment designed to accomplish the same objective. If after a period of no treatment the voice has regressed, initiate a therapy review. Continue with therapy and follow-up until optimal voice for the speaker and his or her mechanism has been maintained.

P. Follow-up assessments are scheduled for 2 weeks, 6 weeks, and 6 months following cessation of treatment. If the voice is normal, the patient is terminated from the program. If the voice has regressed, a review therapy program is instituted and follow-up is done on a more frequent basis until the target voice is maintained to both the clinician's and patient's satisfaction.

# References

Aronson A. Clinical voice disorders. New York: Thieme, 1985.

Baken R. Clinical measurement of speech and voice. San Diego: College Hill Press 1986.

Boone D. The voice and voice therapy. Englewood Cliffs NJ: Prentice-Hall, 1982.

Fritzell B, Fant G, eds. Voice acoustics and dysphonia. J Phonet 1987; 14.

Hirano M. Clinical examination of voice. New York: Springer-Verlag Wien, 1981.

Hirano M, Bless DM. Videostroboscopy of the larynx. San Diego: College Hill Press, 1987.

Moore P. Voice disorders. In: Shames GH, Wiig EH, eds. Human communication disorders: an introduction. Columbus: Charles E Merrill, 1982: 141.

Morrison MD, Nichol H, Rammage LA. Diagnostic criteria in functional dysphonia. Laryngoscope 1986; 94:1.

Tucker HM. The larynx. New York: Thieme, 1987.

# MEASUREMENT OF SUCCESS OF TREATMENT

ELIMINATION OF
  DISORDER _____

BEHAVIORAL
  Normal voice _____
  Improved quality _____
  Pitch improved _____
  Loudness improved _____
  Tension reduced _____

PERCEPTUAL
  Auditory
    voice improved on any
    parameter _____
  Visual
    vibration improved on
    any parameter _____
  Effort level reduced _____
  Patient accepts voice _____

AERODYNAMIC
  Decreased airflow _____
  Increased airflow _____
  Change in $R_G$ _____
  Increase in V _____
  Increased control _____

ACOUSTIC
  Frequency range increased _____
  Habitual frequency age-sex appropriate _____
  Intensity range increased _____
  Habitual intensity situation appropriate _____
  Jitter decreased _____
  Shimmer decreased _____
  SNR increased _____

VOICE EDUCATION
  Know how to best use voice _____
  Know voice limitations _____
  Know how to avoid voice problems _____

**Figure 1** Sample form for measuring success of treatment.

# PROSODY IN THE YOUNG CHILD

*Raymond D. Kent, Ph.D.*

A. Prosodic disorder may be related to insufficiencies in respiratory or laryngeal function, so it is important to exclude impairments in respiratory and phonatory support. Maximal function tests are one means of assessment, but other tests are needed to identify limitations in dynamic function. The vocal control prerequisites for prosody include loudness variation, adequate duration of phonation (for prolonged vowels or repeated syllables), appropriate pitch level, pitch variation, and acceptable voice quality. Insufficiencies or abnormalities in these phonatory dimensions should be ruled out before further assessments of prosodic function are attempted.

B. The evaluation of prosody requires multisyllabic productions. If the client cannot produce accurately the number of syllables in modeled patterns, the target pattern of prosody for a particular syllabic sequence cannot be assessed. This issue is especially important for the severely disordered child who cannot produce multisyllabic patterns fluently.

C. If the child cannot match the syllable number correctly, it is appropriate to test for auditory sequencing ability and/or to train for accuracy in reproducing syllable number. One training procedure is to pair syllable production to an accompanying motor task (e.g., finger tapping or foot tapping) or to a set of objects or pictures (so that the client can produce each syllable as he or she points to the associated object or picture). The accompanying task can be faded if performance improves satisfactorily.

D. As in (C), the vocal response can be paired with a gesture or a visual cue. Such pairing often facilitates sequencing or syllable "flow." In addition, visual cues can be used to symbolize the desired stress pattern; large objects or pictures can be paired with heavy stress and small objects or pictures can be paired with light stress.

E. Severe articulatory impairment may interfere with prosodic features, so an effort should be made to identify any phonetic elements that the client can produce fluently and correctly. To avoid articulatory interference in prosodic assessment, humming or reiterant speech can be used. With humming, the object is to determine if the client can reproduce the cadence, tempo, "melody," or stress pattern of a modeled utterance. Reiterant speech substitutes a recurring syllable, e.g., /ma/, for the phonetically varied syllables of normal speech (Liberman and Streeter, 1978; Nakatani and Shaffer, 1978). A reiterant speech version of "Twinkle, twinkle, little star" is BA ba BA ba BA ba BA, where the upper case letters denote syllables with heavy stress. Reiterant speech should be formed of syllables that are within the child's articulatory competence. The syllables /ma/ and /ba/ are good choices for most children.

F. Use speech materials appropriate for the language development of the child. Even simple expressions such as "bye bye" and "stop that!" can be useful to assess prosodic variation. Age-appropriate materials can be selected for informal assessment. Games offer many opportunities for prosodic variation. If necessary, stress variations can be introduced in sentences of no more than two to three syllables, e.g., "Stop that DOG," "STOP that dog," "Stop THAT dog."

G. Perceptual description may suffice for most needs, but instrumental assessment offers advantages of quantification. Whenever possible, measures should be made of speaking rate; fundamental frequency range, mean and distribution; mean level and range of intensity; and distribution of syllable durations. Stress patterns should be evaluated for different levels of vocal effort and lung volume, whispered and voiced speech, different pitch levels, and different speaking rates.

For general discussions of prosody—its development, description, and role in language—see Allen and Hawkins (1980), Cohen and t'Hart (1982), and Crystal (1973).

## References

Allen GD, Hawkins S. Phonological rhythm: definition and development. In: Yeni-Komshian GH, Kavanagh JF, Ferguson CA, eds. Child phonology. Vol. 1. Production. New York: Academic Press, 1980.

Cohen A, Collier R, t'Hart J. Declination: construct or intrinsic feature of speech pitch? Phonetica 1982; 39:254.

Crystal D. Non-segmental phonology in language acquisition: a review of the issues. Lingua 1973; 32:1.

Liberman MY, Streeter LA. Use of nonsense-syllable mimicry in the study of prosodic phenomena. Acoust Soc Am 1978; 63:231.

Nakatani LH, Shaffer JA. "Hearing" words without words: prosodic cues for word perception. Acoust Soc Am 1978; 63:234.

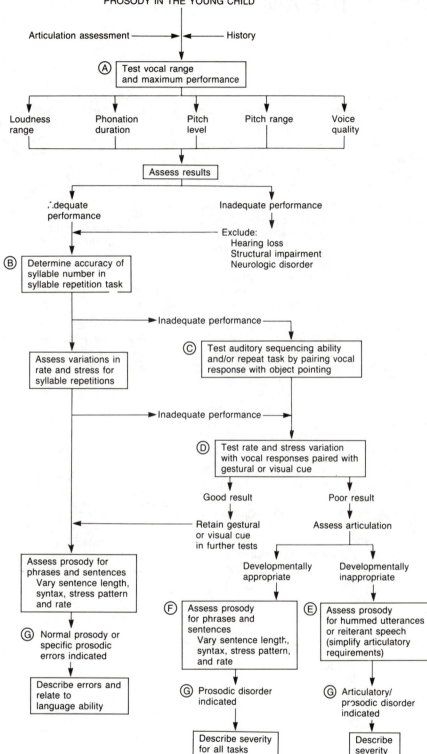

PROSODY IN THE YOUNG CHILD

Articulation assessment ⟶ ⟵ History

Ⓐ Test vocal range and maximum performance

Loudness range | Phonation duration | Pitch level | Pitch range | Voice quality

Assess results

Adequate performance

Inadequate performance

Exclude:
Hearing loss
Structural impairment
Neurologic disorder

Ⓑ Determine accuracy of syllable number in syllable repetition task

Inadequate performance

Assess variations in rate and stress for syllable repetitions

Ⓒ Test auditory sequencing ability and/or repeat task by pairing vocal response with object pointing

Inadequate performance

Ⓓ Test rate and stress variation with vocal responses paired with gestural or visual cue

Good result

Poor result

Retain gestural or visual cue in further tests

Assess articulation

Assess prosody for phrases and sentences
Vary sentence length, syntax, stress pattern and rate

Developmentally appropriate

Developmentally inappropriate

Ⓖ Normal prosody or specific prosodic errors indicated

Ⓕ Assess prosody for phrases and sentences
Vary sentence length, syntax, stress pattern, and rate

Ⓔ Assess prosody for hummed utterances or reiterant speech (simplify articulatory requirements)

Describe errors and relate to language ability

Ⓖ Prosodic disorder indicated

Ⓖ Articulatory/prosodic disorder indicated

Describe severity for all tasks

Describe severity

# PROSODY IN THE ADULT

*Kathryn M. Yorkston, Ph.D.*

The prosodic or melodic aspects of speech include suprasegmental features of stress patterning, intonation, rate, and rhythm.

A.  Because prosodic patterning is used to signal meaning (e.g., declarative vs. interrogative or most prominent word in an utterance) the clinician needs to confirm that speakers understand the meaning that they are to convey.

B.  The breath group theory of intonation (Lieberman, 1967) suggests that words are grouped into units based on breath groups. The breath groups are then marked for intonation and stress. Since respiratory support for speech is a problem for many individuals with neurologic disorders, the clinician must identify the habitual and maximal breath group units produced by the speaker and assess prosodic patterning both within and across these breath group units.

C.  Minimization is the flattening of fundamental frequency and intensity contours seen in parkinsonian speakers and in some individuals with right hemisphere damage (Kent and Rosenbek, 1982). For some parkinsonian speakers with excessively rapid speaking rates, rate control is an effective strategy to encourage more appropriate prosody. For individuals for whom speaking rate is appropriate, training involves heightening the relationship between the meaning and production of an utterance.

D.  An excess-and-equal prosodic pattern is one in which all syllables within an utterance are produced with effort; thus, none stand out as prominent with respect to the others. This is often the case in patients with ataxic dysarthria (Darley et al, 1975). If the speaker is unable to accurately signal stress, treatment involves identifying the suprasegmental features that the speaker can control. If the speaker accurately signals stress but does so

in a bizarre manner, assessment involves identifying the factors that contribute to bizarreness. Training typically involves reducing excessive fundamental frequency and intensity adjustments and increased use of durational adjustment, such as vowel prolongation and pausing (Yorkston et al, 1984).

E.  Monopatterning is characterized by an excessively regular pattern across breath groups. For example, in some mildly ataxic individuals, breath groups may be short and equal in duration each with a similar falling fundamental frequency pattern.

F.  For some dysarthric individuals, respiratory support may be the limiting factor in phrasing. For these speakers, training focuses on increasing respiratory support for speech.

G.  For other speakers, their habitual breath group is shorter than their respiratory control would allow. For these individuals training involves varying the breath group length to coincide with the grammar and meaning of the utterance.

## References

Darley F, Aronson A, Brown J. Motor speech disorders. Philadelphia: WB Saunders, 1975.

Kent R, Rosenbek J. Prosodic disturbance and neurogenic lesions. Brain and Language 1982; 15:259.

Lieberman P. Intonation, perception and language. Cambridge, MA: The MIT Press, 1967.

Yorkston KM, Beukelman DR, Minifie FD, Sapir S. Assessment of stress patterning. In: McNeil MR, Rosenbek JC, Aronson AE, eds. The dysarthrias: physiology, acoustics, perception, and management. San Diego: College-Hill Press, 1984:131.

PATIENT WITH PROSODY DISORDER

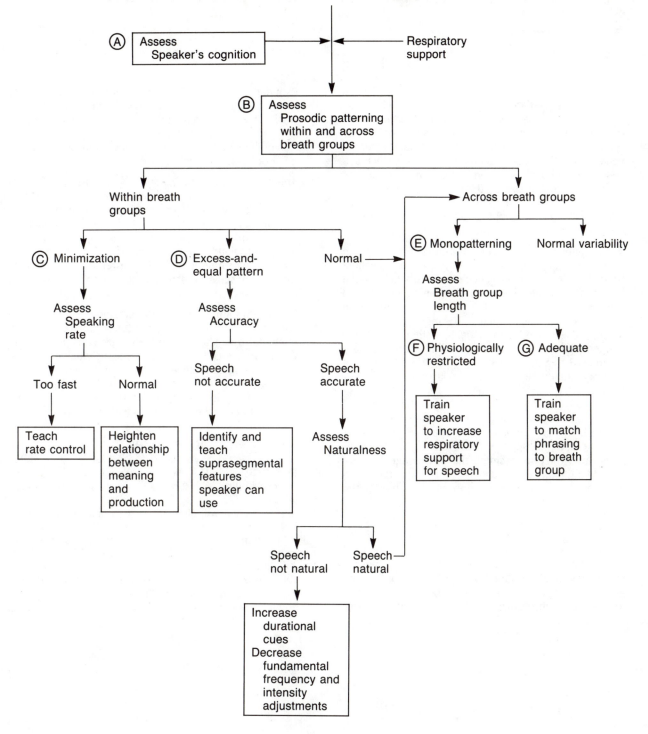

# SPEECH MANAGEMENT IN THE ALARYNGEAL PATIENT

*Bernd Weinberg, Ph.D.*

A. The term speech management is used to emphasize that a fundamental rehabilitation objective following total laryngectomy is the restoration of oral communication or speech (Weinberg, 1983). Speech management is not synonymous with voice restoration, although human voice production is an essential part of the speech act. Treatment approaches that equivocate voice restoration with restoration of speech (Hamaker and Singer et al, 1985; Singer and Blom, 1981) serve to oversimplify the total rehabilitation sought for all laryngectomized patients, i.e., restoration of oral communication.

B. Three major approaches are used to restore speech in alaryngeal patients: teaching the laryngectomized patient (1) to speak with the assistance of a prosthetic artificial larynx or voicing source, (2) to develop esophageal speech, and/or (3) to develop speech with some form of surgical-prosthetic assistance. The most common form of speech developed with surgical-prosthetic assistance is tracheoesophageal speech. The three contemporary approaches to restoring speech for the alaryngeal patient are not mutually exclusive. A given laryngectomized patient may have speech restored by one or all of these methods. For example, the use of a prosthetic artificial larynx by an alaryngeal patient does not preclude or diminish the likelihood of developing esophageal or tracheoesophageal speech. The reverse of this statement is also true. The point is simply that three, mutually complementary, rather than mutually competing or contradictory, forms of speech restoration are available for the alaryngeal patient.

C. Some laryngectomized patients fail to develop satisfactory voicing skills following total laryngectomy and a period of therapy directed to achieve standard esophageal speech; Reexaminations designed to uncover the reasons for this failure are required, and consideration may be given to surgical modification of the voicing source, (e.g., selective myotomy) and/or to completing tracheo-esophageal puncture as a secondary procedure. Some patients fail to develop satisfactory voicing skills following tracheoesophageal puncture; reexaminations are required, and consideration is given to surgical modification of the voicing source (e.g., selective myotomy) if this has not been considered or completed.

D. The return path following selective myotomy indicates that surgical modification of the voicing source in the form of selective myotomy may be considered when a standard esophageal speaker fails to develop satisfactory voicing skills following a period of therapy (Chodosh et al, 1984). Following such modification, the speech management plan for this patient returns to the voice restoration stage of esophageal speech management process.

E. The return path following tracheoesophageal puncture with or without selective myotomy emphasizes that tracheoesophageal puncture may be considered as a secondary procedure and remedial alternative to standard esophageal voice restoration failure. In this circumstance, it is necessary to return to the initial phase of speech restoration management, since this patient must proceed through the entire management tree once again.

## References

Chodosh P, Giancarlo H, Goldstein J. Pharyngeal myotomy for voice rehabilitation post laryngectomy. Laryngoscope 1984; 94:52.

Hamaker RC, Singer MI, Blom ED. Primary voice restoration at laryngectomy. Arch Otolaryngol 1985; III:182.

Singer MI, Blom ED. Selective myotomy for voice restoration after total laryngectomy. Arch Otolaryngol 1981; 107:670.

Weinberg B. Voice and speech restoration following total laryngectomy. In: Perkins WH, ed. Current therapy for communication disorders: voice disorders, New York: Thieme-Stratton, 1983.

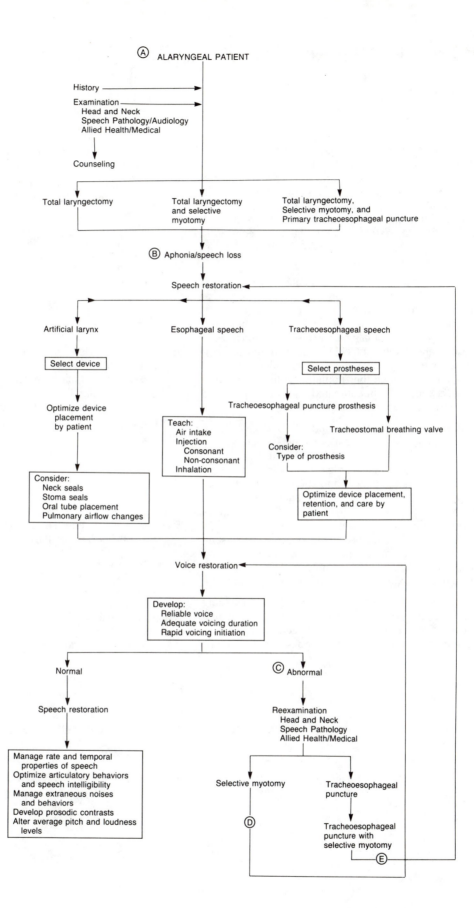

Ⓐ ALARYNGEAL PATIENT

History ⟶

Examination ⟶
  Head and Neck
  Speech Pathology/Audiology
  Allied Health/Medical

Counseling

Total laryngectomy

Total laryngectomy
and selective
myotomy

Total laryngectomy,
Selective myotomy, and
Primary tracheoesophageal puncture

Ⓑ Aphonia/speech loss

Speech restoration

Artificial larynx

Esophageal speech

Tracheoesophageal speech

Select device

Select prostheses

Optimize device
placement
by patient

Tracheoesophageal puncture prosthesis

Tracheostomal breathing valve

Teach:
  Air intake
  Injection
    Consonant
    Non-consonant
  Inhalation

Consider:
Type of prosthesis

Consider:
  Neck seals
  Stoma seals
  Oral tube placement
  Pulmonary airflow changes

Optimize device placement,
retention, and care by
patient

Voice restoration

Develop:
  Reliable voice
  Adequate voicing duration
  Rapid voicing initiation

Normal

Ⓒ Abnormal

Speech restoration

Reexamination
  Head and Neck
  Speech Pathology
  Allied Health/Medical

Manage rate and temporal
  properties of speech
Optimize articulatory behaviors
  and speech intelligibility
Manage extraneous noises
  and behaviors
Develop prosodic contrasts
Alter average pitch and loudness
  levels

Selective myotomy

Tracheoesophageal
puncture

Ⓓ

Tracheoesophageal
puncture with
selective myotomy

Ⓔ

# VELOPHARYNGEAL DYSFUNCTION

*Ronald Netsell, Ph.D.*

Velopharyngeal dysfunction (VPD) during speech results from a variety of causes including: cleft palate, other craniofacial syndromes, neurologic disorders, and faulty learning. The severity of VPD can range from mild-moderate (resulting in perceived nasality and, perhaps, nasal "snorts" without affecting speech intelligibility) to moderate-severe (resulting in reduced intelligibility or totally unintelligible speech). VPD can occur in apparent isolation or in combination with dysfunction in other areas of the vocal tract.

A. The speech evaluation includes an auditory-perceptual estimate of the presence and severity of VPD. The peroral examination may reveal a maxillary or submucous cleft, velar clefting, large tonsils, velopharyngeal asymmetries, or other visible abnormalities. The history should include the onset and duration of VPD, an account of any previous treatment, and a statement of the patient's or guardian's concern about the problem. History of hearing disorders should be documented, and hearing should be tested if a problem is suspected.

B. The medical examination should be conducted by an otolaryngologist, a neurologist, and others as appropriate. If the team suspects that the VPD may require treatment, physiologic tests should be ordered. Aerodynamic evaluation determines the pattern and severity of VPD, nasal cavity resistance, and estimates of subglottal air pressure and laryngeal air flow during speech. Videofiberoptics provide information on the pattern and severity of VPD. Midsagittal and frontal cinefluorography is used to visualize the velopharyngeal anatomy and function during speech, including lateral wall movement and the vertical locus of maximal velopharyngeal movement.

C. VPD can result in consistent nasal air escape to varying degrees or an inconsistent pattern of closure in which the patient demonstrates the ability to achieve full closure at some times, but not others. Establishing the pattern and severity of VPD is critical in deciding if treatment is necessary and, if so, the treatment of choice.

D. Most mild cases of VPD are not treated or quicky respond to a period of speech therapy. Most, but not all, moderate-severe cases require prosthetic or surgical management. When the option is available, a trial period with a prosthesis is helpful in predicting the long-term benefit of surgery. In our experience, patients with moderate-severe VPD secondary to neurologic disorder are best treated with a palatal lift prosthesis.

E. Regardless of etiology, patients receiving prosthetic or surgical management require intensive, and sometimes protracted, periods of speech therapy.

F. If the response to treatment is good, these cases need to be followed for a number of years. Whereas there is a reasonable data base on the long-term outcome of pharyngeal flap surgery with cleft palate, the long-term results of prosthetic and surgical procedures with other populations are lacking. When the response to treatment is poor, the patient should be returned to the "treatment decision" level.

## References

Ewanowski SJ, Saxmon JH. Orofacial disorders. In: Hixon TJ, Shriberg LD, Saxmon JH, eds. Introduction to communication disorders. Englewood Cliffs, NJ: Prentice-Hall, 1980.

Johns DF, Salyer KE. Surgical and prosthetic management of neurogenic speech disorders. In: Johns DF, ed. Clinical management of neurogenic communicative disorders. Boston: Little, Brown, 1978: 311.

Netsell R, Rosenbek JC. Treating the dysarthrias. In: Darby JK ed. Speech and language evaluation in neurology: adult disorders. Orlando, FL: Grune & Stratton, 1985: 363.

## VELOPHARYNGEAL DYSFUNCTION

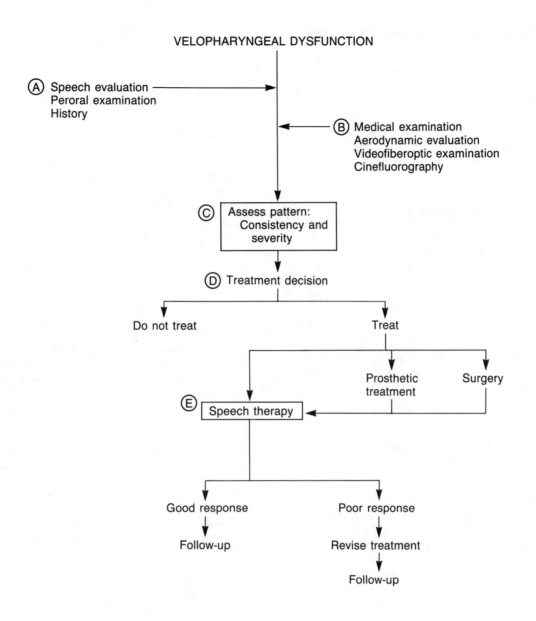

Ⓐ Speech evaluation
Peroral examination
History

Ⓑ Medical examination
Aerodynamic evaluation
Videofiberoptic examination
Cinefluorography

Ⓒ Assess pattern:
Consistency and
severity

Ⓓ Treatment decision

Do not treat          Treat

Prosthetic          Surgery
treatment

Ⓔ Speech therapy

Good response          Poor response

Follow-up          Revise treatment

Follow-up

# CRANIOFACIAL ANOMALIES RELATED TO SPEECH DISORDERS

*Sally J. Peterson-Falzone, Ph.D.*

This decision tree is constructed to accommodate two means of patient ascertainment: (1) presence of a known craniofacial anomaly (CFA) or (2) presence of an articulation or resonance problem leading the speech-language pathologist to suspect such a defect.

A. The majority of craniofacial defects and syndromes directly affect the physical systems of speech and hearing. In addition, intellectual development and psychosocial adjustment often are at risk. Infants and toddlers with known craniofacial defects require early and regular evaluations by the speech-language pathologist who can institute or refer the patient to stimulation programs if development is not age-appropriate.

B. Regardless of age of ascertainment, and often even in cases of extensive previous treatment, the speech-language pathologist should assist the patient and family in determining whether all appropriate medical and allied medical referrals have been made. For example, many families are unaware of the need for regular otolaryngologic care for children with clefts. Others may be unaware of the advisability of a genetic work-up.

C. The traditional dichotomy of "organic" versus "functional" speech problems has become increasingly suspect over recent decades as (1) the development of more sophisticated diagnostic techniques has allowed better exploration of the anatomy and physiology of the speech mechanism in the individual patient, and (2) anatomic dissections in the laboratory have taught us more about variability in structure from specimen to specimen. A classic example of the former was the discovery, chiefly through the use of nasopharyngoscopy, of muscular deficiencies on the nasal surface of the velum in speakers who in earlier times probably would have been given the label of "functional hypernasality" simply because they exhibited no overt cleft or obvious submucous defect (Croft et al, 1978). An example of the latter was the report of Zemlin (1978) of significant interspecimen variation in the lingual musculature responsible for elevation of the lateral margins of the tongue, a finding that he speculated could be responsible for persistent problems in production of consonants requiring such elevation.

D. Children who progress through the speech-learning years with an unrepaired or inadequately repaired craniofacial defect such as a cleft palate often retain certain abnormal speech production patterns even after an intact physical mechanism has been provided. The most common example of this is the persistency of compensatory articulations, such as glottal stops and pharyngeal fricatives (Trost, 1981, for a more complete listing and description).

E. The primary or initial surgical treatment of a craniocial birth defect may not produce the desired result, e.g., a structurally and functionally intact velopharyngeal mechanism following cleft palate repair. The speech-language pathologist evaluating a patient with a "repaired defect" must ascertain whether the physical management (surgical or prosthetic) has in fact accomplished the treatment objective. The task of making this decision is often complicated by the persistence of presurgical speech patterns as mentioned above and the problems that some children and adults have in learning to use a newly adequate mechanism.

F. Anatomic-physiologic defects of the auditory system, larynx, and neuromotor system are frequently seen in congenital craniofacial anomalies, e.g., ear malformations and cranial nerve involvement in hemifacial microsomia, cleft larynx in G syndrome, vocal abuse in cleft palate. Diagnosis and treatment of communication disorders in speakers with craniofacial anomalies requires full assessment of the status of the systems and structures listed, including an estimate of the effect of intellectual function on communication skills. However, discussion of those encased in brackets in the decision tree may be found in other chapters of this book and will not be repeated here.

G. This listing assumes that speech-language pathologists functioning in public schools or other nonmedically based settings will not have access to an armamentarium of sophisticated equipment, and that the initial decisions will be based upon those findings that can be derived with the use of the professional's own eyes, ears, and fingers plus a tongue blade and a small mirror, auditory and language testing notwithstanding. Assessment of phonologic development and articulation skills includes spontaneous speech samples as well as standardized tests. "Screening" procedures for velopharyngeal incompetence (VPI) are rather gross indices, such as checking for fogging on a small mirror held beneath the nose during production of pressure consonants, or the "modified tongue-anchor technique" described by Fox and Johns (1970). The presence of nasal grimacing is not a reliable index of velopharyngeal function, even at this level of assessment, because some speakers persist in such grimacing even when VPI is no longer present and, conversely, many speakers with VPI never show such grimacing.

H. As mentioned above, the presence of compensatory articulations does not necessarily mean that the velopharyngeal mechanism is not intact after physical management. Although an anatomic or physiologic problem *was* present which presumably led to their development (and some other residual structural problem such as a dental malocclusion may still be present), compensatory articulations are learned patterns that typically persist after an intact mechanism has been provided.

I. "Phoneme-specific velopharyngeal inadequacy" refers to the occurrence of nasal emission or posterior nasal frication exclusively on specific consonants, usually the sibilants or sibilants and affricates, with no air loss on the remaining pressure consonants and no hypernasal resonance. This pattern is *not* indicative of true physiologic inadequacy of the velopharyngeal mechanism.

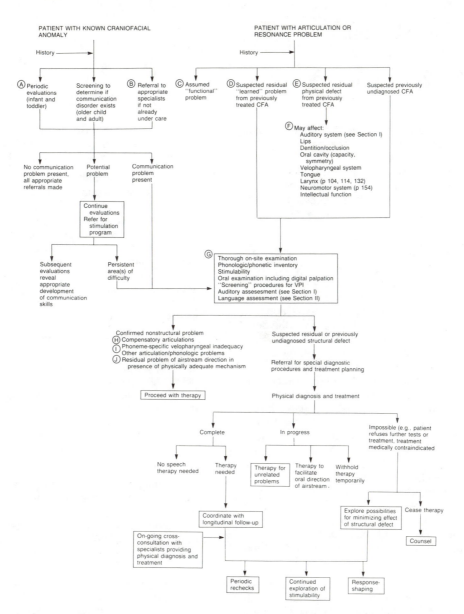

J. Some speakers persist in nasal direction on the airstream, even after an intact velopharyngeal mechanism has been provided. Such speakers are often assisted by the use of simple biofeedback devices, which provide, for example, visual cues that such inappropriate direction of the airstream is taking place. Young children may benefit from the use of simple games that reward appropriate oral direction of the airstream. Such therapy techniques are *not* equivalent to the outdated and unfounded recommendations for various forms of "physical therapy" for the velopharyngeal mechanism such as blowing and sucking exercises, which were formerly believed to strengthen palatal elevation and velopharyngeal closure.

## References

Croft C, Shprintzen R, Daniller A, Lewin M. The occult submucous cleft palate and the musculus uvulae. Cleft Palate J 1978; 15:150.

Fox D, Johns D. Predicting velopharyngeal closure with a modified tongue-anchor technique. J Speech Hear Disord 1970; 35:248.

McWilliams BJ, Morris HL, Shelton RL. Cleft Palate Speech. Toronto: BC Decker, 1984.

Peterson-Falzone S. Articulation disorders in orofacial anomalies. In: Lass N, McReynolds L, Northern J, Yoder D, eds. Speech language, and hearing. Vol II. Philadelphia: WB Saunders, 1982.

Peterson-Falzone S. Resonance disorders in structural defects. In: Lass N, McReynolds L, Northern J. Yoder D, eds. Speech language and hearing. Vol II. Philadelphia: WB Saunders, 1982.

Siegel-Sadewitz V, Shprintzen R. The relationship of communication disorders to syndrome identification. J Speech Hear Disord 1982; 47 (4):338.

Smith DW. Recognizable patterns of human malformation. 3rd ed. Philadelphia: WB Saunders, 1982.

Sparks S. Birth defects and speech-language disorders. San Diego: College-Hill Press, 1984.

Trost JE. Articulatory additions to the classical description of the speech of persons with cleft palate. Cleft Palate J 1981; 18:193.

Zemlin WR. A two-hour time lapse dissection through the respiratory system, the larynx, and articulatory system. Presented before the Seventh Symposium on the Care of the Professional Voice. The Julliard School, New York City, 1978.

# MOTOR SPEECH DISORDERS

*Raymond D. Kent, Ph.D.*
*Jane F. Kent, M.S.*

Dysarthria, dysprosody, apraxia of speech, and oral apraxia comprise the motor speech disorders. These disorders may occur singularly or in combination. The initial clinical objective is to identify the major presenting disorder, but the clinician should be alert to concomitant motor speech impairment; e.g., a dysarthria may partner apraxia of speech. Assessment is complicated by the lack of agreement in the literature on nosology and symptomatology. This problem is particularly serious with apraxia of speech (also known as verbal apraxia). Not all clinicians recognize a syndrome by this name, but regardless of the chosen nosology, the decision tree should serve to distinguish a disorder from a dysarthria and an oral apraxia. Other names for this disorder may be motor aphasia, little Broca's aphasia, phonemic aphasia, or aphemia. Whatever nomenclature is employed, the decisions themselves should constitute a fairly general assessment process. Most descriptions of dysarthria stress the consistency of the motor impairment in both speech and nonspeech tasks; however, the clinician should be aware of some exceptions to the consistency criterion. Oral apraxia affects the performance of nonspeech oral gestures and possibly speech movements as well. Apraxia of speech is an impairment restricted to speech functions and is regarded by different authorities as a motor speech impairment, a phonological impairment, or both. Early descriptions emphasized a predominance of substitution or sequencing errors, but recent studies have shown a variety of "subphonemic" abnormalities (Darley et al, 1975; Rosenbek et al, 1984). Dysprosody may result from: a focal lesion to the right (nondominant) hemisphere, an affective disorder, learning English as a second language, or a motor speech disorder that impairs the rate, rhythm and fluency of speech.

A. Particular attention should be given to indications of neurologic damage or abnormality, or to difficulties with speech and language. If the client is a child, obtaining information on speech and language development, beginning with babbling and early words can be useful (Aram, 1984).

B. A number of standard and nonstandard articulation tests can be used, but tests that sample different places and manners of articulation are especially useful. If the motor impairment is severe, as in the case of unintelligible speech, it may be difficult to assess articulation in anything beyond monosyllables. On the other hand, assessment of apraxia of speech in its milder forms may require difficult or complex speaking tasks. Tests for both dysarthria and apraxia of speech are commercially available, but the enterprising clinician can obtain entirely satisfactory assessments from standard articulation tests supplemented by assessments of articulation in various speaking tasks (Darley et al, 1975; McNeil et al, 1984).

C. Prosodic abnormalities often partner articulatory (segmental) disorders. Their occurrence together can reflect mutual impairment or their nonindependence in speech function. For example, a difficult and labored articulation usually is accompanied by a slow speaking rate and reduced stress contrasts, but these prosodic irregularities may disappear in articulation tasks that are easy for the client (such as reiterated speech, p 144).

D. Performance load variables include phonetic complexity, speaking rate, utterance length, verbal formulation requirements, and word familiarity. These variables may be manipulated singly or in combination to achieve different degrees of performance load. Errors in apraxia of speech are particularly susceptible to performance load variables. One approach to manipulation of performance load is to add prefixes or suffixes to base forms (e.g., jab–jabber––jabbering). It also is useful to compare production of phonetic or syllable targets in monosyllables versus polysyllables.

E. Oral nonverbal gestures include such behaviors as protruding the tongue, pursing the lips, licking the corners of the lips, and maximal openings of the jaw. These behaviors should be evaluated both in isolation and in sequential performance. Nonspeech oral motor tasks are particularly important in the assessment of oral apraxia and dysarthria, for which impairment is likely. The same tasks used to assess oral nonverbal gestures are useful to assess the cranial nerves that innervate the oral structures.

F. Maximum performance tests include measures of maximum duration of vowel phonation, maximum duration of production of [s] versus [z], vital capacity and other ventilatory measures, fundamental frequency range, maximum number of syllables produced on one breath, and maximum diadochokinetic rates. Generally, maximum function tests are most sensitive to reduced strength or capacity. Subnormal performance should alert the clinician to the need for more detailed assessments of structure and function. In addition, subnormal results should be kept in mind in further assessments, and care should be taken that speech samples do not exceed the basic capabilities of the speaker.

G. Dysprosody may result from several different conditions. If dysprosody occurs in isolation, a detailed prosodic assessment should be completed (pp 144, 146). Consideration should be given to respiratory or laryngeal impairment, neuropsychological status, and sociocultural factors.

H. An articulatory disorder in the absence of readily identified motor impairment either may not have a motor basis or the motor impairment is subtle. In either case, a detailed evaluation of articulatory function is in order. Patterns of error should be identified for different tasks (reading, conversation, automatic or reactive speech), and observations should be made of inconsistencies in number and type of errors. Response to intervention should be followed carefully during trial of different intervention strategies.

I. A detailed examination of speech motor function includes, but is not limited to, the tasks mentioned in F

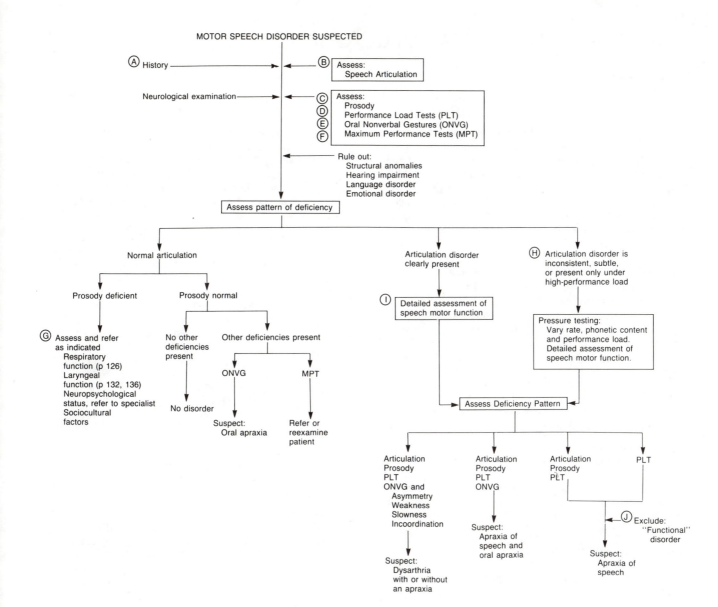

MOTOR SPEECH DISORDER SUSPECTED

(A) History

(B) Assess:
Speech Articulation

Neurological examination

(C) Assess:
(D) Prosody
(E) Performance Load Tests (PLT)
(F) Oral Nonverbal Gestures (ONVG)
Maximum Performance Tests (MPT)

Rule out:
Structural anomalies
Hearing impairment
Language disorder
Emotional disorder

Assess pattern of deficiency

Normal articulation

Prosody deficient

Prosody normal

Articulation disorder
clearly present

(H) Articulation disorder is
inconsistent, subtle,
or present only under
high-performance load

(G) Assess and refer
as indicated
Respiratory
function (p 126)
Laryngeal
function (p 132, 136)
Neuropsychological
status, refer to specialist
Sociocultural
factors

No other
deficiencies
present

Other deficiencies present

(I) Detailed assessment of
speech motor function

Pressure testing:
Vary rate, phonetic content
and performance load.
Detailed assessment of
speech motor function.

ONVG

MPT

No disorder

Suspect:
Oral apraxia

Refer or
reexamine
patient

Assess Deficiency Pattern

Articulation
Prosody
PLT
ONVG and
Asymmetry
Weakness
Slowness
Incoordination

Articulation
Prosody
PLT
ONVG

Articulation
Prosody
PLT

PLT

(J) Exclude:
"Functional"
disorder

Suspect:
Dysarthria
with or without
an apraxia

Suspect:
Apraxia of
speech and
oral apraxia

Suspect:
Apraxia of
speech

and H. The nature of the detailed examination varies with the time available for testing and the resources available to the clinician. Minimally, the clinician should evaluate the major speech subsystems (respiratory, laryngeal, velopharyngeal, and oral articulatory) for symmetry, strength, speed of movement, and coordination. When possible, a speech structure should be tested for range, direction, and speed of movement. It can be informative to examine for rigidity (resistance to passive movement), tremor or other involuntary movement, ability to resist movement on demand (as when pushing against the tongue with a tongue depressor or other object), and ability to perform nonspeech tasks such as bilabial trilling (raspberry), clucking the tongue, panting, or fast repetitive coughing.

J. The so-called "functional" articulation disorders can present a difficult diagnostic challenge and run the risk of becoming a wastebasket category. Strictly speaking, such a disorder has no conceivable structural or motoric basis. As such, the functional disorder can be a default category, i.e., the one that remains after all other possibilities have been excluded. If no evidence can be seen for motor impairment, then the clinician should reevaluate the history, test for stimulability and evaluate the likelihood of faulty learning, dialect, or affective psychiatric disorder.

## References

Aram DM, ed. Assessment and treatment of developmental apraxia. Sem Speech Lang 1984; 5:

Darley FL, Aronson AE, Brown JR. Motor speech disorders. Philadelphia: WB Saunders, 1975.

McNeil MR, Rosenbek JC, Aronson AE, eds. The dysarthrias: physiology, acoustics, perception, management. San Diego: College-Hill, 1984.

Rosenbek JC, McNeil MR, Aronson AE, eds. Apraxia of speech: physiology, acoustics, linguistics, management. San Diego: College-Hill, 1984.

# THE DYSARTHRIC OR APRAXIC CLIENT

*Raymond D. Kent, Ph.D.*

It is impossible to include within one decision-making tree all management strategies that could be considered for the dysarthrias and apraxia of speech. Books could be, and have been, written on this subject (Darley, Aronson et al, 1975; Johns, 1978; McNeil, Rosenbek et al, 1984; Perkins, 1983; Rosenbek, McNeil et al, 1984). However, it is possible to consider the determination of the major management goals for these neurologic speech disorders. Specific treatment procedures vary with the nature of the disorder (e.g., type of dysarthria), severity of the speech disturbance, age of the client, and several other factors. However, other articles in this book present treatments that can be applied to the specific impairments affecting respiration, phonation, and articulation. To set management goals, the clinician should consider the client's history and communicative needs; the results of detailed speech, language, and hearing evaluations; and the results of the neurologic examination. It is particularly important to set management goals and objectives that are consistent with the prognosis for the disorder. For example, very different goals may be established for a client with a stable neurologic condition and for a client who is likely to experience progressive deterioration.

A. The overall plan of management should be defined by social communicative goals, both short term and long term, if appropriate. Relevant considerations include age, educational and vocational status, home environment, and communicative needs (current and future). These factors often can be discussed with the client or with the client's care-giver(s).

B. Global speech goals include improvements in any of the following: intelligibility, rate, quality, prosody, fluency, and loudness (or similar overall characteristics of speech). These goals should be chosen to be consistent with the social communicative goals set in A.

C. Specific management objectives are to be set in three areas: subsystem, phonetic, and sensorimotor. The term "objective" is used here to refer to a narrower aim than that considered within the broader goals established in A and B. The narrower objectives should be consistent with, and are often guided by, the social-communicative and global-speech goals.

D. Speech subsystem objectives should be evaluated for the subsystems illustrated in the tree (Netsell and Daniel, 1979, give some examples of this approach). Objectives can be specified for any subsystem for which abnormal function has been identified. These objectives are coordinated with the phonetic objectives and sensorimotor objectives to be developed in E and F. Subsystems are defined both anatomically and functionally as respiratory, laryngeal, and upper airway.

E. Phonetic objectives are defined in accord with phonetic error patterns or individual phonetic errors. Examples are listed in the tree. Phonetic objectives should be considered relative to the objectives set in D and F.

F. Sensorimotor objectives are defined in terms of motor and sensory variables, such as those listed in the tree. For example, it may be decided (1) to work toward increased strength of a subsystem, (2) to reduce muscle tone in the lips and face, or (3) to promote sensory awareness of an articulatory position or movement. Sensorimotor objectives should be considered relative to the objectives in D and E.

G. Management priorities should be determined by evaluating the objectives defined in D, E, and F relative to the broad social-communicative and global-speech goals set in A and B. For example, it might be judged that a first step toward increasing a client's intelligibility (a speech goal) is to improve the strength, endurance, and timing (motor objectives) of the velopharynx (subsystem) so that nasal-nonnasal consonant distinctions are made (phonetic objective). Particular care should be taken that management objectives in D, E and F are not in conflict at any point in the management plan. For example, a management focus on improving the production of lingual fricatives should be avoided or modified if fricative production causes the client to experience an undesired overflow of tension or effort to another subsystem, thereby by causing speech disruption.

H. Setting priorities for management should recognize factors such as those listed. As an example, the goal of improving velopharyngeal function might be satisfied by prosthetic management.

I. Management of a severe or complex disorder may involve several steps or phases. For instance, improvement of intelligibility in a client with flaccid dysarthria affecting several subsystems might require a management sequence of (1) increasing the strength and endurance of the respiratory system, (2) prosthetic management of the velopharynx, (3) improving the strength and speed of tongue tip movements, (4) developing precision of alveolar consonants in monosyllables, and (5) promoting fluent production of phonetic sequences in which manner variations occur for sounds that share alveolar articulation.

J. The earlier determination of broad goals (A and B) and specific management objectives (D, E, or F) should make explicit the means of evaluation. Some examples are: evaluation of respiratory strength and endurance by recording a client's intraoral air pressure during an air-pressure maintenance task; judging single word intelligibility for monosyllable word lists, and scaling perceived nasality during vowel phonation. Generally, specifying a goal or objective includes, implicitly or explicitly, a means to evaluate whether and when the goal or objective is reached.

K. When one phase of management has satisfied its goal or objective, the clinician can go to the next phase in priority or work to promote carry-over of the modified behavior to various speaking situations.

L. If a phase of management fails to satisfy its goal or ob-

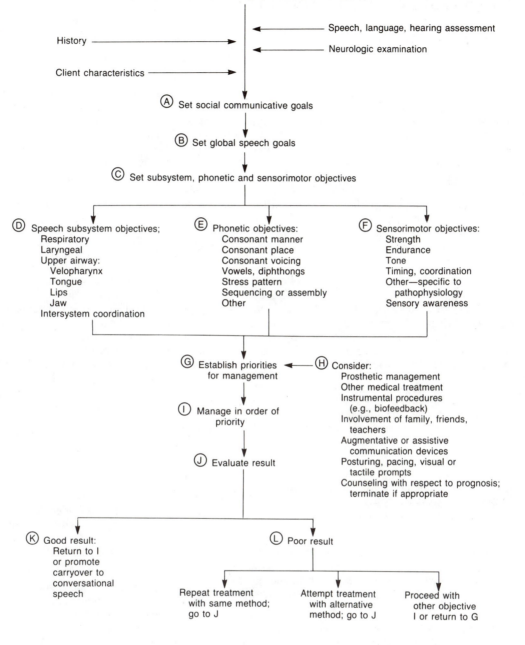

MANAGEMENT GOALS IN DYSARTHRIA AND APRAXIA

History ⟶ Speech, language, hearing assessment
Neurologic examination

Client characteristics ⟶

Ⓐ Set social communicative goals

Ⓑ Set global speech goals

Ⓒ Set subsystem, phonetic and sensorimotor objectives

Ⓓ Speech subsystem objectives;
Respiratory
Laryngeal
Upper airway:
Velopharynx
Tongue
Lips
Jaw
Intersystem coordination

Ⓔ Phonetic objectives:
Consonant manner
Consonant place
Consonant voicing
Vowels, diphthongs
Stress pattern
Sequencing or assembly
Other

Ⓕ Sensorimotor objectives:
Strength
Endurance
Tone
Timing, coordination
Other—specific to
pathophysiology
Sensory awareness

Ⓖ Establish priorities
for management

Ⓗ Consider:
Prosthetic management
Other medical treatment
Instrumental procedures
(e.g., biofeedback)
Involvement of family, friends,
teachers
Augmentative or assistive
communication devices
Posturing, pacing, visual or
tactile prompts
Counseling with respect to prognosis;
terminate if appropriate

Ⓘ Manage in order of
priority

Ⓙ Evaluate result

Ⓚ Good result:
Return to I
or promote
carryover to
conversational
speech

Ⓛ Poor result

Repeat treatment
with same method;
go to J

Attempt treatment
with alternative
method; go to J

Proceed with
other objective
I or return to G

jective, the clinician can repeat treatment with the same or an alternative method, or can proceed to another objective. If a critical management aim cannot be satisfied, the clinician may have to reconsider the overall management goals or objectives and perhaps modify the prognosis. Finally, it is often as important to note a client's strengths and capabilities as to describe weaknesses or deficiencies. Areas of strength or areas of acceptable performance can be central factors in a management plan. It can be helpful to identify strengths that can compensate for uncorrectable weaknesses.

## References

Darley F, Aronson A, Brown J. Motor speech disorders. Philadelphia: WB Saunders, 1975.

Johns DF, ed. Clinical management of neurogenic communicative disorders. Boston: Little, Brown, 1978.

McNeil MR, Rosenbek JC, Aronson A, eds. The dysarthrias. San Diego: College Hill Press, 1984.

Netsell R, Daniel B. Dysarthria in adults: physiologic approach to rehabilitation. Arch Phy Med Rehab, 1979; 60:502.

Netsell R, Rosenbek J. Treating the dysarthrias. In: Darby J, ed. Speech and language evaluation in neurology: adult disorders. Orlando: Grune & Stratton, 1985:363.

Perkins WH, ed. Dysarthria and apraxia. Current therapy of communication disorders. New York: Thieme-Stratton, 1983.

Rosenbek JC, McNeil MR, Aronson A, eds. Apraxia of speech. San Diego: College Hill Press, 1984.

# SPEECH DYSFLUENCY ANALYSIS

*Ruth E. Martin, M.H.Sc.*

Whenever an individual presents with dysfluent speech, a specific dysfluency analysis should be included in the overall communication assessment, because information about the nature of the dysfluency contributes to the formulation of a diagnosis and comprehensive baseline measures of dysfluency are necessary if one is to determine the efficacy of treatment. The general approach to analyzing dysfluency presented here can be applied to a number of different client populations, for example, the young child with a short history of dysfluency (Adams, 1984), the adult whose dysfluency dates back to childhood, or the individual who recently has acquired dysfluency as a consequence of nervous system damage (Rosenbek, 1984).

A. Obtain repeated speech samples (multiple baselines) in order to determine the consistency of the dysfluency across time and across situations. Both audiotaped and videotaped speech samples are suggested, since certain components of the dysfluency pattern such as facial movements and postural changes are difficult or impossible to capture using audiotape alone.

B. The severity and quality of the dysfluency may vary as a function of the speaking task, depending on the etiology of the dysfluency and the individual. Thus, samples should be drawn during a variety of speaking acitivities in which the cognitive-linguistic demands are modified systematically (Ingham, 1984).

C. Obtain at least one covert speech sample, that is, one unbeknownst to the client. This is recommended since some individuals may modify their dysfluencies during an overt speech assessment without the clinician's knowledge.

D. One aim of the dysfluency analysis is to construct a composite profile that reflects the nuances of the dysfluency in a number of everyday situations. This can be achieved by varying the speaking situation in terms of both location and speaking partner.

E. Since dysfluencies are embedded in the ongoing speech pattern, it is important to analyze the other dimensions of speech, such as respiration, phonation, and articulation, and to delineate the relationships between these parameters and the moments of dysfluency. Various methods of acoustic analysis such as speech spectrography can be used to validate and extend one's perceptual findings.

F. The dysfluency macroanalysis yields general information about the frequency of dysfluency, rate of speech, and speech naturalness. The frequency of dysfluency can be expressed as the percentage of dysfluent syllables. The rate of speech is determined by calculating the speaking rate or articulatory rate. (For a detailed description of how these measures are calculated, see Costello and Ingham, 1984). Speech naturalness is rated using a nine point scale, 1 being most natural and 9 being least natural.

G. The dysfluency microanalysis provides more detailed information regarding:

$G_1$. How the dysfluencies are distributed within the discourse structure and within the conversational dynamics.

$G_2$. The frequencies of specific dysfluency types within the overall body of dysfluencies. These can be expressed as percentages by dividing the number of any one dysfluency type by the total number of all dysfluencies and then multiplying by 100.

$G_3$. The durations of dysfluencies and fluent intervals. For example, the average duration of dysfluency, the durations of the three longest dysfluencies, the average duration of fluent intervals, and the durations of the three longest fluent intervals are useful measures. (For details, see Costello and Ingham, 1984).

$G_4$. The nonspeech behaviors that accompany dysfluencies. By analyzing the videotaped speech samples, these behaviors may be described in relation to the corresponding dysfluencies.

H. Since the client's awareness and perception of the dysfluency are important considerations in terms of both diagnosis and treatment, it is recommended that a speech self-analysis be done by the client. Rating scales may be used for this purpose (Table 1).

I. After considering the results of the dysfluency analysis in light of information obtained from the history and from other assessment findings, additional explorations, such as auditory perceptual, language, and motor speech testing, should be considered (Riley and Riley, 1983). Referrals to other disciplines such as neurology, ENT, and psychology may also be indicated.

## References

Adams, MR. The differential assessment and direct treatment of

**TABLE 1   Client's Self-Analysis of Dysfluency**

| Dimension | Rating | | |
|---|---|---|---|
| | | 1 2 3 4 5 6 7 8 9 | |
| Severity | Least severe | | Most severe |
| Speaking rate | Very slow | | Very fast |
| Speech naturalness | Very natural | | Very unnatural |
| Speaking effectiveness | Very effective | | Very ineffective |

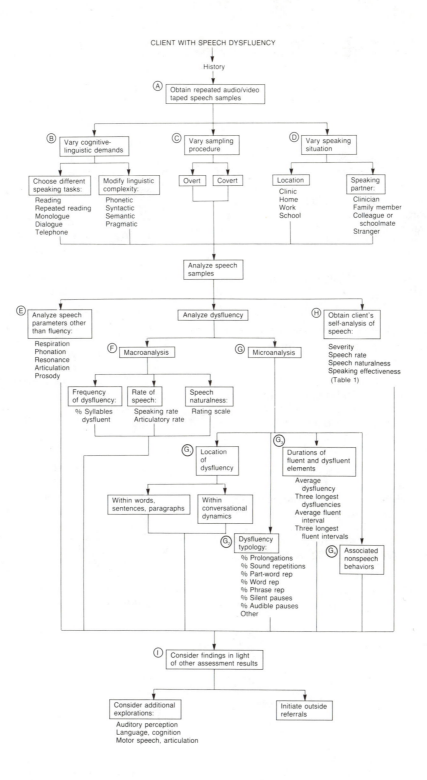

CLIENT WITH SPEECH DYSFLUENCY

History

(A) Obtain repeated audio/video taped speech samples

(B) Vary cognitive-linguistic demands

(C) Vary sampling procedure

(D) Vary speaking situation

Choose different speaking tasks:
Reading
Repeated reading
Monologue
Dialogue
Telephone

Modify linguistic complexity:
Phonetic
Syntactic
Semantic
Pragmatic

Overt   Covert

Location
Clinic
Home
Work
School

Speaking partner:
Clinician
Family member
Colleague or schoolmate
Stranger

Analyze speech samples

(E) Analyze speech parameters other than fluency:
Respiration
Phonation
Resonance
Articulation
Prosody

Analyze dysfluency

(H) Obtain client's self-analysis of speech:
Severity
Speech rate
Speech naturalness
Speaking effectiveness
(Table 1)

(F) Macroanalysis

(G) Microanalysis

Frequency of dysfluency:
% Syllables dysfluent

Rate of speech:
Speaking rate
Articulatory rate

Speech naturalness:
Rating scale

(G₁) Location of dysfluency

(G₃) Durations of fluent and dysfluent elements
Average dysfluency
Three longest dysfluencies
Average fluent interval
Three longest fluent intervals

Within words, sentences, paragraphs

Within conversational dynamics

(G₂) Dysfluency typology:
% Prolongations
% Sound repetitions
% Part-word rep
% Word rep
% Phrase rep
% Silent pauses
% Audible pauses
Other

(G₄) Associated nonspeech behaviors

(I) Consider findings in light of other assessment results

Consider additional explorations:
Auditory perception
Language, cognition
Motor speech, articulation

Initiate outside referrals

stuttering. In: Costello JM, ed. Speech disorders in children: recent advances. San Diego: College-Hill Press, 1984:261.

Costello JM, Ingham RJ. Assessment strategies for stuttering. In: Perkins W, Curlee R, eds. Nature and treatment of stuttering: new directions. San Diego: College-Hill Press, 1984:303.

Ingham RJ. Stuttering and behavior therapy: current status and experimental foundations. San Diego: College-Hill Press, 1984.

Riley GD. Riley J. Evaluation as a basis for intervention. In: Prins D, Ingham RJ, eds. Treatment of stuttering in early childhood: methods and issues. San Diego: College-Hill Press, 1983:43.

Rosenbek JC. Stuttering secondary to nervous system damage. In: Perkins W, Curlee R, eds. Nature and treatment of stuttering: new directions. San Diego: College-Hill Press, 1984:31

# FLUENCY IN THE 2- TO 6-YEAR-OLD CHILD

*Meryl J. Wall, Ph.D.*

A. Assess genetic and medical history. Observe spontaneous speech for external manifestations of aberrant interactions of respiratory, laryngeal, and supralaryngeal components of the speech production system (e.g., speaking on inhalation or on expiratory reserve volume, glottal attack, vocal fry, and articulatory incoordinations). Conduct an oral peripheral speech examination. The child with considerable physiologic involvement may require direct symptomatic intervention.

B. Some stutterers are delayed in language and speech acquisition. The client may require tests of receptive and expressive language, speech skills, and pragmatic use of language. Language-speech therapy is incorporated as indicated. Assess parental speech rate and linguistic complexity as appropriate speech models. Counsel parents regarding rate and complexity, directly treating rate if necessary.

C. Assess the reactions and attitudes of the child, parents, and significant others to the child's speech. Assess the child's general behavioral patterns and interactive abilities. Note reactions of withdrawal from or avoidance of speaking situations.

D. Describe the onset and developmental characteristics of the dysfluencies. Note the existing dysfluencies, such as sound of syllable repetitions, prolongations, hard blocks, accessory behaviors. Measures to assist in differential diagnosis and provide baseline data include frequency of dysfluencies, number of repetitions per unit, and duration of the blocks. (Van Riper, 1982; Adams, 1977).

E. Borderline fluency may involve parent counseling and follow-up only. If there is considerable involvement of factors A, B, and C, such as a strong genetic history of parental pressures regarding linguistic performance, short-term therapeutic intervention and parent counseling are recommended.

F. Fluency facilitation is a method of eliciting short, fluent utterances at slow-normal speech rate and shaping the utterances toward normal conversational speech. It is used with stutterers of any severity and may be sufficient to achieve fluency in borderline or mild-to-moderate stutterers. It is one aspect of a more broadly-based therapy which would include attention to pertinent areas subsumed under A, B, and C.

G. For the moderate-to-severe stutterer, work directed toward modifying the stuttering block may be indicated in addition to fluency facilitation. With young children, this is usually done by contrasting their "hard" speech with "easy" speech, or "bumpy" speech with "smooth" speech. By combining simple explanation with modeling procedures, the child learns to loosen tight articulatory contacts.

## References

Adams MR. A clinical strategy for differentiating the normally non-fluent child and the incipient stutterer. J Fluency Disord 1977; 2:141.

Myers F, Wall M. Toward an integrated approach to early childhood stuttering. J Fluency Disord 1982; 7:47.

Van Riper C. The nature of stuttering, 2nd edition. Englewood Cliffs, NJ: Prentice-Hall, 1982.

Wall MJ, Myers FL. Clinical management of childhood stuttering. Austin: Pro-Ed, 1984.

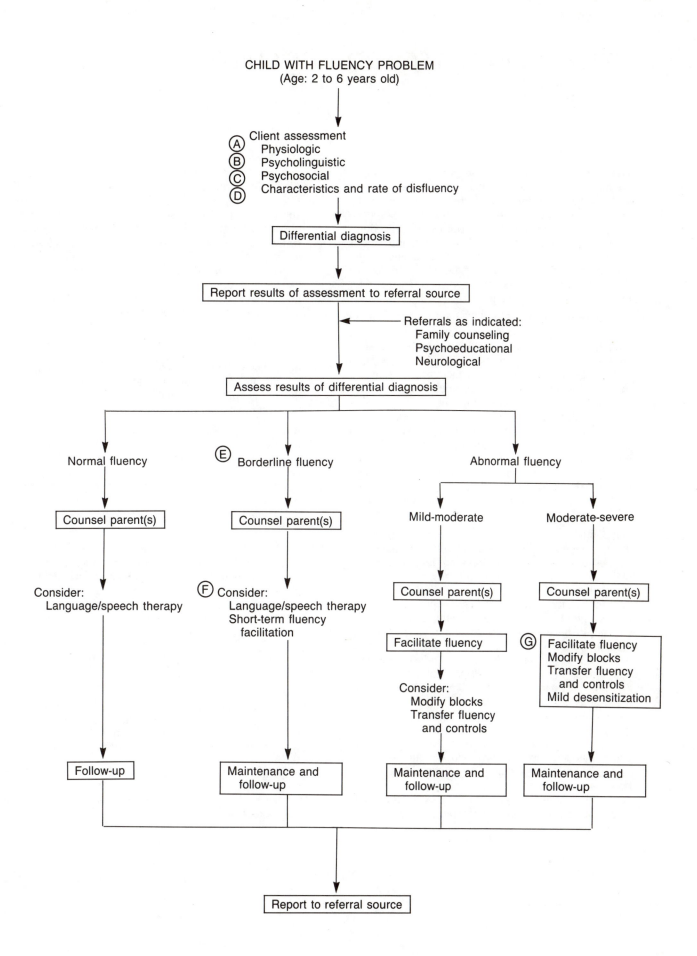

CHILD WITH FLUENCY PROBLEM
(Age: 2 to 6 years old)

Client assessment
Ⓐ   Physiologic
Ⓑ   Psycholinguistic
Ⓒ   Psychosocial
Ⓓ   Characteristics and rate of disfluency

Differential diagnosis

Report results of assessment to referral source

Referrals as indicated:
Family counseling
Psychoeducational
Neurological

Assess results of differential diagnosis

Normal fluency                Ⓔ Borderline fluency                    Abnormal fluency

                                                          Mild-moderate            Moderate-severe

Counsel parent(s)            Counsel parent(s)

                                                          Counsel parent(s)        Counsel parent(s)

Consider:                 Ⓕ Consider:
Language/speech therapy      Language/speech therapy
                             Short-term fluency
                             facilitation

                                                          Facilitate fluency    Ⓖ Facilitate fluency
                                                                                   Modify blocks
                                                                                   Transfer fluency
                                                          Consider:                  and controls
                                                          Modify blocks            Mild desensitization
                                                          Transfer fluency
                                                          and controls

Follow-up                    Maintenance and            Maintenance and          Maintenance and
                             follow-up                  follow-up                follow-up

Report to referral source

# STUTTERING IN THE SCHOOL-AGE CHILD

*Hugo H. Gregory, Ph.D.*
*June Haerle Campbell, M.A.*

A. Whether the referral is from the parents or teacher, or the result of an expression of concern by the child, we seek to clarify the informant's observations by obtaining a description of the problem, both in terms of speech characteristics and attitudes. As appropriate, procedures of evaluation and treatment are described, and reports of previous evaluation and treatment are obtained. If uncertain about the significance of the perceived fluency difference, the child's speech is screened. The need for further evaluation is determined.

B. Evaluation is considered as a differential process aimed toward determining the precise nature of the fluency problem and the factors that may be assumed (based on clinical experience and research) to be contributing to or related to the problem. These factors are designated horizontally across the diagram. The history may suggest that certain factors be emphasized in observations and tests: attitudes of the child, family, and teachers; articulation; language; motor coordination of the speech mechanisms; other behaviors such as attention and learning difficulties; and interpersonal behavior. The psychological evaluation adds information about personality and intellectual functioning that is related to case history findings and informal and formal observations and tests of speech and language.

C. Differential evaluation results in initial decisions about therapy, but evaluation continues throughout treatment. Various factors are focused upon according to the results of the evaluation. For example, a concomitant language or articulation problem may be considered as a possible contributing factor and is managed appropriately. With this age group it is difficult to determine how specific we should be in analyzing and modifying stuttering. Therefore, we always begin with a less specific approach in which the clinician models an easy relaxed approach with smooth movements (ERA-SM) beginning with words and working up to longer more complex utterances. We teach relaxation and point out to the child that an increased feeling of relaxation is being carried over into the coordination of exhalation, phonation, and articulation. If there is a rate problem or a cluttering element, appropriate modifications are made. A more specific approach of analyzing and imitating stuttering and seeing how this can be modified is used only to the extent needed. In our experience, some children need this on only a few sounds, others on several words, and a few chil-

dren need extensive work on many aspects of speech production. Concrete behavioral terminology is used in discussion of speech and attitudes. Combinations of variables (topics, persons present, listener reaction, location, physical activity, and prompts) are manipulated carefully by the clinician throughout the course of therapy so as to progress successfully from easier to more difficult activities. Parents are taught relaxation procedures and, just like their children, learn more easy relaxed speech with longer pause times. The psychological evaluation provides information about psychosocial factors and may reveal a need for the child and the parents to have psychological counseling. (Note on the decision chart that the arrows below the factors focused upon in therapy run horizontally to the left toward speech modification, indicating that all of these variables are assumed to affect fluency. Keep in mind that the factors emphasized differ from person to person.)

D. As therapy progresses, attention is given to planning activities aimed toward the child being able to emit normally fluent speech in progressively more difficult natural environmental situations. Parents and teachers learn how to reinforce the child for appropriate changes. Transfer activities in the classroom should be planned. Recordings made in these situations tell us about the effectiveness of therapy.

E. Just as stuttering is cyclic before therapy, stutterers will find it difficult to maintain steady progress following therapy unless there are rechecks with the speech-language pathologists and unless the family and teachers know how to reward the child for continuing efforts. Monthly rechecks are needed for 12 to 18 months following formal therapy.

## References

Curlee R, Perkins W. Nature and treatment of stuttering: new directions. San Diego: College-Hill Press, 1984.

Gregory H, ed. Stuttering therapy: prevention and intervention with children. Memphis: Speech Foundation of America, 1985.

Gregory H. Stuttering: Differential Evaluation and Therapy. Austin: Pro Ed, 1985.

Wall M, Myers F. Clinical management of childhood stuttering. Baltimore: University Park Press, 1984.

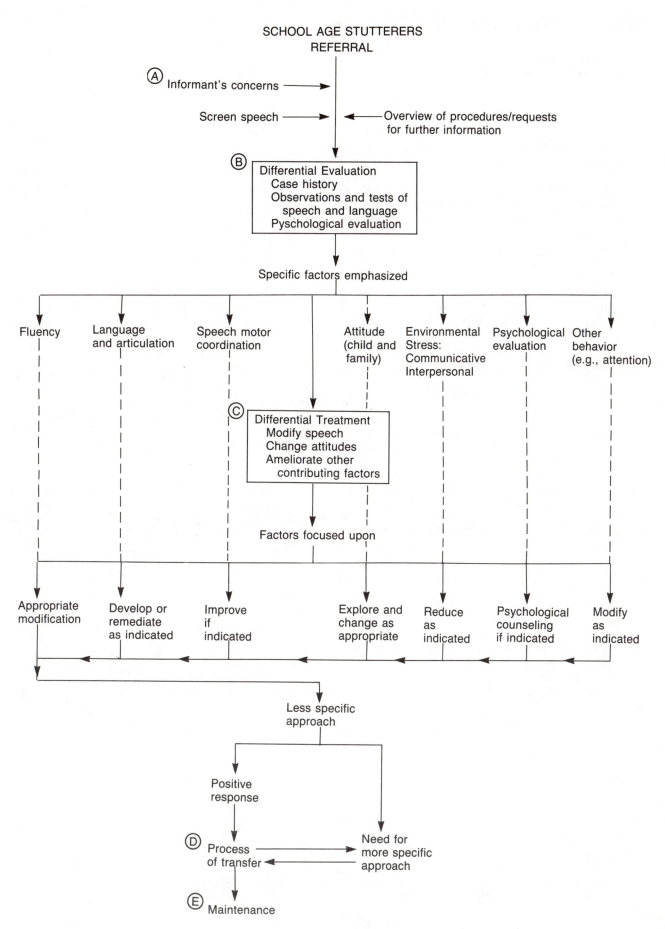

# STUTTERING IN THE ADULT

Hugo H. Gregory, Ph.D.
June Haerle Campbell, M.A.

A. During the initial interview ask the client to describe the present problem, to tell about changes during recent years, and to describe any previous therapy. To observe speech briefly, give the client a passage to read and ask him to describe his job. Ask appropriate questions to evaluate the client's motivation for therapy. If therapy is seen as a probability, describe procedures of evaluation and treatment and obtain reports of previous therapy.

B. Evaluation is aimed toward a thorough understanding of the problem in terms of stuttering behaviors (core and accessory), attitudes about stuttering, and other aspects as indicated horizontally across the diagram. Trial therapy reveals the way in which the person may be expected to respond to analysis and modification of stuttering procedures and to fluency shaping. A small minority of adult stutterers who emit severely tense clonic blocks do not show an ability to modify the behavior readily. To prevent discouragement and increased anxiety, use a fluency shaping approach initially until the person experiences less tension and increased fluency. On the other hand, most adult stutterers experience increased fluency so readily when either modifying stuttering or using fluency enhancing procedures that we believe it important not to allow fluency to emerge without the client first gaining some understanding of the unadaptive stuttering behavior. The psychological evaluation adds information that helps the therapist understand attitudinal aspects more clearly and may indicate the presence of generalized conflicts that should be explored in psychotherapy, either before or concomitant with stuttering therapy.

C. Although the general goals of therapy can be determined by an evaluation such as the one we have outlined, important things are learned about adult clients during the process of therapy. Some findings during therapy confirm initial impressions; other findings add information that indicate new directions to be explored. The initial evaluation may indicate that the person is quite "cognitive" about his problem, thus, a client who requires considerable discussion of the rationale for each step in therapy. As we get to know the client, we may learn that he feels very inadequate about his social skills; therefore, we include social-skills training as therapy proceeds.

In modifying speech, therapy proceeds from shorter to longer utterances, from less meaningful to more meaningful, and from easier to more difficult situations. In our clinic, we combine a stutter-more-fluently model and a speak-more-fluently model by helping the person who stutters to first analyze, monitor, and modify his stuttering and then proceed to build fluency. From the beginning, we tell our clients that we want them to be good speakers. As they learn to modify their speech they learn to vary rate, loudness, inflection, and pause time. Flexibility both in speech and in attitudes is one of the key concepts in our therapy. (Note on the decision chart that the arrows below the factors focused upon in therapy run horizontally to the left toward speech modification, indicating that all of these variables are assumed to affect fluency, keeping in mind that the factors emphasized differ from person to person.)

D. Generalization of change occurs throughout therapy, but as therapy progresses, the clinician and the client plan a hierarchy of speaking situations from easier to more difficult that are role played in the clinic before transfer is attempted in real life. It is our experience that speech change is the crucial characteristic of successful therapy. Recordings made in extratherapy situations are the best indicators of progress.

E. Maintenance refers to the continuations or persistence of speech and attitudinal changes over time. Usually stutterers experience varying degrees of regression or relapse following therapy. We have learned to deal with this by scheduling recheck sessions for 12 to 18 months on a biweekly or monthly basis. Successful clients are those who participate in the recommended maintenance program.

## References

Curlee R, Perkins W. Nature and treatment of stuttering: new directions. San Diego: College-Hill Press, 1984.

Gregory H. Controversies about stuttering therapy. Baltimore: University Park Press, 1979.

Perkins W, ed. Stuttering disorders. New York: Thieme-Stratton, 1984.

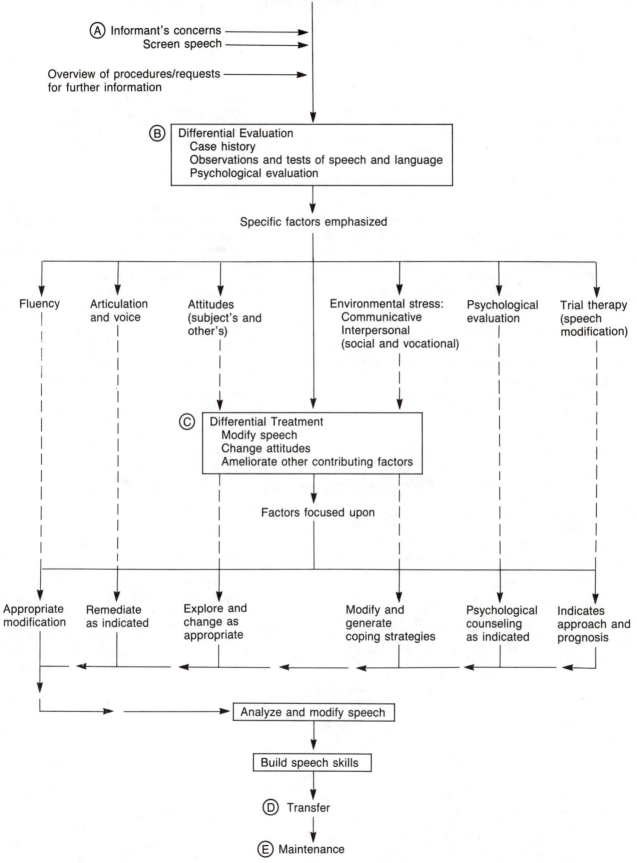

ADULT STUTTERERS

Ⓐ Informant's concerns
Screen speech

Overview of procedures/requests
for further information

Ⓑ Differential Evaluation
Case history
Observations and tests of speech and language
Psychological evaluation

Specific factors emphasized

Fluency

Articulation
and voice

Attitudes
(subject's and
other's)

Environmental stress:
Communicative
Interpersonal
(social and vocational)

Psychological
evaluation

Trial therapy
(speech
modification)

Ⓒ Differential Treatment
Modify speech
Change attitudes
Ameliorate other contributing factors

Factors focused upon

Appropriate
modification

Remediate
as indicated

Explore and
change as
appropriate

Modify and
generate
coping strategies

Psychological
counseling
as indicated

Indicates
approach and
prognosis

Analyze and modify speech

Build speech skills

Ⓓ Transfer

Ⓔ Maintenance

# REFERRAL FOR SPEECH-LANGUAGE PATHOLOGY

*David E. Hartman, Ph.D.*

A rationale for referral for speech-language pathology services has been addressed only anecdotally in the literature. Texts written primarily for physicians concerning the role of and services provided by speech-language pathology have followed a similar trend (Darby 1981a, 1981b, 1985a, 1985b; Metter, 1985).

Generally, referral for speech-language pathology examination assumes that (1) a communicative disorder exists, (2) it can be traced or linked to a recognizable etiology, and (3) the signs of the communicative disorder are potentially treatable. Examination is also sought for screening and baseline purposes prior to, during, and following surgery and trial drug, behavioral, or prosthodontic regimens. Following a careful review of the history and/or reasons for referral and determination of the chief complaints, the examination incorporates perceptual, acoustic, physiologic, and qualitative or quantitative measures to assess communicative function. The proposed referral model outlines the speech-language pathologist's role and responsibilities to the referral source following evaluation and during and following treatment.

A. Communicative disorders can be classified according to neurogenic, psychogenic, structural-mass, iatrogenic, and idiopathic etiologies that may vary from acute and static to chronic and progressive in nature. The etiologies may be multiple and overlap, thereby producing more than one communicative disorder at a time. Therefore, recognition and delineation of presenting symptoms and signs and a healthy skepticism regarding referring diagnosis(es) are tantamount to accurate examination and disposition.

B. Neurogenic disorders are those secondary to focal or multifocal involvement of the neuraxis and include confused language, generalized intellectual impairment (dementia), aphasia, dysarthria, and speech-oral apraxia. Co-occurring neurogenic disorders of mastication and deglutition may be included in this group.

C. Psychogenic disorders include those whose cause rests in psycho-emotional or psychiatric discord and possibly learning. The term "functional" is sometimes used synonymously with psychogenic. Disorders whose primary etiology is psychogenic include conversion reaction and musculoskeletal tension voice disorders, the language of psychoses, as well as many of the development articulation and language disorders of childhood.

D. Structural-mass changes including those secondary to exogenous trauma, cleft lip and palate, tumors, and endocrine dysfunction. Arthritis can produce varying degrees of aberrant speech and deglutition depending upon those structures involved and to what extent.

E. Iatrogenic disorders are those that are clinically induced and as such may produce neurogenic, structural-mass or psychogenic communicative disorders. For example, a dominant hemisphere tumor may produce mild aphasia; resection of the tumor results in exacerbation of the language signs and the presentation of speech-oral apraxia. Laryngectomy produces aphonia, and intubation may produce laryngeal granulomas and dysphonia following extubation. A recommendation for protracted voice rest for nonspecific laryngitis may render a conversion reaction aphonia after the inflammation subsides.

F. Idiopathic disorders are those for which no recognizable etiology can be found. Certain forms of spastic (spasmodic) dysphonia are characteristic of idiopathy.

G. Following evaluation and, if possible, differential diagnosis, the speech-language pathologist should discuss the findings in detail with the referral source. The options following examination are to (1) refer the patient for further evaluation, (2) render a prognosis and institute treatment, or (3) follow for eventual referral, discharge, or prognosis and treatment.

H. If therapy is provided, treatment strategies may include behavioral, prosthodontic, medical, surgical, or combinations thereof. The speech-language pathologist is most directly concerned with providing behavioral and prosthodontic treatment. Whereas the former may incorporate more traditional therapeutic regimens utilizing various learning theories, the latter may implement communication augmentation systems including communication boards, artificial larynges, as well as the computer. The speech-language pathologist may participate in medical therapy by providing measurements concerning changes in a patient's communicative function during a drug regimen. Surgical-prosthetic voice restoration utilizes the speech-language pathologist for counseling preoperatively and postoperatively as well as for ongoing speech therapy.

I. A trial period of therapy is followed by a reevaluation of the patient and the efficacy of the treatment procedures utilized. This information is reported to the referral source. The speech-language pathologist is then faced with the options to (1) continue treatment, (2) discharge the patient, (3) follow-up the treatment, or (4) refer the patient on. If treatment is to be continued, at some time the patient and therapy must be reevaluated and the findings again passed along to the referral source. If the patient is to be followed, a choice at some time must be made to refer on, discharge, or maintain therapy.

## References

Darby JK, ed. Speech evaluation in medicine. New York: Grune & Stratton, 1981a.

Darby JK, ed. Speech evaluation in psychiatry. New York: Grune & Stratton, 1981b.

Darby JK, ed. Speech and language evaluation in neurology: childhood disorders. New York: Grune & Stratton, 1985a.

Darby JK, ed. Speech and language evaluation in neurology: adult disorders. New York: Grune & Stratton, 1985b.

Metter EJ. Speech disorders: clinical evaluation and diagnosis. New York: SP Medical and Scientific Books, 1985.

PATIENT REFERRED FOR SPEECH-LANGUAGE PATHOLOGY

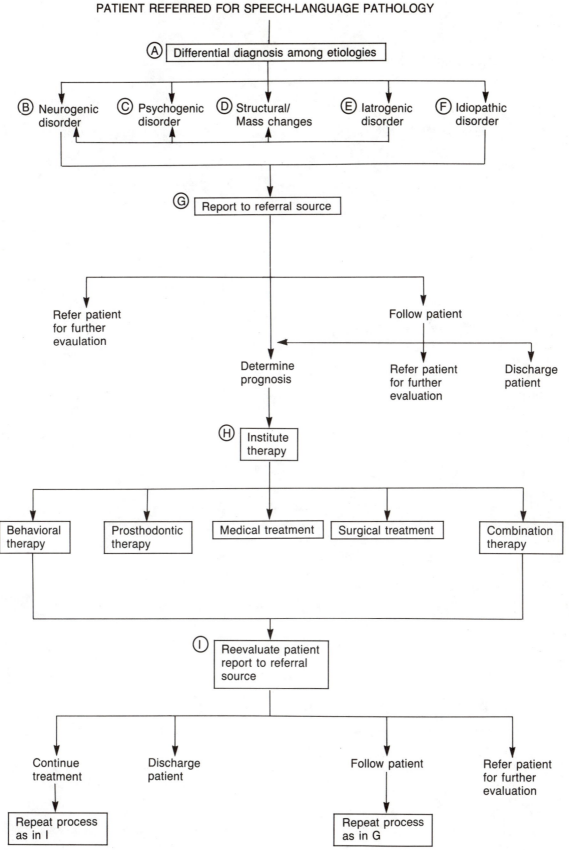

# IV: Related Clinical and Professional Issues

Speech-language and hearing services are provided in a variety of settings. Thus, this section provides decision perspectives covering medical and educational environments as clinical practice sites. This section also provides decision topics related to special issues that clinicians will find useful in some service delivery situations. That is, counseling clients and families related to communicative disorders; consideration in evaluating tests and assessment procedures; decisions to be made in use of statistics in clinical research, and procedures for securing third-party payment for the service offered. Clinicians are asked to perform many duties, and we trust these special topics will be of interest.

# SERVICE DELIVERY SYSTEM IN THE PUBLIC SCHOOL

*Lee J. Gruenewald, Ph.D.*

A. The multidisciplinary team (M-team) in each school comprises two or more individuals skilled in assessment and programming for students with exceptional educational needs. It is district policy that those professionals providing programs and services to students must be involved in the assessment to determine whether special programming is required. Assessment processes and procedures follow an ecologic model. Assessment includes observation, interview, formal and informal testing, and diagnostic teaching.

B. In order to facilitate M-team assessment, the following statements developed by the Madison Metropolitan School District (1981a, 1981b) are used to rule in or rule out the need for exceptional education programming in speech and language.
   1. Articulation disorders (Table 1). Those student's whose speech is characterized by substitutions, distortions, and/or omission.
   2. Voice disorders (Table 2). These students demonstrate disorders of pitch, volume, intensity, and prosody.
   3. Fluency (stuttering) (Table 3). Many young children exhibit nonfluent speech from time to time. Generally, the young child is not aware or concerned about nonfluency. However, parents and teachers are concerned. In these cases, the speech and language clinician may consult only with the parent or teacher to remove the communicative stress in the student's environment or to reduce the adult's expectation of speech fluency at all times.
   4. Language (Table 4). These students have difficulty in comprehending and/or producing language.

C. When the M-team has completed its data gathering, analyses, and syntheses, the M-team findings and recommendations are forwarded to the eligibility review committee (ERC). This committee comprises the administrator for the speech and language program as well as other speech and language program support staff. If the ERC determines that additional data are required for appropriate programing, the M-team findings are returned to the school M-team to complete the additional assessment.

D. The ERC places the student in a speech and language program based on the M-team findings and the development of an Individual Educational Program (IEP). Type and frequency of programing are indicated on the basis of disability and handicapping condition.

E. Although parents are involved in the M-team assessment and IEP development, programing is not implemented until the parents approve the plan.

## References

Madison Metropolitan School District. Perspective and position speech and language program. Madison:1981a.

Madison Metropolitan School District. The multidisciplinary team process handbook. Madison: Integrated Student Services, 1981b.

**TABLE 1   Students with Articulation Disorders**

| Rule In | Rule Out |
| --- | --- |
| Those students whose entire phonologic systems are disordered | Those students whose sound substitutions are developmentally appropriate |
| Those students whose speech is characterized by many substitutions, distortions, and omission, which render it largely unintelligible to the average listener | Those students identified by dentists, parents, and physicians as having tongue thrust; it has long been an accepted policy of Madison Metropolitan School District to enroll these students for therapy only if there is a concomitant handicapping condition and need for an exceptional education program in speech and language |
| Those students whose articulatory competency is affected by motor problems such as dyspraxia or dysarthria | |
| Those students whose actual speech is not judged as largely intelligible, but for whom a relatively mild disability is handicapping socially, emotionally, or academically | |

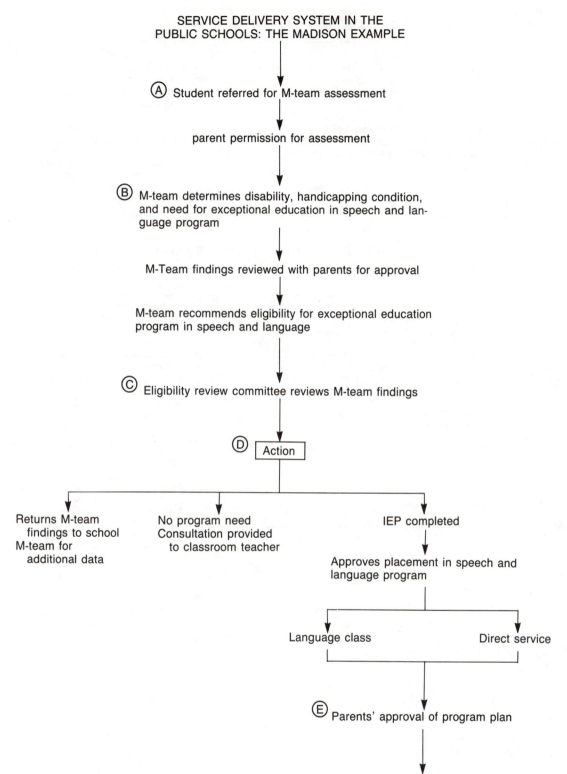

SERVICE DELIVERY SYSTEM IN THE
PUBLIC SCHOOLS: THE MADISON EXAMPLE

(A) Student referred for M-team assessment

parent permission for assessment

(B) M-team determines disability, handicapping condition,
and need for exceptional education in speech and language program

M-Team findings reviewed with parents for approval

M-team recommends eligibility for exceptional education
program in speech and language

(C) Eligibility review committee reviews M-team findings

(D) | Action |

Returns M-team          No program need          IEP completed
findings to school      Consultation provided
M-team for              to classroom teacher
additional data
                                                 Approves placement in speech and
                                                 language program

                                    Language class                    Direct service

                                    (E) Parents' approval of program plan

                                    Student placed and program initiated

**TABLE 2  Students with Voice Disorders**

| Rule In | Rule Out |
|---|---|
| Those students whose physician has provided a written recommendation for voice therapy | Those students who are unwilling or unable to reduce vocal abuse after a period of trial therapy |
| Those students whose deviant voice quality has been persistent and noted by adults and peers as atypical for age and sex | Those students whose parents and teachers are unwilling or unable to modify the student's environment in order to eliminate vocal abuse, and in whom voice quality is unchanged after a period of trial therapy |
| Those students whose degree of disorder is moderate to severe | |

**TABLE 3  Students with Fluency Disorders**

| Rule In | Rule Out |
|---|---|
| Those students whose oral language is characterized by repititions of speech sounds, words, or phrases | Those students whose nonfluent behaviors are not observed across environments |
| Those students for whom communication is an effort and who demonstrate struggle, avoidance, and other maladaptive coping behaviors | Those students whose nonfluency is transitory, and mild and could be viewed as part of the nonfluency that occurs frequently when children begin school |
| Those students who are aware of their nonfluency | Those students who, after a period of trial therapy, do not choose to continue the therapy process; this decision should be made jointly by the student and his parents |

## TABLE 4    Students with Language Disorders

| *Rule In* | *Rule Out* |
|---|---|
| Students who demonstrate significant delay or disorder in comprehension | Students who demonstrate a match between achieved cognitive development and achieved language development even though this achievement is less than would be expected for a student of his or her chronological age |
| Students who demonstrate a mismatch between language development and cognitive development; specifically, language performance that is less than would be expected when compared to cognitive performance | Students who have not achieved symbolic function |
| Significant delay or disorder is defined as minus 1 standard deviation or less than the 15th percentile | Students whose speech and language problems are the result of the lack of desire to communicate within the school environment, rather than the inability to communicate |
| Although a significant delay or disorder may not be present in any one aspect of language or speech pathology, the combinations of delay across syntax, morphology, semantics, pragmatics, or phonology may combine to equal a significant delay or disorder | Students whose problems are related to auditory perception discrimination and memory without evidence that the auditory difficulties also significantly interfere with the comprehension of oral language |
| Evidence of a significant delay or disorder of language is documented by the use of several formal or informal assessment procedures, which are substantiated by observation and interview information and academic performance; the use of language samples collected in natural, spontaneous situations, compared to the student's use of language in academic contexts when necessary, is strongly encouraged to further document the need for intervention | Students whose speech and language problems are not evident in all environments |
|  | Students who are fluent in a language other than English and in whom speech and language problems are the result of second language learning |
| Initial or ongoing training in the use of augmented communication systems may be provided in the context of direct therapy to students demonstrating significant delays in language acquisition, a significant discrepancy between cognitive and linguistic performances, and the need for a nonoral communication system; practice with the system to achieve communicative competency with need to be provided within the student's regular or exceptional education program | Students whose speech and language problems reflect different environmental, cultural, or dialectic influences |
|  | Students whose speech and language problems are the result of inconsistent curriculum methodology and instructional approaches |
|  | Students whose speech and language problems are the result of environmental expectations, which are superior to developmental expectations, and developmental norms |

# CASELOAD SELECTION IN THE PUBLIC SCHOOL SETTING

*Stan Dublinske, Ed.D.*

Prudent professional practice and federal, state, and local polices dictate the selection of clients who are provided services in the schools. Following is a step-by-step process for selecting cases based on those practices and policies.

A. All children are screened for speech, language, and hearing problems during preschool years or at a specified grade level in school to determine possible communication disorders.

B. Assess all children who fail the screening to determine current levels of performance in speech, language, or hearing. Prior to the initial assessment, obtain permission from the parents or guardian. Assessments should include a case history, classroom observation, and data and information from other professionals. At least two procedures must be used to assess each child who is suspected of having a communication disorder (Code of Federal Regulations, 1982). As a result of the assessment referrals may be made to such specialists as psychologists or physicians. Speech-language pathologists or audiologists should conduct primary assessments of speech, language, or hearing.

C. Make the diagnosis only after all data and information collected during the assessment process has been reviewed. The diagnosis should be specific to the speech disorder—articulation, voice, fluency; language disorder—form, content, function; or hearing disorder—deaf, hard of hearing identified (ASHA, 1982).

D. Following the diagnosis determine whether the child is eligible for special education and related services. In making this decision consider the severity of the problem, the child's overall functional communication status, and federal, state, and local policies related to eligibility (Snope et al, 1981).

E. After eligibility has been determined a team of professionals develop an individualized education program (IEP) for the child. That team includes the speech-language pathologist or audiologist, the parents, and another specialist or the classroom teacher (Dublinske, 1978). The IEP must include a statement of the (1) child's current level of performance, (2) annual goals and short-term objectives, (3) specific special education and related services to be provided, (4) projected date for initiation of services and the anticipated duration of services, and (5) objective criteria and evaluation procedures and schedules for determining, at least annually, whether the short-term instructional objectives are being met (Code of Federal Regulations, 1982). The IEP also must indicate if the child will be served individually or in a group, and the frequency and intensity of the services.

F. Decisions regarding the appropriate placement for a child are based on the specific special education and related services indicated in the IEP. Available alternatives may include services in the regular classroom, resource room programs, self-contained classes, day and residential schools, and homebound instruction. Written permission must be obtained from the parent(s) or guardians the first time a child is placed in a special education program.

G. Once appropriate placement has been determined for each communicatively handicapped child with an IEP, scheduling becomes an issue. In scheduling cases, determine appropriate caseload size (ASHA, 1984). Give top priority to the needs of the communicatively handicapped child. Also consider existing professional standards, state mandates, and local policy regarding minimum and maximum caseloads.

H. Intervene as indicated in the IEP. The service provider determines the specific clinical activities and procedures necessary to accomplish the goals and objectives indicated in the IEP.

I. Conduct an annual review and determine the need for additional service.

## References

American Speech-Language Hearing Association. Definitions communicative disorders and variations. ASHA 1982; 24:949.

American Speech-Language-Hearing Association. Guidelines for caseload size for speech-language services in the schools. ASHA 1984; 26:53.

Code of Federal Regulations, Washington, DC: US Government Printing Office, 1982; Sec. 300.532.

Code of Federal Regulations, Washington DC: US Government Printing Office, 1982; Sec. 300.346.

Dublinske S. PL 94-142: Developing the individualized education program (IEP). ASHA 1978; 20:320.

Snope S, Duran J, Dublinske S. Comprehensive assessment and service evaluation. Allen, TX: Developmental Learning Materials, 1981.

CASELOAD SELECTION IN THE PUBLIC SCHOOL SETTING

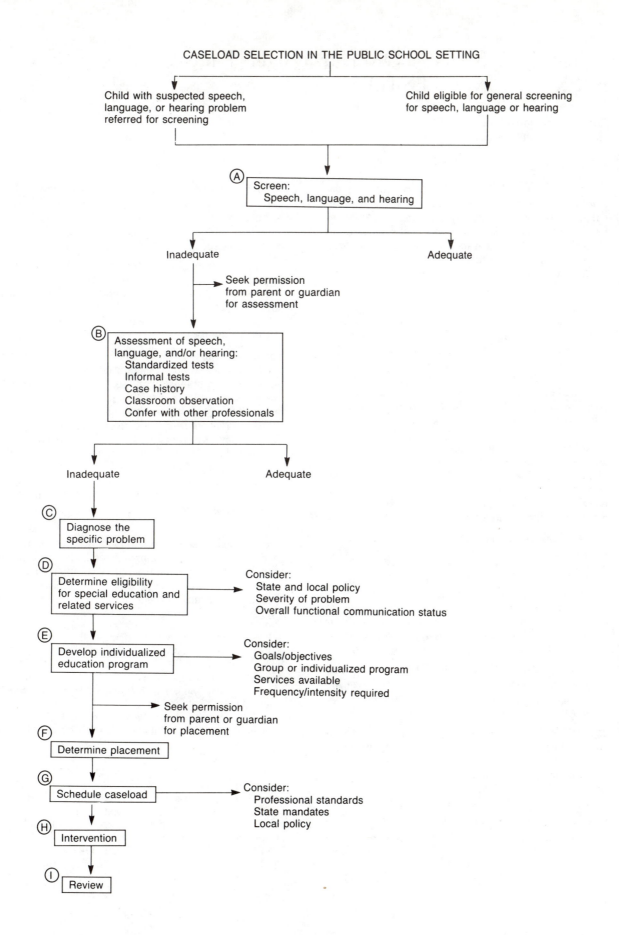

# SERVICE DECISIONS FOR THE PATIENT IN A SHOCK TRAUMA CENTER

*Roberta Schwartz-Cowley, M.Ed.*
*Mark J. Stepanik, M.S.*

A. After a severe traumatically brain-injured (TBI) or spinal-cord-injured (SCI) patient is admitted and receives initial lifesaving therapy, a patient care audit (PCA) is performed routinely to determine caseload selection and clinical service delivery. A speech-language pathologist reviews the patient's history and medical chart, attends medical rounds, and makes informal behavioral observations to determine care priorities.

B. Prioritizing TBI and SCI patients depends largely on neurologic stability (as evidenced by neurosurgical findings, computerized tomography [CT] scan information, the Glasgow Coma Scale [GCS] [Teasdale and Jennett, 1974], and the Ranchos Los Amigos Scale [RLAS] [Hagen and Malkmus, 1979]) and on pertinent behavioral observations made during the PCA. Negative findings that indicate low priority status include unstable intracranial pressure (ICP) and/or the patient having a slim probability of survival or being essentially unresponsive to stimulation. When there is a response to verbal stimulation, an ability to follow commands, or a RLAS of II to III (or higher), a medium-to-high priority status is assigned. Such a patient is scheduled for protocol assessment, whereas a low priority patient is monitored during medical rounds and reaudited.

C. Augmentative communication systems are necessary to investigate cognitive-linguistic (C-L) functioning in a patient who suffers verbal restriction owing to severe dysarthria, orofacial anomalies, tracheostomy, or being ventilator- or respirator-dependant. These systems include electronic larynges, computer-assisted devices, or electronic communication systems that are retained by the patient until no longer necessary. Protocol assessment is indicated if C-L dysfunction is suspected.

D. Because of its high incidence in TBI and SCI patients (Ylvisaker and Longemann, 1985), dysphagia is investigated using radiologic techniques. This condition may be treated in conjunction with C-L deficits.

E. Otologic and audiologic screening are necessary to determine hearing acuity. Rescreening may be necessary because of unreliable test results or inconsistent response patterns. Failing a reliable pure tone screening, complaints of tinnitus, vertigo, or loss of hearing sensitivity indicate further otologic and audiologic procedures.

F. Short protocol assessment should investigate alerting or arousal abilities, attending skills, recall or memory, sequencing, and basic problem-solving abilities in a hierarchal fashion, beginning with low level skills (Adamovich et al, 1985). Any breakdown in performance should warrant further "extended" assessment. Most commonly, memory and attention deficits are found (Hagen, 1984).

G. Extended protocol assessment includes high-level thought processes, including convergent thinking, deductive reasoning, inductive reasoning, divergent thinking, and multiprocess reasoning (Adamovich et al, 1985). A breakdown in performance on this measure should indicate an appropriate place to initiate treatment.

H. In the early stages of recovery, clinical efforts are directed toward eliciting and sustaining responses using a structured program of sensory and sensorimotor stimulation; these efforts progress through more advanced levels of active information processing (Adamovich et al, 1985). Clinical tasks are selected carefully, depending on the level of cognitive function, and clinical goals are then reassessed and modified depending on the amount of cognitive return. Careful attention to the environment, the amount and mode of stimulation, and the carryover of clinical procedures to direct-care staff, family, and other rehabilitation personnel should always be maintained.

I. Protocol reassessment should be performed at the time of discharge from the trauma center. Depending on the patient's placement, information regarding the patient's course of recovery, current cognitive-linguistic status, and response to therapy can be vital to efficient programming within the new setting.

## References

Adamovich B, Henderson J, Averback S. Cognitive rehabilitation of closed head injured patients. San Diego: College-Hill Press, 1985.

Hagen C. Language disorders in head trauma. In: Holland A, ed. Language disorders in adults. San Diego: College-Hill Press, 1984:245.

Hagen C, Malkmus D, Durham P. Levels of cognitive functioning. Head Trauma Rehabilitation Seminar. Ranchos Los Amigos Hospital, Los Angeles, 1977.

Teasdale G, Jennett B. Assessment of coma and impaired consciousness: a practical scale. Lancet 1974; 2:81.

Ylvisaker M, Logemann J. Therapy for feeding and swallowing disorders. In: Ylvisaker M, ed. Head injury rehabilitation. San Diego: College-Hill Press, 1985:195.

TBI OR SCI PATIENT ADMITTED TO TRAUMA CENTER

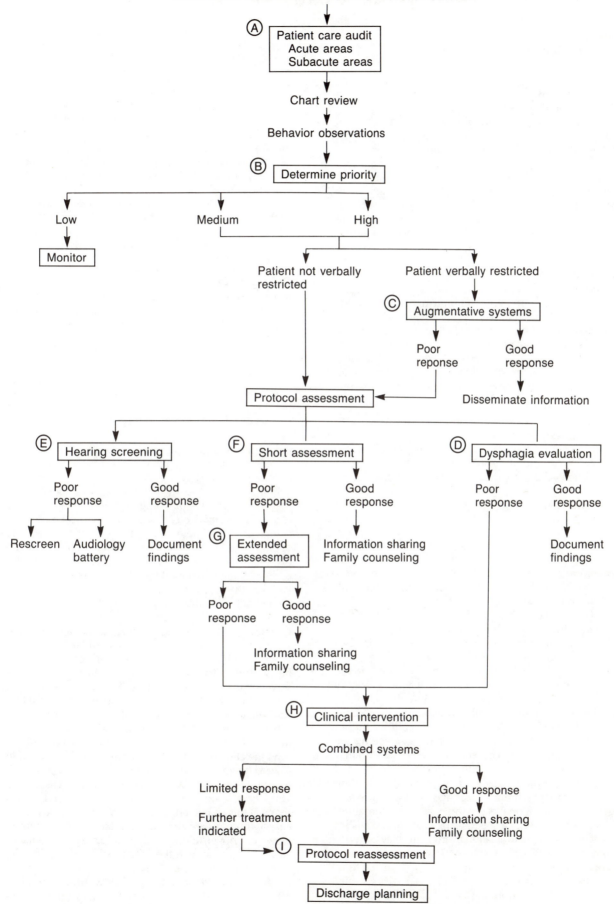

# EVALUATION OF THE AT-RISK INFANT

*Michael J. Clark, Ph.D.*
*Shirley N. Sparks, M.S.*

A. Different kinds of circumstances are presumed to decrease the chance that an infant will develop communication skills normally. Known birth defects often involve cognitive or sensorimotor disabilities, which predictably complicate the development of communication skills. Difficult medical and physiologic circumstances of birth do not lead with the same degree of certainty to communication disorder, but since they usually involve lengthened hospital care in a neonatal intensive care unit, they cause a disruption of the normal context of infant-parent interaction. Of equal importance are a variety of family circumstances that may interfere with parents' ability to deal with infants in a nurturing manner; these circumstances may lead to inadequate caregiving, which has consequences for communication development. The biologic and caregiving risk factors are not mutually exclusive. Biologic difficulties may precipitate familial developments that disrupt care-giving, and stressed family circumstances may contribute to the genesis of biologic difficulties. The majority of infants who are presumed to be at risk for unsatisfactory communication development are at risk for reasons of both kinds.

B. An infant and his caregiver(s) are part of a system of interaction. They affect each other mutually, in complex ways. Therefore a speech-language clinician assessing an infant's communication development must attend to this system—the individual participants and their interaction. The three branches of the decision tree do not represent kinds of assessment to be selected from, but rather foci of attention, that are all necessary.

C. The procedures represented here deal with the infant's communication skills, particularly the ability to respond to communication signals and to initiate communication. For some children, e.g., those with identified birth defects, it is virtually certain that communication skills will be delayed or limited, but for most children presumed to be at risk, delayed or limited skills are a possibility, not a certainty. For screening an infant's communication development, the Early Language Milestone (ELM) Scale (Coplan, 1983) may be used; it surveys a variety of communicative behaviors (auditory receptive, vocalization-speech, and visual) that occur with some reliability in children from 0 to 36 months of age. Failure in any of the three areas calls for further assessment. The criteria for passing the screening are liberal, so failure should be taken seriously. The ELM may be administered by any health professional. In this and all other instruments that compare a child to children of the same age, chronological age must be corrected to allow for gestational age if the infant was premature. If in-depth testing by a speech-language clinician is indicated, a variety of evaluation instruments may be used. Norm-referenced tests, which yield either age equivalency scores or scores showing the extent of deviance from the mean performance expected for given ages, identify children who are performing significantly less well than expected and may need intervention. Scores are not predictive of future skill attainment. Since most such instruments have been standardized on normals and do not permit compensation for impaired sensory or motor skills, using them with infants with known birth defects usually serves no useful purpose; performance is clearly deviant and intervention is required. Criterion-referenced tests identify skill levels in various domains and are useful for guiding formulation of intervention goals. A useful annotated bibliography of infant and child assessment instruments, both norm- and criterion-referenced, is found in Rossetti (1986). Most of these focus on communication behavior.

D. The procedures represented here focus on caregiver attributes. They lead to a characterization of knowledge, skills, and attitudes that may affect how the caregiver(s) approach and respond to the infant. Caregivers may be, in degrees, knowledgeable or ignorant about infants; they may or may not be able to translate their knowledge into action when dealing with their own infants; and they may be emotionally invested in their caregiving situation in helpful or harmful ways. It is important to remember that positive caregiver attributes do not depend on socioeconomic or ethnic status. Especially important here is the question of whether the caregivers make themselves available, physically and emotionally, for interaction with the infant. Another important question concerns the caregivers' expectations about the infant's eventual attainment. The caregivers may expect an unrealistically positive outcome, or they may unfairly disregard the infant's potential. A third question is how the caregiver views interaction with the infant. Caregivers coping with the birth of a handicapped child expectably make some accommodations to their child's individual ways of responding. The clinician should note whether the caregiver is highly directive in attempting to interact with the infant or, on the other hand, is responsive to the infant's communicative signals. Caregiver responsiveness is seen as an advantage in the Transactional Intervention Program (TRIP) (Mahoney and Powell, 1984), which was developed for use in families with handicapped infants. A small number of observation instruments are available to guide the clinician in assessing caregiver attributes. One example is the Parent Behavior Progression (PBP; Bromwich, 1978). (This instrument is also pertinent to assessing the caregiver–infant interaction, discussed in section E.) The PBP allows the clinician to characterize the caregiver's attitude toward the infant, the caregiver's ability to observe and interpret the infant's behavior, and the caregiver's knowledge about the infant's abilities and needs. In arriving at this characterization, the clinician can use both caregiver comments about the infant, as during interviews or conversations, and actual caregiver behavior while interacting with the infant. Another widely used instrument is the Home Observation for Measurement of the Environment (HOME; Caldwell and Bradley, 1978). Other instruments are available to guide the cli-

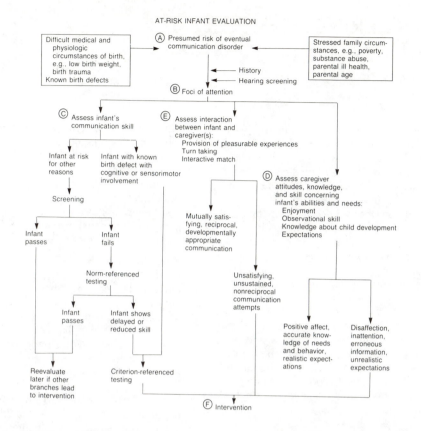

AT-RISK INFANT EVALUATION

nician in observing caregiver attributes in stressful situations or during certain kinds of interaction such as feeding.

E. The procedures represented here deal with the nature of the interaction between infant and caregiver(s). Observation focuses on whether the participants achieve mutually satisfying communication with each other. An infant's communication development takes place via recurring successful interaction with caregiver(s), so it is important for the clinician dealing with an infant at risk to attend to this interaction by actual observation. The assessment objective is to judge whether the interaction is reciprocal, in the sense that the participants easily take turns with each other, and mutually satisfying and enjoyable. An infant who does not participate in this kind of interaction misses a necessary learning experience for developing communication skill. For assessment of the reciprocal nature of the caregiver–infant interaction, one should observe both turn taking and interactive match, which refers to the caregiver's ability to adapt to the infant's behavioral style, interests, and abilities. (These concepts underlie the TRIP [Mahoney and Powell, 1978].) Gaze, vocalization, and movement are the common content of normal infant–caregiver interaction, and the clinician should observe the patterning of these signals. How well does the caregiver read and respond to the infant's communicative signals, e.g., cues of alertness and readiness for interaction versus cues of overstimulation? How does the infant respond to the caregiver's cues of eye contact, facial expression, and vocalizing, which indicate interest in communicating with the infant? The PBP discussed in section D is useful here as well, in that it deals with the caregiver's awareness of the kinds of interaction (and other experiences) the infant finds pleasurable and interesting.

F. This article does not deal with intervention in detail, but several principles of intervention in infant communication development may be mentioned. First, the infant and caregiver(s) compose the critical unit; intervention focuses on the infant in interaction with the caregiver(s) rather than with the clinician. Second, intervention may need to be very extensive and intensive or, on the other hand, brief nonintensive intervention may suffice. In some cases, a caregiver may only need a brief period of developmental guidance (informing about expected infant development), while in other cases knowledge and skills may be grossly insufficient, requiring extensive help. Third, caregivers may be unable or unwilling to accept help from clinicians until their own needs are met; a nonthreatening trusting relationship with the clinician needs to develop. Fourth, intervention directed toward infants' communication skills need not be highly didactic in nature; these skills are best seen as learned through satisfying interaction with caregivers, not as taught by caregivers or clinicians.

## References

Bromwich R. Working with parents and infants: an interactional approach. Baltimore: University Park Press, 1978.

Caldwell B, Bradley R. Home observation for measurement of the environment. Little Rock: University of Arkansas at Little Rock, 1978.

Coplan J. Early language milestone scale. Tulsa: Modern Education Corporation, 1983.

Mahoney G, Powell A. Transactional intervention program: a demonstration early intervention project for birth through three-year-old handicapped infants. Woodhaven, MI: Woodhaven School District, 1984.

Rossetti L. High-risk infants: identification, assessment, and intervention. Boston: Little, Brown, 1986.

# COUNSELING PRINCIPLES FOR FAMILY PARTICIPATION

*James R. Andrews, Ph.D.*
*Mary A. Andrews, M.S.*

A. Family participation and cooperation are elicited by assuming a family perspective. This involves developing an appreciation for the manner in which the communicative disorder manifests itself in the natural environment of the family. An openness to learning about this gives the clinician a broader understanding of the problem than can be derived from the traditional client-clinician dyad alone. Second, communicative disorders both influence and are influenced by family structure and interactive patterns. These may be expected to change with improvement of the problem. Treatment is enhanced by reinforcing those interactive patterns that facilitate change. Third, every family is organized around specific rules, roles for individual members, and a hierarchical power structure. When treatment procedures and suggestions are congruent with these variables and are couched in the language and experience of the family, the potential for successful participation by the family is high. Families will not be able to cooperate when suggestions are incongruent with those variables. Fourth, behaviors are continually being shaped and maintained within the family context. Access to these recurring interactive patterns allows the clinician to broaden the influence of treatment and hasten the process of change.

B. The treatment configuration decision is based upon (1) the clinician's professional setting, (2) the client's specific speech-language disorder, and (3) the interest and availability of the client's family members. Some clinical settings provide the space, time, and support services needed to convene and treat the whole family. Disorders related to language development, stuttering, hearing impairment, and aphasia are particularly amenable to a family approach. Most family members are willing to participate when their help and expertise are actively solicited. When the treatment context, disorder, or family is not amenable to a family approach, the clinician can choose to treat the individual while maintaining contact and developing cooperative interaction with the client's family members.

C. The family systemic intervention choice means that family members will be convened for the speech-language assessment and treatment sessions (Andrews and Andrews, 1986). This is accomplished by contacting a significant family member to arrange a time when all persons can attend. The assessment session should include both parents if the client is a child living in a two-parent family; natural parents and step-parents if the child's parents are separated or divorced and maintain a friendly relationship; siblings and grandparents who are actively involved with the child; or the spouse and adult children of older clients. All these individuals may not be available for every treatment session. However, both parents, when the client is a child, and the spouse, when the client is an adult, should be actively involved in all phases of the treatment process. This treatment choice makes carryover automatic.

D. The individual systemic intervention choice means that the clinician works alone with the client while maintaining contact with significant family members and developing an awareness of the effect of speech-language treatment of the client's interactive environment. Although treated individually, the clinician and client assess treatment goals with an understanding of their impact on contextual variables. This treatment choice makes carryover more likely.

E. When the disorder is assessed with family participation, the first step is to learn (1) how the problem is experienced by each member of the family, (2) what each family member has done in an attempt to improve the problem, (3) which "interventions" were successful, and (4) what each family member believes should be changed (Haley, 1976). During the assessment interview the clinician listens for agreement or disagreement among family members, observes interactive patterns, and listens for techniques that the family believes have been successful or that show promise for improving the communicative disorder. As the clinician conducts the clinical portion of the evaluation, family members assist to the extent possible, and the clinician comments upon the problem as it unfolds in order to share his developing perception of the problem. Together the clinician and the family select appropriate goals and procedures for implementing these goals at home. Throughout the assessment, counseling techniques are used to elicit and maintain family cooperation and to enhance the clinician's understanding of the problem as it is embedded within family interactions. The counseling techniques have been defined and described in detail by Andrews (1986).

F. The clinician assesses the disorder in the usual manner with the exception that this is done with the family in mind. The clinician, for example, may imagine how the problem might manifest itself at home, how family members might react to the problem, and how family members might be involved in assisting at home. Contact with the family is critical in an effort to develop more complete information and confirm or rule out initial assumptions. This may occur through a combination of telephone conversations, parent conferences, and written messages. Family cooperation is elicited by using the counseling techniques listed. These have been defined and described in detail by Andrews (1986).

G. Treatment by and large is implemented by the family through carefully devised treatment assignments given by the speech-language pathologist. Assignments must be phrased in the language and experience of the family, based upon previous family successes in changing the problem, couched in terms that show respect for the family organization and structure, administered through the family spokesperson, be enjoyable and rewarding to the family, and be appropriate from the speech-language pathologist's point of view. Families who understand the

# COUNSELING PRINCIPLES FOR FAMILY PARTICIPATION

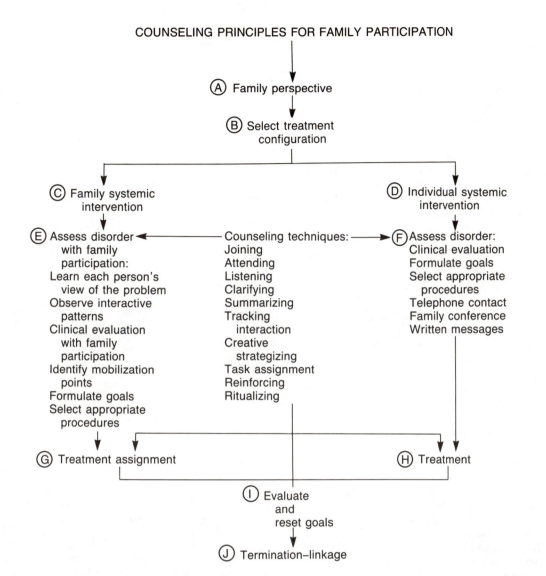

(A) Family perspective

(B) Select treatment configuration

(C) Family systemic intervention

(D) Individual systemic intervention

(E) Assess disorder with family participation:
Learn each person's view of the problem
Observe interactive patterns
Clinical evaluation with family participation
Identify mobilization points
Formulate goals
Select appropriate procedures

Counseling techniques:
Joining
Attending
Listening
Clarifying
Summarizing
Tracking interaction
Creative strategizing
Task assignment
Reinforcing
Ritualizing

(F) Assess disorder:
Clinical evaluation
Formulate goals
Select appropriate procedures
Telephone contact
Family conference
Written messages

(G) Treatment assignment

(H) Treatment

(I) Evaluate and reset goals

(J) Termination–linkage

problem and the purpose of assignments often modify them to make a better fit to their family life style and to the member with the problem. In nearly every case these modifications enhance the effectiveness of the assignments. Treatment occurs as a part of the interactive context of the natural environment and is ongoing and continuous.

H. Treatment is implemented by the speech-language pathologist with an increasing appreciation for the manner in which the problem manifests itself in the environment of the family. Assignments may be given for family members to carry out at home in order to enhance treatment effectiveness. Counseling techniques continue to be used to maintain family cooperation. Contact with the family is made when feasible and possible. Treatment occurs primarily during the session and is administered by the clinician.

I. Progress is evaluated and goals are adjusted to each session. When the family is the unit of treatment, family members demonstrate the intervention techniques that were assigned; describe problems, successes, and modifications; and with the clinician evaluate change. Progress is evaluated as it is observed both in the natural environment and in the session. Each session ends with a new assignment or assignments based upon the new infor-

mation. When the individual is the unit of treatment, progress is assessed and the treatment is modified accordingly. Treatment decisions rest with the clinician, and progress is evaluated as it is observed in the session.

J. Family members collaborate with the clinician in the decision to terminate treatment. The degree to which the family participates in the decision usually is directly proportional to the degree to which they have been part of the habilitative team. When additional or other professional services are to be provided, the clinician should establish links between these professionals and the family. The transition from treatment to either no services or additional or supplemental services may be marked with a ritual of some sort, again depending upon the degree to which the family has been involved.

## References

Andrews MA. Application of family therapy techniques to the treatment of language disorders. Semin Speech and Lang 1986; 7:347.

Andrews JR, Andrews MA. A family based systemic model for speech-language services. Semin Speech and Lang 1986; 7:359.

Haley J. Problem solving therapy. San Francisco: Jossey-Bass, 1976.

# COUNSELING IN COMMUNICATION DISORDERS

Orv C. Karan, Ph.D.
Susan S. Harrington, M.S.
Richard M. Goldstein, M.S.

A. There are many reasons why people with communicative disorders would seek or be referred for counseling. For some, the counselor can provide information for making career decisions or helping to select a job. For others, the counselor can assist in working through the maze of service systems, while still others may be experiencing emotional duress from which they seek relief from the current stressors as well as assistance in preventing the occurrence of future stress.

B. Establishing rapport is an important ingredient in any counseling relationship but becomes critical when counseling persons with communicative disorders. Both the counselor and the counselee must feel comfortable with each other. Counselor patience is essential. The counselor must avoid speaking for the counselee and must be capable of "slowing down" and concentrating on understanding the counselee's message, using aids or cues that are available or that the person is capable of providing.

C. There is wide individual variation among persons with communicative disorders. The counselor must try to learn as much about his or her counselee as possible so as to develop a communication style that will be well suited for the person's particular cognitive, emotional, and experiential level. The counselor must also be willing to spend time in the counselee's natural environment so as to learn how effectively that person relates to others. In some cases, because of the counselee's restricted mobility or the lack of an effective communication system, counseling sessions in the person's natural environment may be considerably more beneficial than in one's office. A potential problem with this approach is that third party payers may not willingly reimburse for therapy or counseling sessions outside a clinic or institution.

D. Counseling is dependent upon the relationship between the counselor and counselee; the essence of this relationship is effective communication. Although counselees with communicative disorders either alone or in combination with other handicapping conditions present challenges for most counselors, those individuals with functional communication systems generally present less of a challenge than those without such systems. For those in the former category, once the counselor and counselee have become comfortable with each other and learn how to successfully communicate (e.g., they become communicatively congruent), the focus of counseling can be directed toward presenting problems and related concerns. For those without functional communication systems the counselor must simultaneously attempt to become more communicatively congruent with the counselee while also addressing those issues for which the person sought counseling in the first place. Not surprisingly, these are usually not mutually exclusive concerns. Standard counseling approaches often must be creatively modified so as to address the individual's unique counseling needs.

## References

Anderson GB, Watson D. Counseling deaf people: research and practice. Little Rock: University of Arkansas Rehabilitation Research and Training Center on Deafness and Hearing Impairment, 1985.

Higgenbotham DJ, Yoder DE. Communication within natural conversational interaction: implications for severe communicatively impaired persons. Top Lang Disord 1982; 2(2):1.

Karan OC, Schalock RL. An ecological approach to assessing vocational and community living skills. In: Karan OC, Gardner WI, eds. Habilitation practices with the developmentally disabled who present behavioral and emotional disorders. Madison: Rehabilitation Research and Training Center in Mental Retardation, 1983:77.

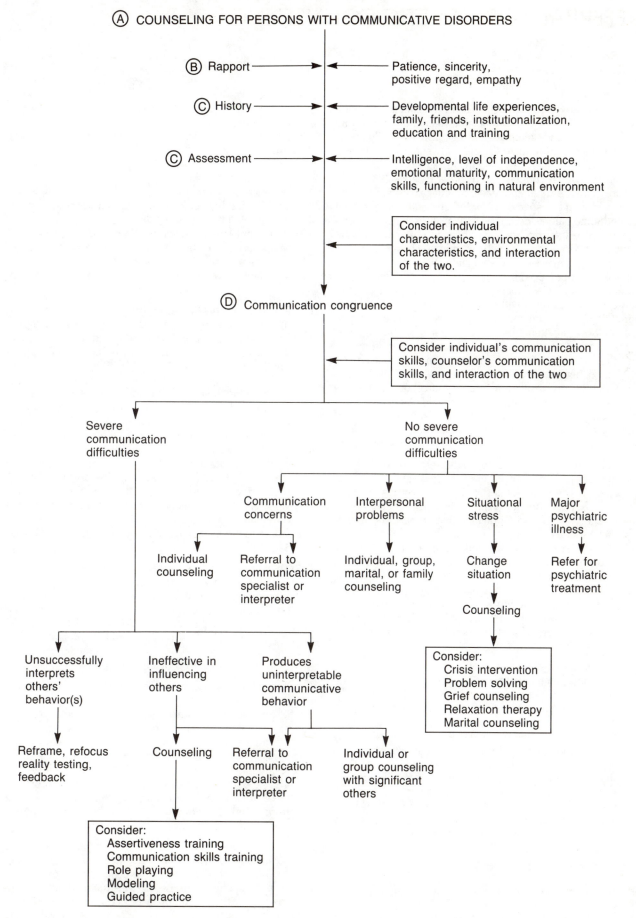

**A** COUNSELING FOR PERSONS WITH COMMUNICATIVE DISORDERS

**B** Rapport — Patience, sincerity, positive regard, empathy

**C** History — Developmental life experiences, family, friends, institutionalization, education and training

**C** Assessment — Intelligence, level of independence, emotional maturity, communication skills, functioning in natural environment

Consider individual characteristics, environmental characteristics, and interaction of the two.

**D** Communication congruence

Consider individual's communication skills, counselor's communication skills, and interaction of the two

Severe communication difficulties

No severe communication difficulties

Communication concerns
- Individual counseling
- Referral to communication specialist or interpreter

Interpersonal problems
- Individual, group, marital, or family counseling

Situational stress
- Change situation
- Counseling

Major psychiatric illness
- Refer for psychiatric treatment

Unsuccessfully interprets others' behavior(s)

Ineffective in influencing others

Produces uninterpretable communicative behavior

Reframe, refocus reality testing, feedback

Counseling

Referral to communication specialist or interpreter

Individual or group counseling with significant others

Consider:
  Crisis intervention
  Problem solving
  Grief counseling
  Relaxation therapy
  Marital counseling

Consider:
  Assertiveness training
  Communication skills training
  Role playing
  Modeling
  Guided practice

183

# REFERRAL FOR GENETIC COUNSELING

*Shirley N. Sparks, M.S.*

There are three reasons for a clinician to consider patient referral to a genetics clinic or physician for genetics counseling: (a) The family needs accurate diagnosis. (b) The family needs accurate information, including risk of occurrence and prognosis. (c) The family needs help in coping with feelings and life situations that concern the disorder (Sparks, 1984). Clinicians who are treating speech, language, or hearing loss in a child with a suspected disorder are appropriate referral agents. Some parents do not avail themselves of genetic services because they do not know how to enter the genetic service network. Others may be intimidated by an unknown system. Parents may feel uncomfortable about seeking genetic services, fearing a possible stigma for having a genetic disorder in the family. A clinician can locate the nearest genetics clinic, provide parents with the name and telephone number of the contact person, and offer an encouraging description of how the genetics clinic operates. Clinicians can explain to parents that diagnosis is the basis for prognosis and that understanding the cause and nature of a child's problem is beneficial to the child. Reports of the visit to the genetics clinic are sent to the referral source, unless the parents ask that the information not be shared. A genetics clinic is a diagnostic and information clinic and does not give ongoing therapy or service. Patients may receive many follow-up contacts, but they usually visit the clinic just once.

A. There are two reasons for low birth weight. (1) The premature baby is an infant of the expected size for its fetal age. (2) The small-for-gestational-age infant is born on time but did not grow properly in utero. The latter category can be further divided into primary and secondary growth deficiencies. Primary growth deficiency includes chromosomal and genetic disorders and inborn errors of metabolism; the growth failure is intrinsic to the fetus. In secondary growth deficiency, the fetus is affected by its environment, and although the genetic coding is normal, the growth deficiency is secondary to a problem outside the fetus that limits its capacity for growth: delivery of nutrients, hormones, or oxygen to the cells (Smith, 1982).

B. Dysmorphology means an impaired or abnormal structure. Fifteen percent of the general population have minor anomalies. Three minor anomalies or a major anomaly with many minor anomalies are found in 3 percent of the population. The important considerations for the clinician to determine in a child suspected of exhibiting dysmorphology are the pattern of anomalies and overall growth retardation. If more than one of the following signs appear, there has been some dysmorphology:

1. Epicanthic folds of the eyes: a prominent fold of skin in the inner corner of the eye. Minor folds are normal and frequent in early infancy but disappear as the nasal bridge develops.
2. Hypertelorism: wide spacing of the eyes.
3. Ears low set or rotated.
4. Preauricular tags or pits just anterior to the ear.
5. Genitalia unusually formed or small.
6. Unusual hair distribution. A very low hairline and heavy eyebrow growth denote abnormal growth in the upper face; unusual hair whorls; hirsutism.
7. Simian palm creases. Four percent of normal babies have simian creases.
8. Curving fingers; stiff joints.
9. Webbing of feet and hands.
10. Absence of fingernails.
11. Wide space between the first toe and others.
12. Hypotonia of all muscles.
13. Prominent lateral ridges on the palate.
14. Malproportion of the body.
15. Asymmetry, especially in the face.
16. Postnatal growth at a consistently slow pace (Smith, 1982).

C. The prenatal history should include the health of the mother during pregnancy (diabetes, viral infections, toxemia, high blood pressure, heart or kidney disease, anemia, or other chronic disease); the age of the parents (mother younger than 18 or older than 35; father older than 55); drugs, radiation, medication, or substances taken during pregnancy (includes alcohol and smoking); and work place exposures. The perinatal history should include labor that was unusually fast or prolonged; birth weight and head circumference; the presence of jaundice, seizures, tremor, or problems with the umbilical cord; resuscitation; Apgar score; and presentation (caesarean, head first, or breech). The postnatal history should include feeding difficulties, weight gain (locate weight and height on charts of normal development), the duration of stay in the hospital (special care or return for failure to thrive), and developmental milestones (Sparks, 1984).

D. There are predictable speech and language abnormalities and cognitive strengths and weaknesses, as well as physical signs, in some syndromes. Treatment plans must be flexible to accommodate a progressive disorder. The clinician and other care providers need to know the manifestations of a disorder in order to separate the organic aspects from those that may be functional or coincidental in order to provide appropriate treatment.

E. A careful history, called a pedigree, of the child's extended family is taken to rule out inheritance patterns of anomalies. In some cases, blood is taken from the child for karyotyping (examination of the chromosomes by microscope to rule out anomalies of the chromosomes, such as Down syndrome). Parents may also be tested for carrier status. More complex blood tests may also be done for some genetic disorders. In the absence of positive laboratory results, diagnosis is often made from examination of physical and behavioral symptoms and family history.

F. Genetic counseling deals with the human problems associated with the occurrence, or risk of occurrence, of a birth defect in a family. The process is an attempt to help the family (a) comprehend the medical facts, including the diagnosis, the probable course of the disorder, and available management; (b) appreciate the way heredity

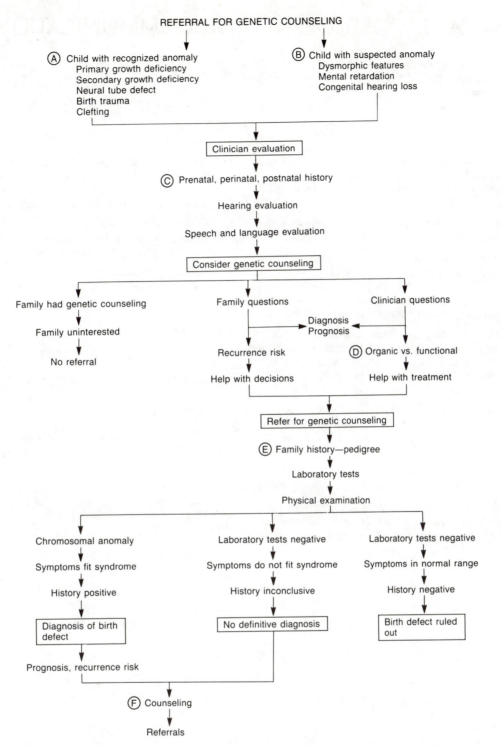

REFERRAL FOR GENETIC COUNSELING

Ⓐ Child with recognized anomaly
Primary growth deficiency
Secondary growth deficiency
Neural tube defect
Birth trauma
Clefting

Ⓑ Child with suspected anomaly
Dysmorphic features
Mental retardation
Congenital hearing loss

Clinician evaluation

Ⓒ Prenatal, perinatal, postnatal history

Hearing evaluation

Speech and language evaluation

Consider genetic counseling

Family had genetic counseling

Family uninterested

No referral

Family questions

Diagnosis
Prognosis

Recurrence risk

Help with decisions

Clinician questions

Ⓓ Organic vs. functional

Help with treatment

Refer for genetic counseling

Ⓔ Family history—pedigree

Laboratory tests

Physical examination

Chromosomal anomaly

Symptoms fit syndrome

History positive

Diagnosis of birth defect

Prognosis, recurrence risk

Laboratory tests negative

Symptoms do not fit syndrome

History inconclusive

No definitive diagnosis

Laboratory tests negative

Symptoms in normal range

History negative

Birth defect ruled out

Ⓕ Counseling

Referrals

contributes to the disorder and the risk of recurrence in relatives; (c) understand the options for dealing with the risk of recurrence; (d) choose the course of action that seems appropriate to them in view of their risk and their family goals and to act in accordance with that decision; and (e) make the best possible adjustment to the disorder in an affected family member or to the risk of recurrence of that disorder. The counseling process aims to help families through their problems, their decision making, their grief, and their adjustments (Ad Hoc Committee on Genetic Counseling, 1975). An essential service provided by the genetics clinic is referral to community agencies, such as mental health agencies, agencies for financial help and family planning, parent support groups, or intervention services for an affected child.

## References

Ad Hoc Committee on Genetic Counseling. Genetic counseling. Am J Hum Genet 1975; 27:240.

Hall JG. Genetic counseling. JAMA 1986; 256:2091.

Smith DW. Recognizable patterns of human malformation, genetic embryologic and clinical aspects. 3rd ed. Philadelphia: WB Saunders, 1982.

Sparks SN. Birth defects and speech-language disorders. Boston: Little, Brown, 1984.

# SEATING AND POSITIONING FOR COMMUNICATION

*Patricia B. Porter, Ph.D.*
*Barbara Wurth, M.S., L.P.T.*
*Shelley Stowers, M.S.P.H., O.T.R.*

A. Watch for contraindications to sitting and history of problems such as fractures, dislocations, scoliosis, and decubitus ulcers that could interfere with client's ability to sit.

B. Evaluate range of motion, muscle tone, strength, reflex development, gross and fine motor abilities.

C. Establish seated position to maximize upper extremity function, head control, eye contact, and vocalizations. Client will be seated most of the time. Goals for proper positioning include prevention of contractures and deformities and maximizing strength (Doherty, 1978).

D. It is essential that the pelvis be in a neutral position with the client sitting on the ischial tuberosities, not the sacrum. A properly aligned pelvis is essential to rest of seating. The seat belt of the chair should be fastened securely to help maintain the pelvis in a correct position.

E. Hips should be flexed and slightly abducted. Angling the seat of the chair so that there is less than 90 degrees between the seat and back of the chair helps prevent the client from arching up out of chair.

F. These lists are suggestions for positioning modification and should not be viewed as all-inclusive (Trefler, 1986).

G. The trunk should be as symmetrical as possible. Side supports can be adjusted to correct scoliosis. Strapping systems can help prevent kyphosis or lordosis.

H. The position of the pelvis or trunk can affect the shoulder girdle, i.e., arching out of chair, scapular retraction, flexion of upper extremities, rounded sitting posture, protracted scapula; may also have flexed upper extremities.

I. Frequently the easiest way to significantly improve head control is to tilt the chair back slightly. It is very easy to test this by propping up the front wheels of the chair.

J. In all of these areas, the first step is to reevaluate the position of the pelvis, hips, and trunk (Porter et al, 1985).

## References

Doherty JM. Handling, positioning and adaptive equipment. In: McDonald ET, ed. Treating cerebral palsy: for clinicians by clinicians. Austin: PRO-ED, 1978.

Porter PB, Carter S, Goolsby E, Martin N, Reed M, Stowers S, Wurth B. Prerequisites to the use of augmentative communication systems. Chapel Hill: Center for Development and Learning, 1985.

Trefler E. Seating for children with cerebral palsy: a resource manual. Memphis: The University of Tennessee Center for the Health Sciences, Rehabilitation Engineering Program, 1986.

POSITIONING AND SEATING: DEVELOPMENT AND USE

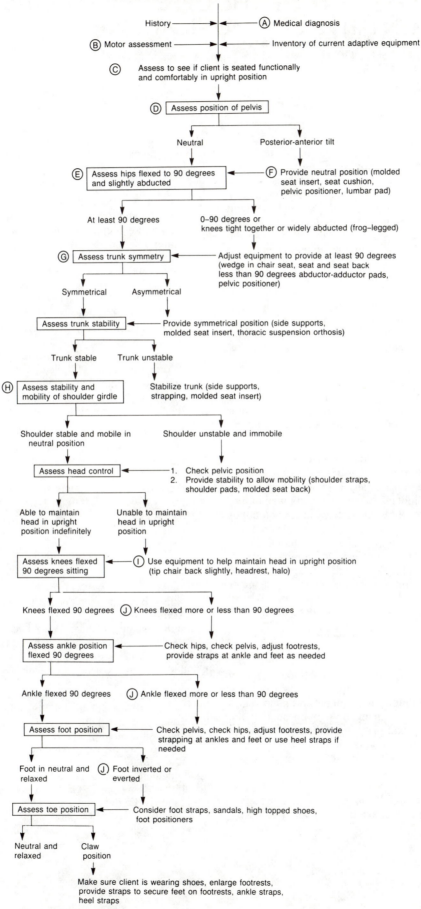

# MOTOR ASSESSMENT OF THE UPPER EXTREMITIES FOR AUGMENTATIVE COMMUNICATION

Shelley Stowers, M.S.P.H., O.T.R.
Mary Ruth Altheide, O.T.R.
Patricia B. Porter, Ph.D.

A. Current practice in the selection of an augmentative communication system emphasizes the use of several augmentative techniques to provide a means of communication for an individual in as many settings as possible, with and without equipment. A match between the client's motor abilities and the motoric requirements of the communication system is a major factor in the selection of the most appropriate system. Therefore, a thorough motor assessment is an integral part of the overall augmentative communication evaluation. Many systems include both unaided and aided techniques to meet the individual communication needs. Motor assessment of the upper extremities should include specific evaluation of the necessary motor abilities required for unaided and aided augmentative communication techniques.

B. Information regarding the client's cognitive abilities and communication needs should be integrated with the motor assessment to ascertain if the evaluated motor components will support the vocabulary and/or communication needs.

C. Evaluation in this area should assist the examiner in determining whether the client has the motor abilities to support a repertoire of signs. Previously gathered information on voluntary movements and range of motion provides gross motor skill data which now requires refinement. Special attention should be placed on motor movements necessary to produce signs (Dennis, 1982). Dunn identified three main areas requiring assessment: (1) the relationship of the sign to the body, (2) hand use patterns (unilateral and bilateral movement, dominant or assistor and reciprocal movement patterns, and (3) hand shapes (position of fingers) (Dunn, 1982).

D. The dominant hand requires special attention because of the motor requirements of signs. Documentation of specific movements of flexion, extension, abduction, adduction, supination, and pronation of upper extremity joints is necessary. Because signing is a dynamic process, the performance of motor movements and handshapes and the speed and accuracy of sign production are directly related to motor planning abilities. A sequence of motor movements is required in the sign production of more than one word. The number of motor sequences an individual can produce successfully provides information about the ability of the motor system to support the number of signs needed for expression of thoughts. If the individual does not exhibit adequate motor skills for a repertoire of signs, an unaided response for yes and no should be explored.

E. The primary purpose of the motor assessment in aided communication is the identification of a mode of indication and the range of indication. A mode of indication is the method an individual utilizes to access a communication technique. It may be a voluntary motor movement such as finger pointing or a voluntary movement used with a piece of adaptive equipment such as a headpointer. The movement selected for use as a mode of indication should be the most accurate, efficient, and reliable movement available to the individual (Coleman, 1980; Vanderheiden, 1977). When evaluating this area, the examiner should be alert to all possible modes of indication available. An individual should not be limited to only one mode of indication if his or her motor and cognitive abilities will support more than one, since each mode may allow the individual access to a different augmentative technique (Stowers, 1987).

F. If exploring alternative modes of indication such as headstick, hand splint or pointer, headlight and/or optical pointer, the aided motor assessment components should be evaluated for each alternative. Use of a keyguard and the angle and placement of materials and devices are also variables which can have impact on motor performance.

## References

Coleman C, Cook A, Meyers L. Assessing non-oral clients for assistive communication devices. J Speech Hear Disord 1980; XLV:515.

Dennis R, Reichle J, Williams W, et al. Motoric factors influencing the selection of vocabulary for sign production programs. TASH Journal 1982; 7:20.

Dunn M. Presign language motor skills. Tucson, AZ: Communication Skill Builders, 1982.

Goossens C, Crain S. Augmentative communication assessment resource. Lake Zurich, IL: Don Johnson Developmental Equipment, Inc, 1986.

Stowers S, Altheide MR, Shea V. Motor assessment for unaided and aided augmentative communication. J Phys Occup Ther Ped 1987; 7 (2):61.

Vanderheiden G. Providing the child with a means to indicate. In: Vanderheiden G, Grilley K, eds. Non-vocal communication techniques and aids for the severely physically handicapped. Austin, TX: Pro-Ed, 1977:20.

# MOTOR ASSESSMENT OF THE UPPER EXTREMITIES FOR AUGMENTATIVE COMMUNICATION

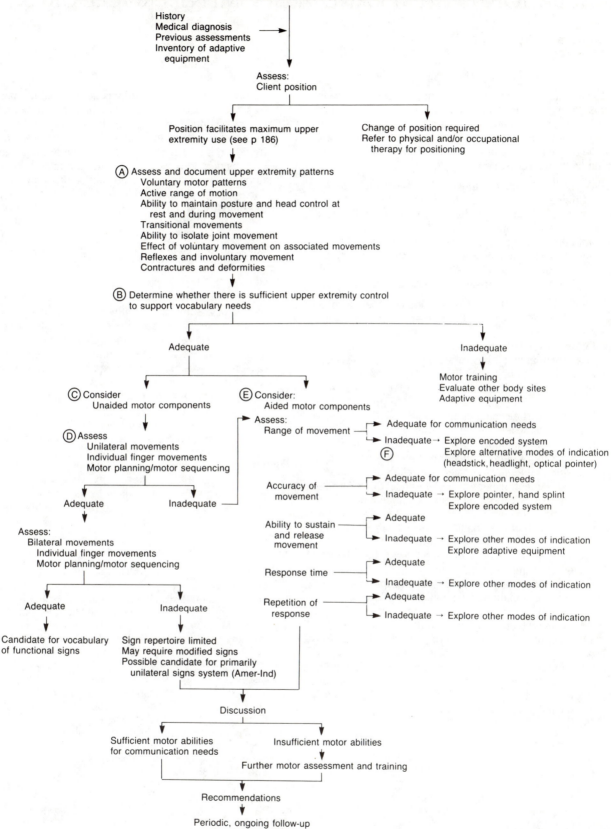

History
Medical diagnosis
Previous assessments
Inventory of adaptive
  equipment

Assess:
Client position

Position facilitates maximum upper
extremity use (see p 186)

Change of position required
Refer to physical and/or occupational
therapy for positioning

(A) Assess and document upper extremity patterns
  Voluntary motor patterns
  Active range of motion
  Ability to maintain posture and head control at
    rest and during movement
  Transitional movements
  Ability to isolate joint movement
  Effect of voluntary movement on associated movements
  Reflexes and involuntary movement
  Contractures and deformities

(B) Determine whether there is sufficient upper extremity control
  to support vocabulary needs

Adequate

Inadequate

Motor training
Evaluate other body sites
Adaptive equipment

(C) Consider
  Unaided motor components

(E) Consider:
  Aided motor components

Assess:
Range of movement → Adequate for communication needs
                   → Inadequate → Explore encoded system
(F) Explore alternative modes of indication
    (headstick, headlight, optical pointer)

(D) Assess
  Unilateral movements
  Individual finger movements
  Motor planning/motor sequencing

Adequate          Inadequate

Assess:
  Bilateral movements
  Individual finger movements
  Motor planning/motor sequencing

Accuracy of → Adequate for communication needs
movement    → Inadequate → Explore pointer, hand splint
                            Explore encoded system

Ability to sustain → Adequate
and release        → Inadequate → Explore other modes of indication
movement                         Explore adaptive equipment

Response time → Adequate
              → Inadequate → Explore other modes of indication

Repetition of → Adequate
response      → Inadequate → Explore other modes of indication

Adequate          Inadequate

Candidate for vocabulary
of functional signs

Sign repertoire limited
May require modified signs
Possible candidate for primarily
  unilateral signs system (Amer-Ind)

Discussion

Sufficient motor abilities
for communication needs

Insufficient motor abilities

Further motor assessment and training

Recommendations

Periodic, ongoing follow-up

# EVALUATION OF TESTS AND ASSESSMENT PROCEDURES

*Dolores Kluppel Vetter, Ph.D.*

The evaluation of a test or assessment procedure for use for a specific purpose is distinct from its psychometric characteristics. A test may have excellent psychometric properties and yet not be appropriate to determine the specific information needed, or the consequences of administering it may be ethically questionable (Messick, 1980).

A. When a standardized test is administered to a person who does not have the same characteristics as the standardization population, there is no assurance the test is measuring the same constructs. Therefore, if the test has not been validated on persons similar to the client being evaluated, care must be taken in interpreting the test scores (Anastasi, 1985). Local or specific norms should be used whenever possible (APA, AERA, NCME, 1985).

B. The type of reliability required for confidence to be placed in the findings of the assessment procedure depends upon the specific questions to be answered (Anastasi, 1982). If the question relates to the assessment of a construct that is basically unitary (e.g., vocabulary), a reported split-half reliability coefficient would be appropriate. Split-half reliabilities are most useful in demonstrating the internal consistency of a measurement instrument. Their magnitude is not usually great when the items of the test are heterogeneous. When the question to be answered by the assessment device relates to the stability of performance over time, a reported test-retest reliability, or alternate-form reliability would be desired. Perfect or near perfect test-retest or alternate-form reliability cannot be expected, since a number of factors may influence performance at either test administration and reliability coefficients may change as a function of the time between administrations. Neither test-retest nor alternate-form reliability may be of interest for tests that·measure attributes or characteristics of a client that are transient in nature, for example, the degree of language impairment immediately following severe head injury. Then a coefficient of internal consistency would be preferable. A score on a test is composed of a true component or attribute of interest and error components that are unrelated to the attribute of interest. Reported standard errors of measurement and a presentation of the sources of error are essential since their consideration helps determine the appropriate use of a test and the interpretation of a test score (APA, AERA, NCME, 1985).

C. The measurements used for validation must be taken into consideration since different interpretations of test scores require different evidence of validity (Guion, 1980). Information on content validity is necessary, but may not be sufficient to determine the usefulness of a device. The test must contain an adequate sampling of relevant items to assess the behavior domain of interest. Procedures used to ensure content coverage and relevance should be considered, particularly for criterion-referenced tests, since face validity alone is not sufficient for these. Concurrent (criterion) validity is essential for tests used in the diagnosis of the existing status or condition of the client, and predictive validity is relevant for tests forecasting a specific outcome in the client. Construct validity, an objective of all tests, provides the basis for determining theoretically derived relationships (APA, AERA, NCME, 1985).

D. Constructs measured by an assessment device have social values; some are positive (e.g., intelligence) and others are negative (e.g., anxiety). Scientists and clinicians have started to focus on the social consequences of administering and interpreting a test to a particular person. Impetus has been added to the consideration of the ethics of administering a test by the concerns for fair testing of minority and handicapped persons. To administer a test that could be interpreted in such a way that a client is stigmatized must make the examiner seriously question its appropriateness. For example, simply knowing that a child was administered the "Test of Deviant Behavior" might be sufficient for uninformed persons to judge the child negatively without knowing the score or what the score meant. In such a case, a different standardized test or an informal procedure should be considered (Messick, 1980).

## References

American Education Research Association, American Psychological Association, National Council on Measurement in Education. Standards for education and psychological testing. Washington, DC: American Psychological Association, 1985.

Anastasi A. Psychological testing. 5th ed. New York: Macmillan, 1982.

Anastasi A. Mental measurement: Some emerging trends. In: Mitchell JV Jr, ed. The ninth mental measurements yearbook. Lincoln, NE: Buros Institute of Mental Measurements of the University of Nebraska-Lincoln, 1985.

Guion RM. On trinitarian doctrines of validity. Prof Psychol 1980; 11:385.

Messick S. Test validity and the ethics of assessment. Am Psychol 1980; 35:1012.

# EVALUATING TESTS AND ASSESSMENT PROCEDURES FOR USEFULNESS

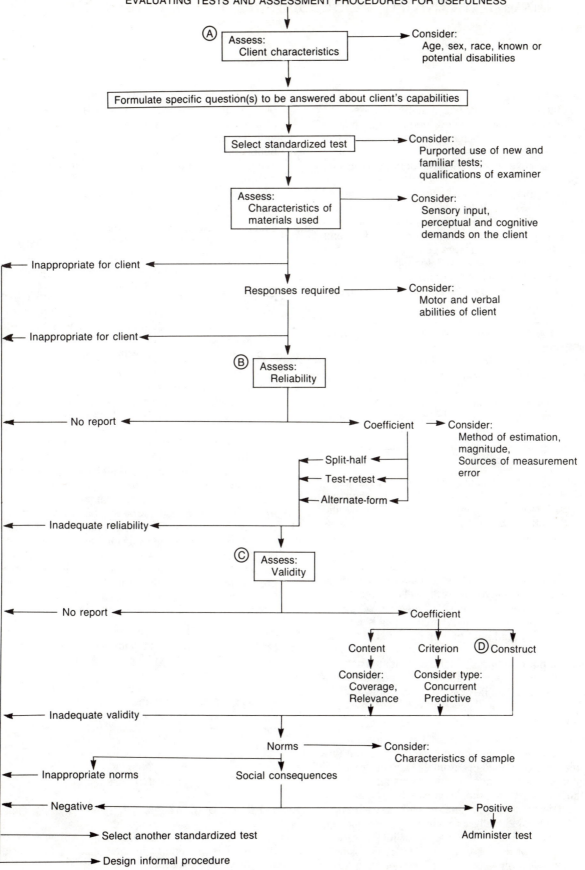

# DESIGNING INFORMAL ASSESSMENT PROCEDURES

*Dolores Kluppel Vetter, Ph.D.*

A. While there may be several circumstances for which an informal assessment procedure may be indicated, the most likely circumstance for developing an informal assessment procedure is when a criterion-referenced standardized test does not exist, that is, when information is needed relative to a client's performance within a specified domain or ability and a standardized means for obtaining the information is not available. The use of norm-referenced tests for describing specific performance or for planning intervention is entirely inappropriate, since norm-referenced tests are constructed of items designed to discriminate among people, not within performance or ability. It is not possible to specify strengths and weaknesses in the client's performance from items administered as part of a norm-referenced test, since the development of items and the test's standardization preclude a valid estimate of performance level. In the absence of a criterion-referenced test, an informal assessment procedure may be the means of obtaining the information needed about the client (McCauley and Swisher, 1984). An informal assessment procedure may also be indicated when the social consequence of administering a standardized test to a client is negative. In this situation, data may be obtained through the use of an informal assessment procedure designed specifically to obtain needed information without the undesirable social consequences.

B. Criterion-referenced data may aid in defining the scope of the attribute to be evaluated; however, the choice of assessment items should be based upon the specific questions to be answered. Sufficient numbers of items must be developed and administered to insure adequate opportunity for occurrence of behavior and adequate sampling of optimum performance (Anastasi, 1982). The difficulty level should be varied among the items if an inference is to be drawn about the level of performance proficiency, since the presence or absence of correct responses to items with a fixed difficulty level is not sufficient. An item should be chosen or designed to have an expected response. An open-ended item usually does not have a place in an informal assessment procedure because the specification of appropriate and inappropriate responses may not be possible. When specification of responses is not possible, an item will be of little value in the evaluation of the client.

C. Because of potential examiner bias in interpreting responses, a specific response for each item should be identified and described in advance of administration of the informal assessment procedure. Items that allow for more than one response should have each response identified and described and the relative merits of each evaluated in advance. Normally items allowing more than one response pose substantial problems for interpretation, and they are not desirable in an informal assessment procedure unless all responses can be identified. Consistent criteria applied to responses increase the poten-

tial replicability of the findings and increase the reliability of clinical judgments based on informal assessment procedures. Whether to reinforce responses or to provide feedback to the client regarding performance depends on the nature of the questions the informal assessment procedure is designed to answer. As an integral part of the procedure and with the potential for affecting the outcome, this should be decided in advance of administration.

D. Comprehension of the instructions has a direct effect on the performance of the client and hence on the validity of the data gathered with an informal assessment procedure. Prior consideration of the selection of vocabulary and of syntactic complexity of oral or written instructions, or of the familiarity of signs or gestures, increases the potential that the understanding of the instructions has not had an adverse influence on performance. When possible, practice items allowing the client to demonstrate understanding of the instructions are desirable.

E. Establishing the guidelines for decision making in advance of administering the informal assessment procedure usually aids in formulating a more dispassionate and objective decision. Since decisions will be related to the circumstances under which the informal assessment procedure was designed, it is important to decide how the client's performance will influence the clinical decisions made. For example, does failure to perform correctly on several items mean that the client is performing as expected? Does it mean that the content domain from which these items came will be the focus of intervention? Or does it mean that a particular placement recommendation will be made for the client? The process of establishing guidelines for relating client performance to clinical decisions results in the informal assessment procedure's being evaluated for both validity and reliability of what is measured. These are essential attributes for the fair evaluation of a client.

F. An evaluation of the effectiveness of the informal assessment procedure forces the examiner to make a judgment about the degree of confidence to be placed in the findings. If this judgment indicates that the informal assessment procedure has not achieved its goals, a modification should be undertaken. If the informal assessment procedure is judged effective, records should be maintained for future reference.

## References

Anastasi A. Psychological testing. 5th ed. New York: Macmillan, 1982.

McCauley RJ, Swisher L. Use and misuse of norm-referenced tests in clinical assessment: a hypothetical case. J Speech Hearing Disord 1984; 49:338.

## DESIGNING INFORMAL ASSESSMENT PROCEDURES

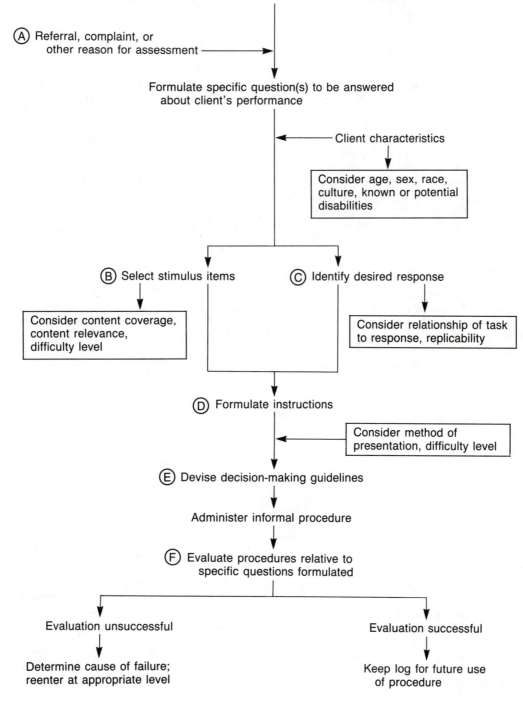

Ⓐ Referral, complaint, or other reason for assessment

Formulate specific question(s) to be answered about client's performance

Client characteristics

Consider age, sex, race, culture, known or potential disabilities

Ⓑ Select stimulus items

Consider content coverage, content relevance, difficulty level

Ⓒ Identify desired response

Consider relationship of task to response, replicability

Ⓓ Formulate instructions

Consider method of presentation, difficulty level

Ⓔ Devise decision-making guidelines

Administer informal procedure

Ⓕ Evaluate procedures relative to specific questions formulated

Evaluation unsuccessful

Determine cause of failure; reenter at appropriate level

Evaluation successful

Keep log for future use of procedure

# UTILITY DESCRIPTIVE STATISTICS

*Michael R. Chial, Ph.D.*

A. Descriptive statistics are useful for summarizing groups of data expressed as numbers. "Data" are reports of observations of events or phenomena (a single report is a "datum"). Summaries of data are valuable because they succinctly convey information that otherwise might be obscured by the detail implicit in a group of numbers. A set of quantitative data can be regarded as a distribution of numbers. Most distributions can be summarized adequately through two types of information: central tendency (e.g., the median and mean) and dispersion (e.g., the range and standard deviation). Specific indexes of either type are called "statistics." (Strictly speaking, a "statistic" is a characteristic or index of a sample of data taken from some larger population of events; analogous characteristics of populations are called "parameters." In the shorthand of mathematics, sample statistics are indicated with English letters, while population parameters are indicated with Greek letters.) Another purpose of descriptive statistics is to compare the similarity or co-relationship of two or more distributions. Williams (1986) provides relatively nontechnical explanations of these and other statistical concepts. Hays (1973) offers more detailed explanations. Many contemporary electronic calculators and a large number of microcomputer programs make computation of descriptive statistics very easy. Kerlinger (1973), Linton and Gallo, (1975), Silverman (1985), and Williams (1986) offer computational details for these and other statistical methods.

B. Goals of descriptive summaries include (1) describing a sample of data (central tendency and dispersion), (2) describing how a single datum (score) relates to an entire sample (standard score), and (3) describing the amount and direction of association between two samples of data. Each goal requires different methods and allows different interpretations.

C. Descriptive statistics cannot be applied indiscriminantly: appropriateness depends upon the scale of measurement achieved by the logical operations that produced the data in the first place. Four scales of measurement account for most (not all) of these operations. They are: nominal (simple classifications such as male and female or social security numbers), ordinal (ranking classifications such as grades of meat or degrees of perceived nasality), equal-interval ("intensive" classifications such as

length, time, and temperature with arbitrary definitions of zero), and ratio (such as percentages for which zero represents the absence of a quantity). These represent a continuum ranging from "weak" nominal scales to "strong" ratio scales. An example will illustrate the four scales just noted. Consider a 100 meter foot-race with five competitors. Runners are identified by numbers attached to their shirts. These numbers (say, 23, 12, 36, 69, and 43) are nominal values. A timekeeper is assigned to each runner. The starting gun is fired and four runners leave their starting blocks (the fifth falls on his face). The timekeepers start their stopwatches as the gun is fired and stop them as their respective runners cross the finish line. Results are as follows: first place—runner 36 (13 seconds), second place—runner 43 (14 seconds), third place—runner 12 (18 seconds), last place—runner 69 (20 seconds). Order of finish constitutes ordinal measurement. Finish times exemplify interval measurement (designation of zero time at the beginning of the race was arbitrary). All four finishers covered the same distance, but at different speeds, a ratio measurement (speed = distance divided by time). Note the rational zero for speed: the runner who fell covered no distance in an infinite amount of time had a speed of zero. Stevens (1951), Siegel (1959), and Williams (1986) offer additional information about scaling and scales of measurement. Table 1 summarizes the logical properties and allowable descriptive statistics for each scale of measurement.

D. Measures of central tendency describe commonalities in a group of data: the way events cluster together. Examples of central tendency include the mode (most common score), the median (middle-most score), and several averages (e.g., arithmetic, geometric, and harmonic means). A common average, the arithmetic mean is usually given the symbol "M" and is calculated by (1) adding the scores and then (2) dividing the sum by the number of scores (N). Arithmetic means adequately estimate the population mean $\mu$(mu) from sample data, assuming random sampling and normal distributions. If either distribution is nonsymmetrical, the median is a better index of central tendency than the mean. Generally, the median should be used for ordinal-scale data and the arithmetic mean for interval- or ratio-scale data. Other indexes

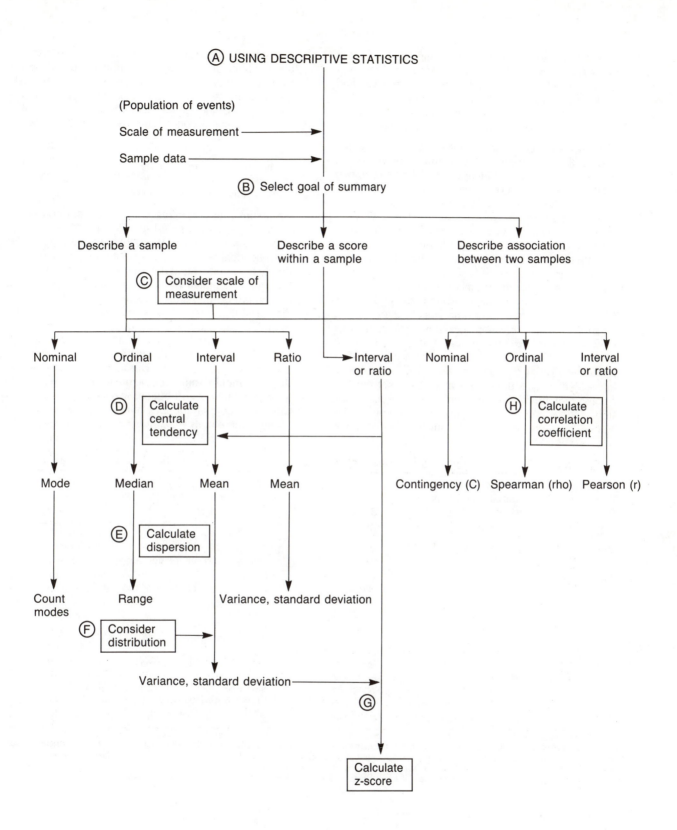

of central tendency include the weighted mean (for interval-scale data), the absolute mean and the root-mean-square (for symmetrical, signed interval data), and the harmonic and geometric means (for ratio-scale data). Central tendency alone is insufficient to describe a set of data; it also is necessary to describe dispersion.

E. Measures of dispersion describe dissimilarities in a group of data: the way events scatter. Examples of dispersion include the number of different events, the range between smallest and largest events, the variance and standard deviation, and the standard error of the mean. The variance ($S^2$) is calculated by (1) finding the mean, (2) finding the difference between each datum and the mean, (3) squaring each difference, (4) adding the squares, and then (5) dividing the sum by the number of scores (N). The standard deviation (S) is simply the square root of the variance. This is the most common index of dispersion for interval-scale data, of value because the units of S are the same as those for individual scores and the mean. (The range is preferred for ordinal-scale data.) This form of standard deviation is appropriate only if we are describing a sample with no real interest in the parent population (or if we actually measured all of the events in a population). More often we want to infer the dispersion of population from sample data. In such cases, step 5 above is modified by subtracting one from the number of scores (N−1). The resulting unbiased variance

and standard deviation are more accurate estimates of the true population parameters. Another index of dispersion, the standard error of the mean (SEM), is the estimated population standard deviation divided by the square root of the sample size. Because the SEM takes sample size into account, it is a "normalized" index that allows direct comparison of the amount of dispersion associated with different sized samples. In the footrace example, the finish times can be summarized as: M = 16.3 seconds, biased SD = 2.9 seconds, unbiased SD = 3.3 seconds, and SEM = 1.8 seconds.

F. Populations are defined as all the events or phenomena of interest. A sample is a subset of a population. We often want to talk about populations, but as a practical matter we must deal with samples. If samples are drawn randomly from populations, the shape and nature of the distribution of sampled values will be similar to the shape and nature of the parent population. Distributions are discussed in terms of shapes because images are easier to understand than equations, but the only methods for assessing the normality of distributions involve calculations. We often assume that distributions of samples and populations are "normal." This amounts to an assumption of particular values for the mean and standard deviation of the parent distribution: specifically, a population mean $\mu$ of zero and a population standard deviation $\sigma$ of one, where both are expressed as standard scores to

**TABLE 1  Allowable Logical Operations and Descriptive Statistics for Four Measurement Scales***

| Measurement Scale | Allowable Logical Operations | | | Central Tendency | Allowable Descriptive Statistics | Correlation |
|---|---|---|---|---|---|---|
| | =, ≠ | >, Tr | + | | Dispersion | |
| Nominal | X | | | Mode§ | No. of modes | Contingency C§ |
| Ordinal | X | X | | Mode<br>Median§ | Range§<br>Quartiles, deciles, percentiles | Spearman $\rho$§ |
| Interval | X | X | X | Mode<br>Median<br>Arith. mean§<br>Weighted mean | Range<br>Quartiles, deciles, percentiles<br><br>Variance§<br>Standard deviation§<br>Stnd. error of mean | Pearson r§ |
| Ratio | X | X | X | Mode<br>Median<br>Arith. mean§<br>Weighted mean<br>Harmonic mean<br>Geometric mean | Range<br>Quartiles, deciles, percentiles<br><br>Variance§<br>Standard deviation§<br>Stnd. error of mean | |

* Scaling is the act of assigning numbers or other symbols to events. Manipulations of symbols respresenting events cannot exceed reasonable manipulations of the events themselves. A group of manipulations (logical operations) is designated symbolically in the table. The symbols = and ≠ refer to equivalence and non equivalence, respectively. ">" ("greater than") implies the ability to order from lesser to greater. "Tr" denotes the property of transitivity (e.g., if A > B and if B > C, then A > C). "+" refers to additivity, the property arising from equality of intervals by which events (hence, numbers) can be added. "Preferred" statistics (designated by §) are those that retain the greatest amount of information implicit in scaled quantities.

be discussed. Normal distributions are "bell shaped," but not all "bell shaped" distributions are statistically normal: the definition of normality derives from numerical values for the parameters $\mu$ and $\sigma$; a bell-like shape is simply a consequence of those values. Other consequences of normality include symmetry of the distribution reflected by (1) medians and means of equal values, and (2) skewness values approximating zero. Skewness is calculated in a manner similar to the standard deviation, except that differences between individual scores and the mean are cubed (raised to the third power) rather than squared. The sum of cubed differences is taken to the third root, rather than to the square root. Near-zero values for skewness suggest symmetry in the underlying distribution. If a distribution is "positively skewed," the mean will be greater than the median; if the distribution is "negatively skewed," the mean will be less than the median.

G. Standard scores express the relation of a single score to the central tendency and dispersion of a group of scores. The standard score or z-score is computed by (1) finding the algebraic (signed) difference between a particular raw score and the mean and then (2) dividing that difference by the standard deviation of the distribution. Thus, a z-score tells where a particular raw score is placed in a set of scores. A standard score of zero indicates that a particular raw score equals the mean. Positive z-scores occur when a particular score exceeds the mean; negative z-scores occur when a particular score is less than the mean. The magnitude of a standard score tells how far (in units of standard deviation) a raw score is from the mean. The z-scores are "standardized" or "normalized" in the sense that they allow direct comparison of distributions having different means, ranges, and dispersions (e.g., results of tests that differ in number of test items). For example, the winner of the foot-race noted earlier had a finish time of 13 seconds, or a z-score of +0.98. Standard scores are valid only if based upon "large" distributions (i.e., 30 or more) of interval- or ratio-scale numbers for which the mean and median are very similar (i.e., "normally" distributed).

H. Correlation coefficients describe the degree of similarity between distributions. In other words, they index the extent to which two or more distributions are statistically associated with each other. Commonly used correlation coefficients include the Pearson product-moment correlation coefficient r (for interval- or ratio-scale numbers), the Spearman rank-order correlation coefficient $\delta$ (for ordinal-scale numbers), and the contingency coefficient C (for nominal-scale numbers). If two data sets differ in measurement scale, the weaker scale should be assumed for both. Pearson and Spearman correlations range in magnitude from −1.0 to +1.0; the contingency coefficient approaches (but cannot reach) unity. A correlation of zero indicates that two sets of data are unrelated. A positive value indicates a direct relation between two distributions: as the values of one distribution get larger, so do those of the other distribution. A negative value indicates an inverse relation: as the values of one distribution get larger, the values of the other get smaller. The numerical size of a correlation coefficient indexes the amount of association between two distributions. Magnitudes of correlations can be described as follows: less than 0.20, "negligible" relation; 0.20 to 0.40, "weak" relation; 0.40 to 0.70, "moderate" relation; 0.70 to 0.90 "strong" relation; more than 0.90, "very strong" relation. The square of the correlation coefficient (called the "coefficient of determination") indicates the strength of association between two sets of data expressed as a percentage of total variation in scores attributable to whatever the distributions (hence, the underlying events) have in common. Imagine that two forms of a vocabulary test produce a Pearson correlation coefficient of r = +0.80 and a coefficient of determination of $r^2 \times 100 = 64$ percent. This indicates a "strong" relationship between the test forms, accounting for 64 percent of the variance in scores from both tests. The remaining variance (36 percent) is due to other factors. Specialized correlation coefficients have been developed for a variety of purposes (see Siegel, 1959; Kerlinger, 1973; and Silverman, 1985).

# References

Hays W. Statistics for the social sciences. 2nd ed. New York: Holt, Rinehart & Winston, 1973.

Kerlinger F. Foundations of behavioral research 2nd ed. New York: Holt, Rinehart & Winston, 1973.

Linton M, Gallo P. The practical statistician: simplified handbook of statistics. Monterey: Brooks/Cole, 1975.

Siegel S. Non-parametric statistics for the behavioral sciences. New York: McGraw-Hill, 1959.

Silverman F. Research design and evaluation in speech-language pathology and audiology 2nd ed. Englewood Cliffs NJ: Prentice-Hall, 1985.

Stevens S. Mathematics, measurement and psychophysics. In: Stevens S, ed. Handbook of experimental psychology. New York: John Wiley, 1951:1.

Williams F. Reasoning with statistics. 3rd ed. New York: Holt, Rinehart & Winston, 1986.

# UTILITY INFERENTIAL STATISTICS

*Michael R. Chial, Ph.D.*

A. Inferential statistics is a branch of applied mathematics used to compare quantitative observations of events or phenomena (data). Data may be drawn or sampled from a larger population of events. A sample of data can be regarded as a distribution in which different events occur with various frequencies. Two or more sets of sampled data can be compared to determine whether they differ with respect to some specific index (e.g., the median, mean, or variance) or with respect to the entire distribution. This is referred to as hypothesis testing. Sometimes the ultimate goal is to make a statement about the differences in underlying populations from which samples were drawn; at other times the goal is limited to the particular samples at hand. In the former case (parametric statistics), inferences are made linking sample statistics to population parameters. In the latter case (nonparametric statistics), there is no special interest in population parameters. (A "statistic" is a characteristic or index of a sample drawn from some larger population; analogous characteristics of populations are called "parameters." Sample statistics are symbolized with English letters and population parameters with Greek letters.) For both parametric and nonparametric statistics, inference is possible because of abstract mathematical knowledge of the relations among distributions of sampled data, distributions of sample statistics, and distributions of population events. The central goal of inferential statistics in the behavioral sciences is to determine whether observed differences between groups are great enough to justify the conclusion that they are real and not due simply to random errors of measurement, or variations among individuals. This goal is most often pursued for the purpose of determining cause-effect relations between independent variables (selected or manipulated by an experimenter) and dependent variables (measured results). The central assumption underlying inferential statistics is that samples have been drawn randomly from populations of people or events of interest (i.e., all possible observations have an equal chance of being selected). Williams (1986) discusses these and other statistical concepts in nontechnical language. Kerlinger (1973), Linton and Gallo (1975), Silverman (1985), and Williams (1986) offer examples and computational details for a number of parametric and nonparametric inferential methods. Many microcomputer programs make computation of inferential statistics fairly easy, but virtually none is capable of selecting a statistical procedure for the user.

B. Inferential statistics permit testing hypotheses about differences among groups as a consequence of independent variables selected or controlled by a researcher. The null hypothesis ($H_0$) is a "default" supposition that two or more groups do not differ. Alternate or "research" hypotheses ($H_r$) may be directional (e.g., group A is greater than group B, or group B is greater than group A) or nondirectional (e.g., group A is not equal to group B). Directional tests are called "one-tailed" and nondirectional tests are called two-tailed." Hypotheses are tested with attention to the probability of making mistakes about decision outcomes. A type I error says that a difference exists when it does not. A type II error says that no difference exists when it really does. The probability of a type I error is symbolized by $\alpha$ (alpha) and is referred to as significance level. Typical values for $\alpha$ are 0.05 and 0.01. "$P_\alpha \leq 0.05$" means that we will be wrong 5 percent of the time when we say that a difference exists. The value of $\alpha$ specified by a researcher reflects that person's views about the costs and benefits associated with being right and being wrong. The probability of a type II error is symbolized by $\beta$ (beta). In any given case, $\alpha$ and $\beta$ are inversely related. The difference between 1.0

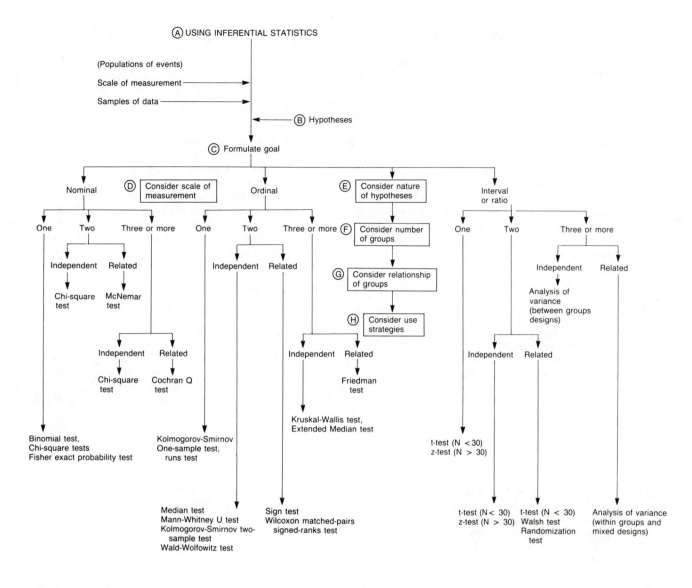

(A) USING INFERENTIAL STATISTICS

(Populations of events)

Scale of measurement ————————→

Samples of data ————————→

(B) Hypotheses

(C) Formulate goal

Nominal

(D) Consider scale of measurement

Ordinal

(E) Consider nature of hypotheses

Interval or ratio

One | Two | Three or more

Independent | Related

Chi-square test | McNemar test

Independent | Related

Chi-square test | Cochran Q test

One | Two | Three or more

(F) Consider number of groups

Independent | Related

(G) Consider relationship of groups

(H) Consider use strategies

Independent | Related

Friedman test

Kruskal-Wallis test, Extended Median test

One | Two | Three or more

Independent | Related

Analysis of variance (between groups designs)

Independent | Related

Binomial test, Chi-square tests Fisher exact probability test

Kolmogorov-Smirnov One-sample test, runs test

t-test (N < 30) z-test (N > 30)

Median test Mann-Whitney U test Kolmogorov-Smirnov two-sample test Wald-Wolfowitz test

Sign test Wilcoxon matched-pairs signed-ranks test

t-test (N< 30) z-test (N > 30)

t-test (N < 30) Walsh test Randomization test

Analysis of variance (within groups and mixed designs)

and $\beta$ is called statistical power: the probability of saying that a difference exists when indeed it does. Users of inferential statistics typically deal with $\beta$ indirectly, maximizing power through selection of (1) sample size (as N increases, so does power), (2) statistical methods (some tests are more powerful than others), and (3) the research hypothesis (one-tailed hypotheses are more powerful than two-tailed hypotheses). Thus, statistical decisions are always based in relative (rather than absolute) certainty: it is possible to accept a research hypothesis, but not to "prove" it beyond all doubt. Further, inferential statistics cannot "prove" that two or more groups are the same, only that they fail to differ in relation to some criterion. Hypothesis testing formally constrains decision outcomes to two: there was a difference (i.e., "reject the null hypothesis") or there was not (i.e., "fail to reject the null hypothesis"). A third option is to suspend decision-making pending additional evidence. Hays (1973) and Siegel (1956) offer excellent discussions of statistical hypothesis testing.

C.  The goal of inferential statistics is to ascertain whether data drawn from two (or more) groups differ with respect to some specified characteristic such that differences may be considered "statistically significant," i.e., are great enough to accept a research hypothesis with no more than a specified probability of a type I error. Such methods can be applied to a wide range of activities in speech-language pathology, including efforts to assess the effectiveness and efficiency of alternative diagnostic and therapeutic strategies. Purposive use of inferential statistics requires several preliminary decisions, the outcomes of which identify a particular statistical procedure.

D.  Choice of a statistical test depends in large part upon the scale of measurement achieved by the operations that originally produced data. Generally, stronger scales of measurement offer greater statistical power. See the previous chapter for discussion of nominal, ordinal, interval, and ratio scales.

E.  Null and research hypotheses may be about medians, means, variances, or entire distributions. Further, hypotheses may be about samples or about underlying populations. The nature of hypotheses excludes certain tests and includes others.

F.  Some inferential tests are designed to compare one empirical group to a population already known; others are designed to compare two empirical groups; still others allow comparison of three or more groups.

G.  Most inferential tests assume that the groups to be compared to each other are statistically independent; i.e., subjects have been measured only once. Because individuals are more like themselves than each other, experimental or evaluation procedures involving repeated observations systematically constrain the variance of events. For this reason, statistical tests of groups not independent of each other (e.g., test-retest measures) entail different calculations. The formal assumptions of some tests preclude multiple observations of the same subjects; other tests have been developed for precisely such purposes.

H.  Use strategies for inferential statistics are very similar, despite a large number of available tests. The following summary of steps involved in practical applications of statistical tests is a modification of that presented by Siegel (1956):
1.  State a null hypothesis ($H_0$) and a research hypothesis ($H_r$). The research hypothesis may be one-tailed (directional) or two-tailed (nondirectional). Most hypotheses are about measures of central tendency, measures of dispersion, or entire distributions.
2.  Select a statistical test that conforms to (a) the scale of measurement implicit in data acquisition, (b) the nature of $H_0$ and $H_r$ (what the hypotheses are about), (c) the number of groups being compared, and (d) whether the groups are statistically independent or related. If all else is equal, choose the alternative test offering the greatest statistical power. Selection of a statistical test in turn specifies a statistical model, a test statistic, and a sampling distribution for that test statistic (e.g., $X^2$, t, z, F).
3.  Specify a sample size (N) and some acceptable probability of a Type I error ($P_\alpha$). Some computer programs calculate exact values of $P_\alpha$, given empirical results;

even so, the experimenter must state a criterion for the type I error.

4.  The previous steps define a critical value of the test statistic, a number that must be equaled or exceeded before $H_0$ can be rejected in favor of $H_r$. Textbooks give critical values of test statistics in tabular form (criteria for statistical significance are defined by degrees of freedom. $P_\alpha$, and—in some cases—whether $H_r$ is one- or two-tailed). Computer programs typically store critical values in the form of equations that are recalculated each time the program is run.

5.  Collect data and perform any preliminary analyses necessary to verify formal assumptions for the statistical model specified in step 2. (Assumptions vary with particular models—those for parametric tests are more restrictive. Common assumptions include normal distributions of underlying population events and equivalent variances among groups.) Next, compute the empirical value of the test statistic. Computational details for many tests are offered by Siegel (1956) and by Linton and Gallo (1975).

6.  Compare the empirical value of the test statistic to the critical value defined in step 4. If the empirical value equals or exceeds the critical value, reject $H_0$ in favor of $H_r$ at the level of significance specified by $P_\alpha$, the probability of a type I error. Do any subsequent tests required to specify (a) the location of significant differences among particular groups (e.g., means comparison tests following analysis of variance) and (b) the strength of experimental effects (e.g., $\omega^2$ or $\eta^2$ strength of association indexes). If the empirical value of the test statistic is less than the critical value, do not reject $H_0$. Remember, you can "prove" that groups differ, but you cannot "prove" that they are the same.

A simplified example will illustrate this strategy. Imagine a new variation of the pharyngeal flap procedure for reducing nasal emissions in cleft palate speakers. A speech clinician wants to determine whether, on the average, the new procedure actually reduces emissions during production of the plosive /p/ in the context /ipipi/. The independent variable is the surgical method (old vs. new), and the dependent variable is nasal air flow measured in cubic centimeters per second (a ratio-scale). The clinician is willing to be wrong 10 percent of the time in saying that the new method is really better (type I error is set at $P_\alpha$ less than or equal to 0.10). The research hypothesis is directional, stating "mean nasal emission is less for the new method than for the old." In other words, $\mu_{new} < \mu_{old}$. The null hypothesis is "no difference"; in other words, $\mu_{new} = \mu_{old}$. Eight clients in each of two groups are tested 6 months after surgery (assume multiple trials contributing to a single mean score for each subject). The t-test for independent means is selected because hypotheses are about two population means, because measurements are interval-scale or stronger, because the groups are statistically independent, and because the sample size is small. Silverman (1985) is consulted for the critical value of the t-statistic: 1.345 (one-tailed, $P_\alpha \leq 0.10$ for 14 degrees of freedom). The observed mean for the "old" method is 0.45 cc per second and the mean for the "new" method is 0.35 cc per second. The empirical t-statistic is calculated to be 1.248. Because this value is less than the critical value, the null hypothesis cannot be rejected. The clinician concludes that the new method does not significantly reduce average nasal emissions in the task noted.

# References

Hays W. Statistics for the social sciences. 2nd ed. New York: Holt, Rinehart & Winston, 1973.

Kerlinger F. Foundations of behavioral research. 2nd ed. New York: Holt, Rinehart & Winston, 1973.

Linton M, Gallo P. The practical statistician: simplified handbook of statistics. Monterey: Brooks/Cole, 1975.

Siegel S. Nonparametric statistics for the behavioral sciences. New York: McGraw-Hill, 1956.

Silverman F. Research design and evaluation in speech-language pathology and audiology. 2nd ed. Englewood Cliffs: Prentice-Hall, 1985.

Stevens S. Mathematics, measurement and psychophysics. In: Stevens S, ed. Handbook of experimental psychology New York: John Wiley, 1951:1.

Williams F. Reasoning with statistics. 3rd ed. New York: Holt, Rinehart & Winston, 1986.

# THIRD PARTY PAYMENT

*Mariana Newton, Ph.D.*

A. Careful attention to this activity before service is initiated is the best insurance for both parties against nonpayment and misunderstanding about money. Mutual understanding provides the foundation for the resolution of subsequent problems in the business aspects.

B. Evaluate terms of private insurance. The best source of information is the supervisor in the claims department of the local or regional office of the insurer (Downey, White et al, 1984). Write down the wording in the plan that supports coverage of speech-language pathology and audiology service. Note the services covered (congenital, acquired, functional disorders, including both evaluation and treatment), the bases for allowing or disallowing coverage, specific provider settings covered, deductible expenses, documentation required, who should file the claim, rules governing billing of the patient for charges not covered and amounts of copayment, service provider requirements, and requirements for physician signature (Downey, White et al, 1984).

C. Some insurance companies require determination of coverage by the insured prior to services for which claims may be made; other carriers may recommend predetermination, especially on services for which coverage may not be routine. Predetermination is advisable for services not carried out by a physician, e.g., speech-language pathology and audiology services, orthognathic surgery, dental care. A description of the proposed services, including the referral source, justification of need, qualifications of the provider, and cost, should be sent on a standard claim form. Label the form boldly to indicate that the submission is for predetermination. Some private insurance carriers and most public-fund reimbursement agencies (e.g., vocational rehabilitation, crippled children's services) require prior authorization of services before they will reimburse. A request (some have particular forms) includes the same information as for predetermination and the authorization received before services are rendered for which reimbursement is expected.

D. Submit a copy of the claim and the responses to the insurer's reason for denial. In a separate letter, address the medical necessity of the services (physician's referral, previous allowed treatment for communication disorder, relationship of communication disorder to medical condition, impairment in health and welfare due to communication disorder), the qualifications of the provider (in states that have licensure, note that the provider is a licensed "practitioner of the healing arts" and the license number; with or without licensure, note that the provider holds the ASHA certificate of clinical competence), the appropriateness of services to patient needs, and the prognosis for improvement. (For specific language in the letter, see Downey, White et al, 1984).

E. The request for review is an appeal for reconsideration after denial; the request is made to the insurance company. That failing, another appeal is available to the state insurance commissioner. Most insurance law is state law, and all states have an insurance commissioner or counterpart (Downey, White et al, 1984). The appeal to the insurance commissioner should include copies of all claim materials submitted previously plus a letter or letters from the insured, the service provider, or the professional expert who has reviewed the case and the claim. (For examples, see Downey, White et al, 1984).

F. If the request for review and the appeals process fails, the final step is judicial review, since the courts constitute the forum for settlement of contract disputes. When the language of the insurance contract is unambiguous, the courts are obliged to follow the language. Most disputes, however, arise because of the ambiguous language used in describing coverage for speech-language pathology and audiology services. Most court decisions are made on the basis of two doctrines. One is the principle of reasonable expectation, relying on the court's determination of the intent of the parties to the contract. Another principle is the doctrine of "adhesion," which suggests that because the insured and insurer do not enjoy equal bargaining power in negotiating the terms of a contract, all ambiguities should be resolved against the insurer. These and other approaches to solving contract disputes, with examples, are reviewed in Downey, White et al, 1984.

G. Include medical diagnosis, ICD–9–CM codes (Downey, White et al, 1984); CPT–4 codes (Physician's Current Procedural Terminology, 1977), the nature of the communication disorder(s), the relationship of the communication disorder to the physical or mental condition, the name of the physician who referred or requested services, the dates when services were rendered, a description of services and charges, and whether assignment will be accepted. Use correct terms in describing needs and services. In describing treatment, indicate what was done. In documenting progress, show change in objective measurable terms as well as how the patient has transferred treatment progress to other situations for practical purposes (Downey, White et al, 1984).

H. When third party reimbursement is denied through private and public sources, referral to specialized agencies may be the best option. Such agencies are not actually third part reimbursers in the usual sense, but they do rely on nonpatient sources of funding for the care of particular conditions and persons of certain ages or in certain circumstances. The public schools, specialized private schools for the mentally or physically impaired, veterans' hospitals, and mental health agencies are some examples. Subsidization of services from outside sources allows fees based on the ability to pay, sliding scales, and in some instances services without any fee to the patient.

THIRD PARTY PAYMENT

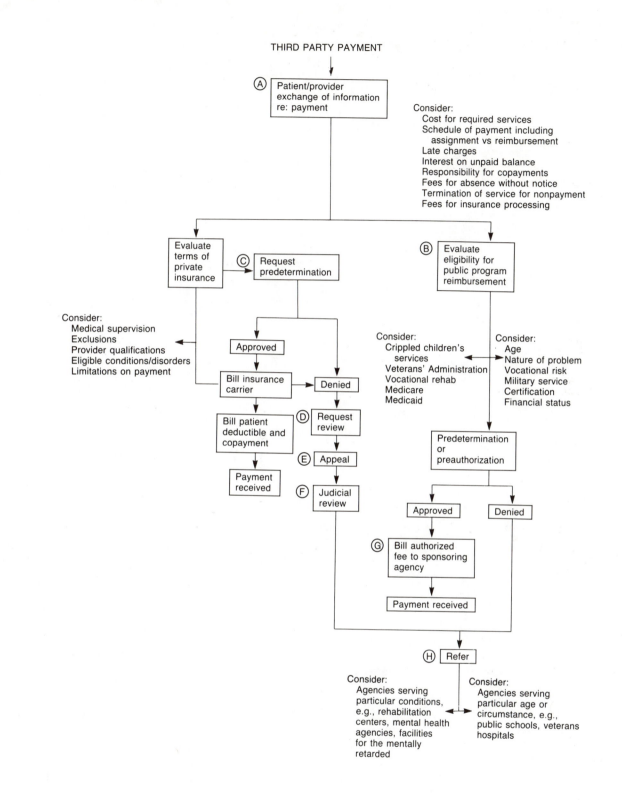

**References**

Downey M, White SC, Karr S. Health insurance manual for speech-language pathologists and audiologists. Rockville, MD: American Speech-Language-Hearing Association, 1984.

Flower R. Delivery of speech-language pathology and audiology services. Baltimore: Williams & Wilkins, 1984.

Physician's current procedural terminology. 4th ed. Chicago: American Medical Association, 1977.

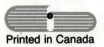